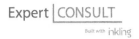 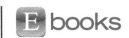

Any screen.
Any time.
Anywhere.

Activate the eBook version
of this title at no additional charge.

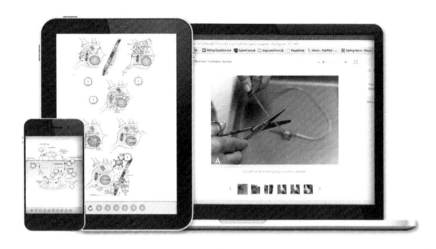

Expert Consult eBooks give you the power to browse and find content,
view enhanced images, share notes and highlights—both online and offline.

Unlock your eBook today.

1 Visit **expertconsult.inkling.com/redeem**

2 Scratch off your code

3 Type code into "Enter Code" box

4 Click "Redeem"

5 Log in or Sign up

6 Go to "My Library"

It's that easy!

Scan this QR code to redeem your
eBook through your mobile device:

**Place Peel Off
Sticker Here**

For technical assistance:
email expertconsult.help@elsevier.com
call 1-800-401-9962 (inside the US)
call +1-314-447-8200 (outside the US)

ELSEVIER

CASE COMPETENCIES in
ORTHOPAEDIC SURGERY

CASE COMPETENCIES in ORTHOPAEDIC SURGERY

Rachel M. Frank, MD
Department of Orthopaedic Surgery
Rush University Medical Center
Chicago, Illinois

Brian Forsythe, MD
Assistant Professor, Division of Sports Medicine
Midwest Orthopaedics at Rush, Rush University Medical Center
Chicago, Illinois

Matthew T. Provencher, MD CAPT (Sel) MC USNR
Chief of Sports Medicine and Surgery, Massachusetts General Hospital
Head Team Physician and Medical Director New England Patriots
Professor of Surgery, USUHS
Visiting Professor, Harvard University
Boston, Massachusetts

ELSEVIER

ELSEVIER

1600 John F. Kennedy Blvd.
Ste 1800
Philadelphia, PA 19103-2899

CASE COMPETENCIES IN ORTHOPAEDIC SURGERY　　　　　ISBN: 978-0-323-39038-5

Notices

Knowledge and best practice in this field are constantly changing. As new research and experience broaden our understanding, changes in research methods, professional practices, or medical treatment may become necessary.

Practitioners and researchers must always rely on their own experience and knowledge in evaluating and using any information, methods, compounds, or experiments described herein. In using such information or methods they should be mindful of their own safety and the safety of others, including parties for whom they have a professional responsibility.

With respect to any drug or pharmaceutical products identified, readers are advised to check the most current information provided (i) on procedures featured or (ii) by the manufacturer of each product to be administered, to verify the recommended dose or formula, the method and duration of administration, and contraindications. It is the responsibility of practitioners, relying on their own experience and knowledge of their patients, to make diagnoses, to determine dosages and the best treatment for each individual patient, and to take all appropriate safety precautions.

To the fullest extent of the law, neither the Publisher nor the authors, contributors, or editors, assume any liability for any injury and/or damage to persons or property as a matter of products liability, negligence or otherwise, or from any use or operation of any methods, products, instructions, or ideas contained in the material herein.

Library of Congress Cataloging-in-Publication Data

Names: Frank, Rachel M., editor. | Forsythe, Brian, editor. | Provencher,
　　Matthew T., editor.
Title: Case competencies in orthopaedic surgery / [edited by] Rachel M.
　　Frank, Brian Forsythe, Matthew T. Provencher.
Description: Philadelphia, PA : Elsevier, [2017] | Includes bibliographical
　　references and index.
Identifiers: LCCN 2015049620 | ISBN 9780323390385 (pbk. : alk. paper)
Subjects: | MESH: Orthopedic Procedures—methods | Musculoskeletal
　　System—surgery | Orthopedics—methods | Clinical Competence | Case Reports
Classification: LCC RD731 | NLM WE 168 | DDC 617.4/7—dc23
LC record available at http://lccn.loc.gov/2015049620

Executive Content Strategist: Dolores Meloni
Content Development Specialist: Laura Schmidt
Senior Content Development Manager: Taylor Ball
Publishing Services Manager: Catherine Jackson
Senior Project Manager: Daniel Fitzgerald
Designer: Renee Duenow

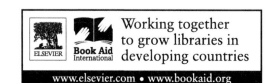

This book aims to educate young surgeons on how to achieve excellence in the operating room. To my mentors, teachers, and coaches—thank you for having the patience to teach me your tips, tricks, pearls, and above all else, passion. To my family and friends—thank you for your love, support, and inspiration— this book would not be possible without you.

Rachel M. Frank

To my family, Jennifer, Abigail, Robert, and Cameron, for providing inspiration and support; to my mentors and colleagues for creating this opportunity; and to the study and practice of orthopaedics for fulfilling a passion for lifelong education.

Brian Forsythe

This book is dedicated to my family for their loving support and to my mentors, fellows, residents, and students, who all have taught me so much.

Matthew T. Provencher

CONTRIBUTORS

Alexander W. Aleem
Resident
Department of Orthopaedic Surgery
Washington University in St. Louis
St. Louis, Missouri

Laith M. Al-Shihabi, MD
Resident, Department of Orthopaedic Surgery
Rush University Medical Center
Chicago, Illinois

Howard S. An, MD
Professor, Department of Orthopaedic Surgery
Rush University Medical Center
Chicago, Illinois

Bernard R. Bach, Jr., MD
The Claude Lambert-Susam Thomsen Professor of
    Orthopaedic Surgery
Director of the Division of Sports Medicine
Director Sports Medicine Fellowship
Orthopaedic Surgery
Rush University Medical Center
Chicago, Illinois

John P. Begly, MD
Resident, Department of Orthopaedics
NYU Hospital for Joint Diseases
New York, New York

Sanjeev Bhatia, MD
Fellow
The Steadman Clinic and The Steadman Philippon
    Research Institute
Vail, Colorado

Randip Bindra, MCh, Orth, FRCS
Professor of Orthopaedic Surgery
Griffith University and Gold Coast University Hospital
Gold Coast, Australia

Nicholas M. Brown, MD
Resident, Department of Orthopaedic Surgery
Rush University Medical Center
Chicago, Illinois

Lisa K. Cannada, MD
Associate Professor
Orthopaedic Surgery
Saint Louis University
St. Louis, Missouri

Emily E. Carmody, MD
Assistant Professor Orthopaedic Oncology and Metabolic
    Bone Disease
Department of Orthopaedics and Rehabilitation
University of Rochester Medical Center and Wilmot
    Cancer Center
Rochester, New York

Peter N. Chalmers, MD
Orthopaedic Resident
Orthopaedic Surgery
Rush University Medical Center
Chicago, Illinois

Peter Chimenti, MD
Orthopaedic Surgery Resident
Department of Orthopaedics and Rehabilitation
University of Rochester Medical Center
Rochester, New York

Cara A. Cipriano, MD
Assistant Professor
Department of Orthopaedic Surgery
Division of Musculoskeletal Oncology
Washington University in St. Louis
St. Louis, Missouri

Mark S. Cohen, MD
Professor, Department of Orthopaedic Surgery
Rush University Medical Center
Chicago, Illinois

Brian J. Cole, MD, MBA
Professor
Department of Orthopaedics
Department of Anatomy and Cell Biology
Section Head, Cartilage Restoration Center at Rush
Rush University Medical Center
Chicago, Illinois

Michael Collins, MD
Research Fellow
Midwest Orthopaedics at RUSH
RUSH University Medical Center
Chicago, Illinois

Gregory L. Cvetanovich, MD
Orthopaedic Surgery Resident
Rush University
Department of Orthopaedic Surgery
Chicago, Illinois

Miguel S. Daccarett, MD
Assistant Professor of Orthopaedic Trauma and Sports
    Medicine
Department of Orthopaedic Surgery
University of Nebraska
Omaha, Nebraska

Matthew B. Dobbs, MD
Professor and Director of Strategic Planning
Department of Orthopaedic Surgery
Washington University School of Medicine
St. Louis, Missouri

Scott M. Doroshow, DO
Orthopaedic Surgery Resident
Philadelphia College of Osteopathic Medicine
Philadelphia, Pennsylvania

Kenneth A. Egol, MD
Vice Chair and Professor
Division of Orthopaedic Trauma, Department of
    Orthopaedic Trauma
NYU Hospital for Joint Diseases
New York, New York

Brandon J. Erickson, MD
Orthopaedic Surgery Resident
Rush University
Department of Orthopaedic Surgery
Chicago, Illinois

Yale A. Fillingham, MD
Orthopaedic Surgery Resident
Rush University Medical Center
Department of Orthopaedic Surgery
Chicago, Ilinois

Brian Forsythe, MD
Assistant Professor, Division of Sports Medicine
Midwest Orthopaedics at Rush, Rush University Medical
    Center
Chicago, Illinois

Rachel M. Frank, MD
Department of Orthopaedic Surgery
Rush University Medical Center
Chicago, Illinois

Nicole A. Friel, MD, MS
Resident, Department of Orthopaedic Surgery
University of Pittsburgh Medical Center
Pittsburgh, Pennsylvania

Todd Gaddie, MD
Resident, Orthopaedic Surgery
University of Nebraska Medical Center
Omaha, Nebraska

Leesa M. Galatz, MD
Professor, Orthopaedic Surgery
Department of Orthopaedic Surgery
Washington University in St. Louis
St. Louis, Missouri

Tad Gerlinger, MD
Associate Professor, Department of Orthopaedic Surgery
Rush University Medical Center
Chicago, Illinois

Hilton Phillip Gottschalk, MD
Vice-Chief
Pediatric Orthopaedic Surgery
Central Texas Pediatric Orthopaedics
Hand and Upper Extremity Program
Pediatric Orthopaedics
Dell Children's Medical Center
Austin, Texas

Joshua A. Greenspoon, BSc
Research Assistant
Steadman Philippon Research Institute
Vail, Colorado

Christopher E. Gross, MD
Assistant Professor
Department of Orthopaedic Surgery
Medical University of South Carolina
Charleston, South Carolina

Steven L. Haddad, MD
Senior Attending Physician
Department of Orthopaedic Surgery
Illinois Bone and Joint Institute, LLC
Glenview, Illinois

Erik Nathan Hansen, MD
Assistant Clinical Professor of Orthopaedic Surgery
Department of Orthopaedic Surgery
University of California, San Francisco
San Francisco, California

Bryan D. Haughom, MD
Resident
Orthopaedic Surgery
Rush University
Chicago, Illinois

Michael D. Hellman, MD
Resident, Department of Orthopaedic Surgery
Rush University Medical Center
Chicago, Illinois

Martin J. Herman, MD
Associate Professor of Orthopaedic Surgery and Pediatrics
Drexel University College of Medicine
Attending Physician at St. Christopher's Hospital for
    Children
Philadelphia, Pennsylvania

Jesse B. Jupiter, MD
AO/Hans-Joerg Wyss Professor
Department of Orthopaedic Surgery
Harvard Medical School
Massachusetts General Hospital
Boston, Massachusetts

Matthew Karam, MD
Assistant Clinical Professor
Department of Orthopaedic Surgery and Rehabilitation
University of Iowa Hospitals and Clinics
Iowa City, Iowa

Monica Kogan, MD
Assistant Professor of Orthopaedic Surgery
Residency Program Director
Director of Pediatric Orthopaedic Surgery
Rush University Medical Center
Department of Orthopaedic Surgery
Chicago, Illinois

Dawn M. LaPorte, MD
Associate Professor, Hand Division
Vice-Director, Education
Department of Orthopaedic Surgery
Johns Hopkins Hospital
Baltimore, Maryland

William N. Levine, MD
Frank E. Stinchfield Professor and Chairman of
    Orthopaedic Surgery
Head Team Physician, Columbia University Athletics
Chief, Shoulder Service
Co-Director, Center for Shoulder, Elbow and Sports
    Medicine
New York Presbyterian/Columbia University Medical
    Center
New York, New York

Joseph Marchese, MD
Resident Physician
Department of Orthopaedic Surgery
University of Connecticut Health Center
New England Musculoskeletal Institute
Farmington, Connecticut

J. Lawrence Marsh, MD
Chair and Department Executive Officer
Department of Orthopaedic Surgery and Rehabilitation
University of Iowa Hospitals and Clinics
Iowa City, Iowa

Robert Nelson Mead, MD, MBA
Resident, Department of Orthopaedic Surgery
Tulane School of Medicine
New Orleans, Louisiana

Samir Mehta, MD
Chief, Orthopaedic Trauma & Fracture Service
Department of Orthopaedic Surgery
University of Pennsylvania Health System
Philadelphia, Pennsylvania

Peter J. Millett, MD, MSc
Director of Shoulder Surgery
The Steadman Clinic and The Steadman Philippon
    Research Institute
Vail, Colorado

Daniel K. Moon, MD, MS, MBA
Massachusetts General Hospital
Assistant in Orthopaedic Surgery
Boston, Massachusetts

Justin T. Newman, MD
Orthopaedic Surgeon
Advanced Orthopaedics and Sports Medicine Specialists
Denver, Colorado

James Albert Nunley, MS, MD
J. Leonard Goldner Endowed Professor
Orthopaedic Surgery
Duke University
Durham, North Carolina

Michael J. O'Brien, MD
Assistant Professor of Clinical Orthopaedics
Division of Sports Medicine
Department of Orthopaedic Surgery
Tulane School of Medicine
New Orleans, Louisiana

Andrew Park, MD
Resident
Department of Orthopaedic Surgery
Washington University in St. Louis
St. Louis, Missouri

Amar Arun Patel, MD
Resident, Orthopaedic Surgery
University of Miami/Jackson Memorial Hospital
Miami, Florida

Maximilian Petri, MD
Research Fellow
The Steadman Clinic and Steadman Philippon Research
    Institute
Vail, Colorado

Marc J. Philippon, MD
Managing Partner, The Steadman Clinic
Co-Chairman, The Steadman Philippon Research Institute
Vail, Colorado

Matthew T. Provencher, MD CAPT (Sel) MC USNR
Chief of Sports Medicine and Surgery, Massachusetts
    General Hospital
Head Team Physician and Medical Director New England
    Patriots
Professor of Surgery, USUHS
Visiting Professor, Harvard University
Boston, Massachusetts

Stephen M. Quinnan, MD
Associate Professor of Orthopaedic Surgery
Miller School of Medicine
University of Miami
Miami, Florida

Andrew Joseph Riff, MD
Resident Physician
Orthopaedic Surgery
Rush University Medical Center
Chicago, Illinois

Jeffery A. Rihn, MD
Associate Professor
Thomas Jefferson University Hospital
The Rothman Institute
Philadelphia, Pennsylvania

James W. Roach, MD
Professor of Orthopaedic Surgery
Department of Orthopaedics
University of Pittsburgh
Pittsburgh, Pennsylvania

Anthony A. Romeo, MD
Professor and Director of Section of Shoulder & Elbow
Midwest Orthopaedics at Rush
Department of Orthopaedic Surgery
Chicago, Illinois

Aaron G. Rosenberg, MD
Professor of Surgery
Department of Orthopaedic Surgery
Rush University Medical College
Chicago, Illinois

Felix H. Savoie, III, MD
Chairman, Department of Orthopaedic Surgery
Tulane School of Medicine
New Orleans, Louisiana

Jesse Seamon, MD
Orthopaedic Trauma Fellow
Department of Orthopaedic Surgery
Saint Louis University
St. Louis, Missouri

Daniel J. Stinner, MD
Orthopaedic Trauma Surgeon
Medical Director, The Center for the Intrepid
Department of Orthopaedics and Rehabilitation
San Antonio Military Medical Center
San Antonio, Texas

Philipp N. Streubel, MD
Assistant Professor
Department of Orthopaedic Surgery
University of Nebraska Medical Center
Omaha, Nebraska

Sophia A. Strike, MD
Resident, Department of Orthopaedic Surgery
Johns Hopkins Hospital
Baltimore, Maryland

Matthew P. Sullivan, MD
Resident
Orthopaedic Surgery
University of Pennsylvania
Philadelphia, Pennsylvania

Stephanie J. Swensen, MD
Resident Physician
Department of Orthopaedic Surgery
NYU Hospital for Joint Diseases
New York, New York

Ivan S. Tarkin, MD
Chief of Orthopaedic Trauma
Department of Orthopaedic Surgery
University of Pittsburgh Medical Center
Pittsburgh, Pennsylvania

Brandon M. Tauberg, MD
Resident, Department of Orthopaedic Surgery
Albert Einstein College of Medicine/Montefiore Medical
    Center
Bronx, New York

Nikhil N. Verma, MD
Orthopaedics Sports Medicine Physician
Midwest Orthopaedics at Rush
Professor, Department of Orthopaedic Surgery, Rush
    University Medical Center
Chicago, Illinois

Arvind von Keudell, MD
Resident
Harvard Combined Orthopaedic Surgery Residency
    Program
Harvard Medical School
Boston, Massachusetts

David Walton, MD
Foot and Ankle Fellow, Department of Orthopaedics
Duke University Medical Center
Durham, North Carolina

Jonathan P. Watling, MD
Resident Physician
New York Presbyterian/Columbia University Medical Center
Department of Orthopaedic Surgery
New York, New York

Michael C. Willey, MD
Clinical Associate Professor
Department of Orthopaedics and Rehabilitation
University of Iowa Hospitals and Clinics
Iowa City, Iowa

Jennifer Moriatis Wolf, MD
Professor
Department of Orthopaedic Surgery
University of Connecticut Health Center
New England Musculoskeletal Institute
Farmington, Connecticut

Paul Hyunsoo Yi, MD
Resident Physician
Department of Orthopaedic Surgery
University of California, San Francisco
San Francisco, California

Marc A. Zussman, MD
Assistant Professor, Department of Orthopaedic Surgery,
    Rush University Medical Center
Clinical Assistant Professor, Department of Surgery,
    University of Illinois
OrthoIllinois
Rockford, Illinois

INTRODUCTION

In 2012, the Accreditation Council for Graduate Medical Education (ACGME)'s Residency Review Committee (RRC) for orthopaedic surgery released a list of 15 case categories "that are representative of broader procedural experiences of a non-fellowship-educated surgeon in the specialty, as well as expectations for minimum numbers in each case category." The purpose of this textbook is simple: to give orthopaedic trainees an efficient reference to prepare for the cases most commonly encountered during training. While all of the techniques described may be found within the literature, never before have they been centralized into a single resource. Notably, this text does not aim to replace or reproduce the content provided by other excellent review sources for in-training and board examinations. Rather, it elaborates on the technical pearls necessary to actually perform the cases. Overall, this text aims to function as a standalone reference that will allow the resident to prepare for a case and perform the relevant surgical steps with confidence and competence.

We have expanded the 15 categories of "orthopaedic surgery case minimums" as determined by the ACGME into 40 technique-based chapters. There are more chapters than categories because some of the categories (i.e., operative treatment of femoral and tibial shaft fractures and all pediatric procedures) cover multiple important procedures commonly performed throughout the duration of orthopaedic training. In addition, several additional chapters cover other categories of commonly utilized surgical techniques (i.e., fasciotomies for compartment syndrome, traction pin placement, etc.) that are often encountered during orthopaedic training but do not fall into the categories defined by the ACGME case minimums.

Each chapter will contain a brief introduction to the case, including the minimum number of cases needed to satisfy ACGME requirements, as well as the commonly used CPT and ICD9 and ICD10 codes relevant to the procedure. Each procedure is described in detail, from room set-up and patient positioning, to surgical steps and postoperative protocols. Surgical steps are accompanied by intraoperative photographs so that the reader has a visual understanding of exactly how each case is performed. Each chapter also contains tables that outline the surgical steps, equipment needed, technical pearls, and common pitfalls. The goal of each chapter is to highlight schematics and photographs, while minimizing text to only essential information, in order to allow the reader to visualize each step of the case before scrubbing in. Finally, intraoperative videos supplement multiple chapters, demonstrating the surgical steps of the specified procedure in real time.

The intended audience of this book includes orthopaedic surgery interns, orthopaedic surgery residents, and orthopaedic surgery fellows. In addition, orthopaedic surgery physician extenders as well as rotating students will benefit from the step-by-step approaches provided in each chapter to prepare for cases. Certainly, this book will not substitute for the content provided by subspecialty textbooks and/or journals with surgical technique sections dedicated to specific cases. Rather, the aim of this textbook is to provide orthopaedic residents and other trainees with a quick, go-to, easy-access reference to prepare for the cases that the ACGME has deemed most appropriate to represent the breadth of surgical experience obtained and required during residency.

FOREWORD

t is an honor to be asked to craft the "Foreword" for this textbook, *Core Competencies in Orthopaedic Surgery,* edited by Drs. Rachel Frank, Brian Forsythe, and Matt Provencher. Reflecting back on a 40-year adventure in orthopaedic surgery and now in my 30th year as a clinician, educator, researcher, and leader in orthopaedic sports medicine, I recall the paucity of textbooks that were available to us as residents in the early 1980s. In this digital and informational age, we have experienced an explosion of high-quality orthopaedic education opportunities. Our CME courses are better, the industry provides focused educational formats on their products, numerous motor skills courses are accessible, and podcasts are provided by the AAOS and most orthopaedic surgical subspecialties. In addition, resources such as VuMedi provide an opportunity to teach techniques in a way we could have only dreamed of 30 years ago! The quality of our association journals are superb with exceedingly high-impact factors for the *American Journal of Sports Medicine, Journal of Bone and Joint Surgery,* and the *Arthroscopy* journal, among many others. Collaboratively, the AAOS, AOSSM, AANA, and multiple other specialty societies have partnered with a tremendous philanthropic effort by its members to build an outstanding new motor skills facility at the new AAOS building in Rosemont, Illinois. Textbooks are the backbone of education and have grown almost exponentially. All areas of orthopaedics are well represented with outstanding textbooks. In sports medicine alone, I recently donated a significant portion of my personal library to our residents' library with over 100 textbooks represented!

So where does this new textbook, *Core Competencies in Orthopaedic Surgery,* fit into our educational buffet? The organizational structure of this text fills a void for our trainees. The ACGME has designated "core competencies" in many pertinent areas of orthopaedics. For example, in how many cases does a resident have to participate to develop a reasonable level of competence? The general organizational format is easily palatable and digestible for residents of all levels. Introductory paragraphs on a topic are followed by common-related CPT and ICD codes. This in itself is quite unique in textbooks. The pertinent aspect of a specific procedure are defined in easily readable bullet point fashion. Room preparation, patient positioning, patient prepping, and specifics regarding the selected procedures focus on fundamental, pearls, and avoiding pitfalls. Tables, photographs, and videos and postoperative protocols complement the concise, efficiently presented material.

I believe this textbook will be well received and on most residents personal libraries. The book is an adjunct to other many outstanding textbooks but its value is in the concise fashion in which materials are presented. One can quickly "skim the icing" off the cake preparing for a case and focus on the essentials of the technical exercise at hand. Kudos to the authors for identifying an important niche for this textbook. I am thrilled to see this textbook prepared by division partner (Brian Forsythe), former fellow (Matthew Provencher), and current chief resident and future fellow (Rachel Frank) come to fruition.

Bernard R. Bach, Jr., MD

CONTENTS

VIDEO CONTENTS

CHAPTER 1

DIAGNOSTIC KNEE ARTHROSCOPY
SURGICAL TECHNIQUE

Rachel M. Frank | Bernard R. Bach, Jr.

The ability to perform a basic diagnostic knee arthroscopy is a critical skill for orthopaedic surgeons. With few exceptions, knee arthroscopy is likely to be performed multiple times per year, regardless of the field in which an orthopaedic surgeon ultimately decides to specialize. In many instances, especially for surgeons who specialize in sports medicine or practice general orthopaedic surgery, knee arthroscopy is the cornerstone of the surgical practice. The surgical skills necessary for thorough, accurate, and efficient knee arthroscopy are typically developed early in residency training. With limitations in work hours, combined with the 2013 Accreditation Council for Graduate Medical Education (ACGME) implementation of skills training requirements for junior residents, development of excellent habits during initial training sessions is now, more than ever, imperative to build a foundation on which to expand one's ability to treat different knee pathologies arthroscopically. The purpose of this chapter is to provide up-to-date technical pearls for performing a thorough, accurate, and efficient diagnostic knee arthroscopy. Of note, many different techniques are used to effectively navigate through the knee, and the technique presented here represents just one of these techniques. As such, the authors wish to emphasize that the reader understand the importance of learning and developing a specific routine for performing a diagnostic knee arthroscopy in order to perform the procedure in a routine fashion for every single knee.

SURGICAL TECHNIQUE

Room Set-Up

- Ensure that all appropriate equipment is in the room.
- Ensure that all implants and instruments are available and sterile.
- Confirm that the monitors are ergonomically positioned.
- Confirm that the video monitor, pump, and shaver systems are functional.
- The video monitor should be placed opposite the surgeon at head level.

Patient Positioning

- The patient is placed in a supine position on the operating table, with the knee at or below the break of the bed.
- A tourniquet is placed high on the thigh, even if inflation is not planned, so that one is prepared in the case of unexpected bleeding; padding around the thigh before placement of the tourniquet is advised. The tourniquet is typically set to 250 to 300 mm Hg.
- A plastic drape (sticky-u) is then placed around the tourniquet to create a barrier between the preparation solution and the tourniquet.

CASE MINIMUM REQUIREMENTS
- N = 30 (knee arthroscopy)

COMMONLY USED CPT CODES
- CPT Code: 29850—Arthroscopically aided treatment of intercondylar spine(s) and/or tuberosity fracture(s) of the knee, with or without manipulation; without internal or external fixation (includes arthroscopy)
- CPT Code: 29851—Arthroscopically aided treatment of intercondylar spine(s) and/or tuberosity fracture(s) of the knee, with or without manipulation; with internal or external fixation (includes arthroscopy)
- CPT Code: 29855—Arthroscopically aided treatment of tibial fracture, proximal (plateau); unicondylar, includes internal fixation, when performed (includes arthroscopy)
- CPT Code: 29856—Arthroscopically aided treatment of tibial fracture, proximal (plateau); bicondylar, includes internal fixation, when performed (includes arthroscopy)
- CPT Code: 29860—Arthroscopy, hip, diagnostic with or without synovial biopsy (separate procedure)
- CPT Code: 29866—Arthroscopy, knee, surgical; osteochondral autograft(s) (e.g., mosaicplasty; includes harvesting of the autograft[s])
- CPT Code: 29867—Arthroscopy, knee, surgical; osteochondral allograft (e.g., mosaicplasty)
- CPT Code: 29868—Arthroscopy, knee, surgical; meniscal transplantation (includes arthrotomy for meniscal insertion), medial or lateral
- CPT Code: 29870—Arthroscopy, knee, diagnostic, with or without synovial biopsy (separate procedure)

Continued

- CPT Code: 29871—Arthroscopy, knee, surgical; for infection, lavage and drainage
- CPT Code: 29873—Arthroscopy, knee, surgical; with lateral release
- CPT Code: 29874—Arthroscopy, knee, surgical; for removal of loose body or foreign body (e.g., osteochondritis dissecans fragmentation, chondral fragmentation)
- CPT Code: 29875—Arthroscopy, knee, surgical; synovectomy, limited (e.g., plica or shelf resection; separate procedure)
- CPT Code: 29876—Arthroscopy, knee, surgical; synovectomy, major, two or more compartments (e.g., medial or lateral)
- CPT Code: 29877—Arthroscopy, knee, surgical; débridement/shaving of articular cartilage (chondroplasty)
- CPT Code: 29879—Arthroscopy, knee, surgical; abrasion arthroplasty (includes chondroplasty where necessary) or multiple drilling or microfracture
- CPT Code: 29880—Arthroscopy, knee, surgical; with meniscectomy (medial *and* lateral, including any meniscal shaving)
- CPT Code: 29881—Arthroscopy, knee, surgical; with meniscectomy (medial *or* lateral, including any meniscal shaving)
- CPT Code: 29882—Arthroscopy, knee, surgical; with meniscus repair (medial *or* lateral)
- CPT Code: 29883—Arthroscopy, knee, surgical; with meniscus repair (medial *and* lateral)
- CPT Code: 29884—Arthroscopy, knee, surgical; with lysis of adhesions, with or without manipulation (separate procedure)
- CPT Code: 29885—Arthroscopy, knee, surgical; drilling for osteochondritis dissecans with bone grafting, with or without internal fixation (including débridement of base of lesion)
- CPT Code: 29886—Arthroscopy, knee, surgical; drilling for intact osteochondritis dissecans lesion
- CPT Code: 29887—Arthroscopy, knee, surgical; drilling for intact osteochondritis dissecans lesion with internal fixation
- CPT Code: 29888—Arthroscopically aided anterior cruciate ligament repair/augmentation or reconstruction
- CPT Code: 29889—Arthroscopically aided posterior cruciate ligament repair/augmentation or reconstruction

- A lateral leg post is placed on the outside of the operating table at the level of the midthigh and is positioned so a valgus stress can be applied to allow improved access to the medial compartment. The post should allow the surgeon to stand between the bed and the patient's ankle (as the thigh is pressed against the leg post); often surgeons may need to use their hip against the patient's leg if no assistance is available.
  - Alternatively, a circumferential leg holder can be used, with placement in the same position along the thigh as the leg post. This leg holder is typically placed at the level of the tourniquet.
- An examination of the knee with anesthesia should be performed after appropriate patient positioning, and various motions, including varus/valgus stress, should be performed to confirm that the position is adequate to permit a thorough examination of the knee.
- A time-out should be performed to ensure patient safety and to confirm the procedure to be performed.

Prepping and Draping

- Skin preparation is performed per surgeon/institution preference; the authors typically use alcohol followed by a chlorhexidine preparation solution while the assistant holds the foot in sterile fashion.
- The extremity is then draped in layers, as follows:
  - Down sheet under the operative leg, over the contralateral leg
  - Sticky-u drape with tails aimed proximally around the thigh, just distal to the plastic drape applied before prepping
  - Impervious stockinette applied over the foot to the midcalf, followed by Coban wrapping (3M, Minneapolis, MN) around the stockinette
  - Arthroscopy extremity drape over the leg to the level of the midthigh, creating the final sterile field; this drape typically has a hole in the center that creates a seal
  - The arthroscopy extremity drape is used by anesthesia to create a barrier to the surgical field.
  - Before draping, a mayo stand can be placed near the head of the bed over the patient's torso; after draping, this can be used to hold some of the arthroscopic equipment that is needed during the case.

Landmarks and Portal Placement

- Helpful landmarks are the patella, patellar tendon, and femoral condyles.
- Standard portals used for diagnostic arthroscopy include the anterolateral (AL), anteromedial (AM), superomedial (SM), and superolateral (SL) portals (Fig. 1-1).
  - With the knee flexed to 90 degrees, the landmarks become more visible.
- The AL and AM portals are primarily used for diagnostic knee arthroscopy; the SM and SL portals are often but not always used.
- The AL and AM portals are located in the "soft spot" on either side of the inferior pole of the patella.
  - AL portal: Between the lateral femoral condyle and lateral proximal tibia (AL); primary viewing portal
  - AM portal: Between the medial femoral condyle and medial proximal tibia (AM); primary working portal
- SM and SL portals are made approximately 4 cm proximal to the medial and lateral poles of the patella, respectively.
  - The SM and SL portals are often used for water flow; although these portals are not always created, they can be helpful in cases that involve extensive synovectomies and procedures within the patellofemoral joint.
- Additional portals: The posteromedial (PM) and posterolateral (PL) portals also occasionally are used in diagnostic knee arthroscopy, although these portals tend

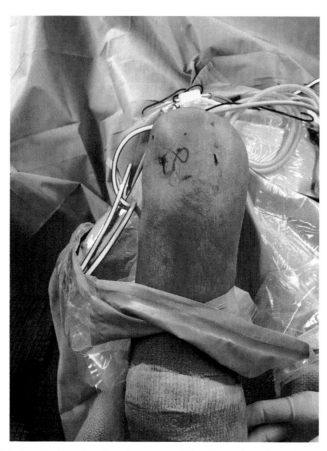

Figure 1-1 Right knee indicates locations for anteromedial and anterolateral portals before a diagnostic knee arthroscopy.

to be used more often for procedure-specific arthroscopies, such as posterior cruciate ligament (PCL) reconstruction (Fig. 1-2).

- The PM and PL portals are made with direct arthroscopic visualization, typically with the knee flexed to 90 degrees.
- The PM portal is created 1 cm proximal to the joint line, at the posteromedial margin of the medial femoral condyle.
  - This portal is helpful for visualization of the PCL and the posterior horn of the medial meniscus.
- The PL portal is created approximately 1 cm proximal to the joint line and 1 cm posterior to the lateral femoral condyle. Care must be taken to avoid injuring the biceps femoris muscle and the common peroneal nerve during creation of the PL portal.
  - This portal is helpful for visualization of the PCL and the posterior horn of the lateral meniscus.
- Other portals occasionally used in diagnostic knee arthroscopy include the transpatellar portal, the proximal superomedial portal, and accessory (far) medial/lateral portals.

Diagnostic Arthroscopic Examination

- If an SM or SL portal is to be used as an outflow, this portal is created first (Fig. 1-3).
- With the knee extended, a #11 scalpel is used to create a 5-mm incision in the SM or SL position, as described previously.
- Next, an outflow cannula with a blunt trocar is inserted into the suprapatellar pouch through the portal.

- Once inserted, the cannula can be swept proximally and distally to release any attached synovium.
- Once the trocar is removed, joint fluid typically is expressed, which confirms the intraarticular position.
- Next, with the knee in 90 degrees of flexion, the AL portal is established, first with a #11 scalpel to make a 5-mm incision in the soft spot lateral to the inferior pole of the patella, as described previously.
  - Vertical, horizontal, or oblique (along Langer's lines) incisions can be used depending on surgeon preference.
  - With vertical incisions, the blade should be directed cephalad to avoid injury to the meniscus.
- After incision, a straight hemostat is inserted through the incision to open up the capsule, with the jaws opening both superior-inferior and medial-lateral.
- Next, the arthroscope cannula with a blunt trocar is inserted through the portal and aimed toward the intercondylar notch.
- The knee is then extended fully, and the trocar is advanced under the patella into the suprapatellar pouch.
- A rotating motion of the hand can be used to gently advance the cannula into the pouch; this motion reduces the risk of iatrogenic cartilage damage.
- The inflow tubing is then attached to the cannula, the trocar is removed from the cannula, and the 30-degree arthroscope is inserted into the cannula and locked into place.
- At this point, the surgeon should ensure the outflow portal is truly in the joint (as opposed to stuck in the synovium) and reinsert if necessary.
- Finally, the surgeon should assess the camera's focus and adjust as appropriate. In the suprapatellar pouch, one can assess for loose bodies, a suprapatellar plica, or synovial hypertrophy.
- The arthroscope is then slightly withdrawn, and the patellofemoral joint is visualized (Figs. 1-4 and 1-5).
- The eyes should be oriented superiorly and then rotated medially and laterally to assess the articular cartilage of the medial and lateral facets of the patella.
- The arthroscope can then be directed laterally, with the camera aiming 30 degrees offset and slightly withdrawn to assess the relationship of the patella in the trochlear groove. The assistant should slowly flex the knee from extension to allow visualization of the entire trochlear groove.
- The superior-most aspect of the femoral condyles is visible at this point.
- The knee is then brought back into full extension, and the arthroscope is driven inward past the patella and directed laterally to enter the lateral gutter. The eyes should be directed medially.
- The surgeon raises the hand and slightly withdraws the arthroscope to access the gutter.
- The arthroscope passes over synovial folds in the gutter and continues to move inferiorly until the popliteus tendon is visualized in the popliteus hiatus.
- Once the synovial folds are identified, the surgeon should raise the camera to visualize the popliteal hiatus.
- Femoral condyle osteophytes or a tight lateral retinaculum can make this visualization difficult.
- The examiner can "tap" the posterolateral aspect of the knee from the outside to visualize any loose bodies.
- Assessment of the PCL in instability cases is recommended.
- With the knee still in extension, the arthroscope is brought back to the suprapatellar pouch and then directed medially to enter the medial gutter.
- The eyes should be directed inferiorly.
- The surgeon raises the hand and slightly withdraws the arthroscope to enter the gutter.
- Synovial folds again are visualized, and a plica may be seen.
- Next, the arthroscope enters the medial compartment.

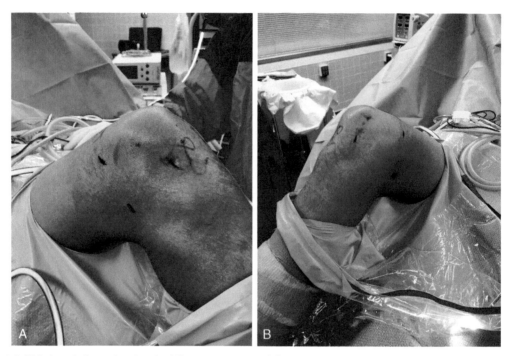

Figure 1-2 Right knee indicates locations for **(A)** posterolateral and **(B)** posteromedial portals before a diagnostic knee arthroscopy.

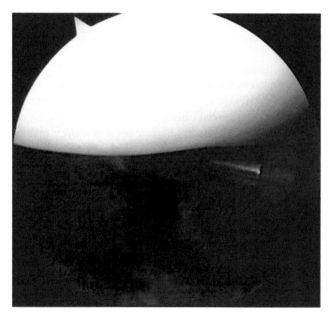

Figure 1-3 Arthroscopic photograph of the left knee shows the patello-femoral joint with the outflow cannula placed superomedially.

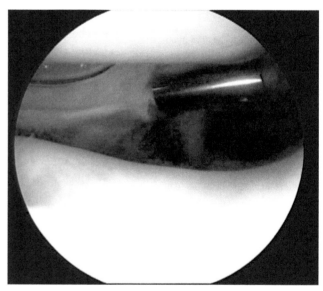

Figure 1-4 Arthroscopic photograph of the left knee shows the patello-femoral joint in extension.

- From the medial gutter, the arthroscope is slightly withdrawn and moved laterally as the knee is placed into flexion with approximately 10 degrees of external rotation.
- A valgus force is applied to the leg, and the camera is directed posterior to visualize the medial compartment from within the notch.
- At this point, an 18-gauge spinal needle is placed into the portal site for the AM portal and is visualized arthroscopically (Fig. 1-6).

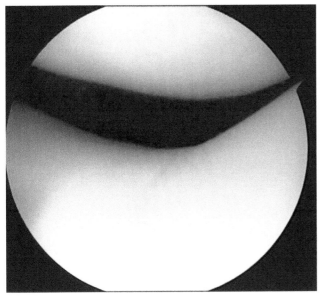

Figure 1-5 Arthroscopic photograph of the left knee shows the patello-femoral joint in slight flexion.

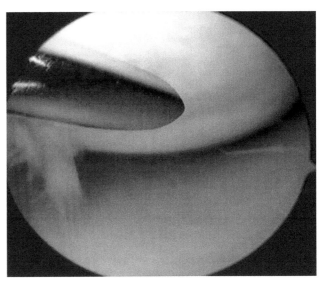

Figure 1-6 Arthroscopic photograph of the left knee shows needle localization for establishing the anteromedial portal.

- The AM portal is then established with a #11 scalpel to make a 5-mm incision, again orientated vertically, horizontally, or obliquely.
- For known lateral meniscus tears, placement of the portal in a more superior position than for a medial meniscus repair can be helpful.
- After creation of the AM portal, a probe is inserted through it into the medial compartment (Fig. 1-7).
- To facilitate this, the surgeon should lift the hand and aim the probe toward the floor to reach the posterior horn of the medial meniscus.
- If the probe does not pass easily into the medial compartment, the knee is brought into flexion and the arthroscope is used to look into the notch and triangulate the location of the probe. Both hands should be at the same vertical level.
- Remember that the eyes of the camera are aimed 30 degrees from the trajectory of the arthroscope.
- Once the probe is visualized, the maneuvers mentioned previously are used to reenter the medial compartment.
- The medial meniscus should be probed along both the superior and the inferior surfaces to assess for tears.
- Placement of the knee into full extension with a valgus force and raising of the hand holding the arthroscope superiorly while pushing inward allows for improved visualization of the posterior horn.
- The eyes can be rotated while in the medial compartment to visualize and inspect the entire meniscus.
- The posterior horn is best visualized looking inward to the notch.
- The eyes should be rotated inferiorly to assess the status of the tibial plateau articular cartilage. The medial femoral condyle is assessed by moving the arthroscope superiorly while flexing the knee from extension.
- Next, the intercondylar notch is visualized.
- The knee is brought into 90 degrees of flexion with the leg hanging off the table.
- The camera is directed from the medial compartment into the notch.
- The entire arch of the notch can be visualized by sweeping the camera superiorly and laterally.
- Once on the lateral side of the notch, the arthroscope can be withdrawn slightly and the anterior cruciate ligament (ACL) is visible.

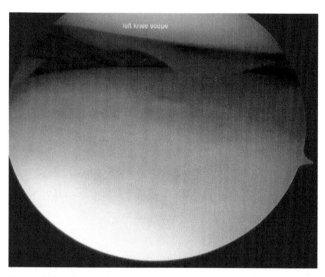

Figure 1-7 Arthroscopic photograph of the left knee shows assessment of the medial meniscus.

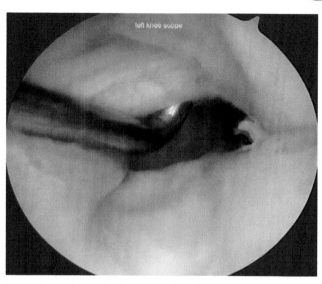

Figure 1-8 Arthroscopic photograph of the left knee shows assessment of the anterior cruciate ligament.

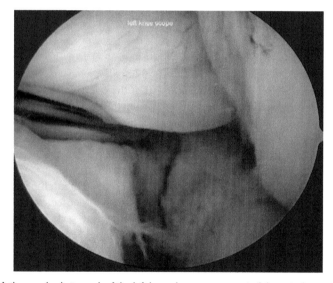

Figure 1-9 Arthroscopic photograph of the left knee shows assessment of the anterior cruciate ligament under mild tension with the probe.

- The probe can be inserted via the AM portal at this time and used to assess the ACL.
- The attachment of the ACL on the lateral femoral condyle should be intact (Fig. 1-8).
- The probe can be used to retract the ACL laterally for visualization of the PCL (Fig. 1-9).
- If visualization of the notch is difficult because of what may appear to be the retropatellar fat pad, this can be débrided with the shaver.
- Next, the lateral compartment is visualized.
- To move from the notch to the lateral compartment, the arthroscope is parked at the level of the inferior aspect of the lateral femoral condyle and the probe is placed in the "parking spot" triangle formed by the lateral border of the ACL, the medial border of the lateral femoral condyle, and the anterior horn of the lateral meniscus.

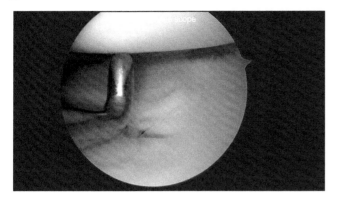

Figure 1-10 Arthroscopic photograph of the left knee shows assessment of the lateral compartment.

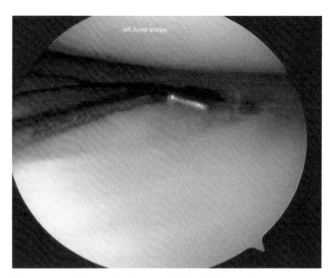

Figure 1-11 Arthroscopic photograph of the left knee shows assessment of the lateral meniscus.

- The knee is brought into the figure-four position with flexion and application of a varus load with internal rotation.
- The foot of the operative leg is rested on the anterior tibia of the contralateral leg.
- As the leg is brought up into the figure-four position, the hand holding the arthroscope should supinate to rotate approximately 90 degrees while aiming posterior with the camera.
- Thus, the correct visual orientation of the lateral compartment is maintained. The entire lateral meniscus should be probed and inspected, especially the posterior horn where tears are often missed (Figs. 1-10 and 1-11).
- The hand holding the arthroscope should be raised toward the ceiling and pushed posterior to facilitate adequate visualization. Gentle increases in varus stress help open up this area.
- The popliteus hiatus should be well visualized.
- The posterior horn of the lateral meniscus is naturally more lax than the posterior horn of the medial meniscus.
- The camera should be gently moved laterally, with the eyes oriented laterally to view the midbody of the meniscus followed by the anterior horn.
- To truly visualize the anterior horn, the camera is slowly and gently withdrawn.
- The anterior horn is sometimes better visualized with the arthroscope through the AM portal.
- The tibial plateau and lateral femoral condyle articular surfaces are subsequently assessed.

Posterior Diagnostic Knee Arthroscopy (Video 1-1)

Posterior Compartments (Fig. 1-12)
- Although many authors agree that posterior knee arthroscopy should be performed as part of most, if not all, diagnostic arthroscopic procedures, visualization of the posterior compartments of the knee is especially helpful in evaluation for loose bodies and in repair of meniscus root tears.
- For access to the posteromedial and posterolateral compartments of the knee, the modified Gillquist maneuver is typically performed.
  - This maneuver is referred to as a contralateral drive-through maneuver.
- For visualization of the posteromedial compartment, the knee is flexed to 90 degrees and a blunt trocar is placed through the AL portal toward the anterolateral wall of the medial femoral condyle.

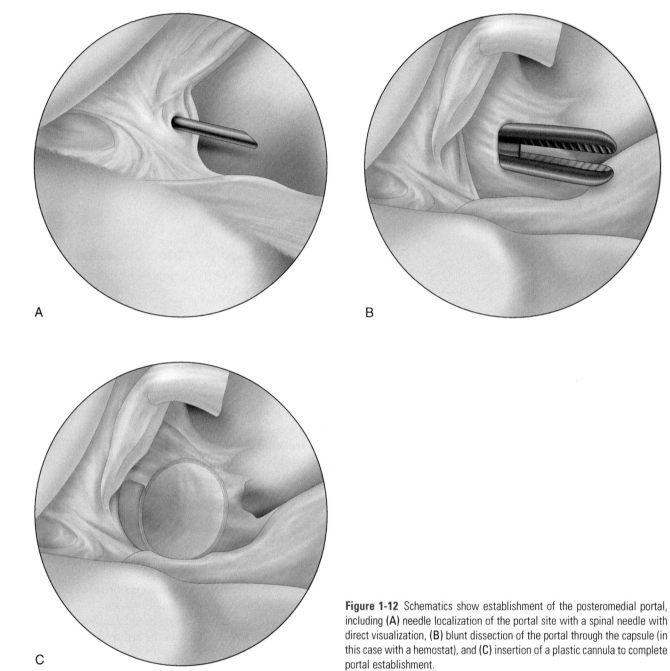

A

B

C

Figure 1-12 Schematics show establishment of the posteromedial portal, including **(A)** needle localization of the portal site with a spinal needle with direct visualization, **(B)** blunt dissection of the portal through the capsule (in this case with a hemostat), and **(C)** insertion of a plastic cannula to complete portal establishment.

- The obturator is slowly advanced posteriorly while the knee is slowly extended until it "pops" through the interval between the medial femoral condyle and the PCL; a valgus stress is applied to help facilitate access.
- Care should be taken to avoid injury to either the PCL or the medial wall of the intercondylar notch.
- The arthroscope is advanced over the trocar. The same technique is used to access the posterolateral compartment, with the trocar inserted into the AM portal and gently pushed and advanced through the interval between the medial aspect of the lateral femoral condyle and the ACL; a varus stress is applied to help facilitate access. Pending surgeon comfort, the arthroscope can be used directly instead of the blunt trocar. Often, the use of a 70-degree arthroscope is helpful for visualization of the posterior compartments of the knee.

- The authors have also found that an ipsilateral drive-through maneuver can be helpful for accessing the posterior compartments.
- When this maneuver is performed, the arthroscope is placed from the AL portal and slid in the interval between the ACL origin and the lateral wall of the intercondylar notch; conversely the AL portal may be used to slide into the posteromedial portal between the PCL and the medial wall of the intercondylar notch.
- Dependent on the visualization and relative joint tightness, varying degrees of knee flexion from 70 degrees (i.e., figure 2-4 position) to 30 degrees may facilitate this maneuver.
- Although the contralateral drive-through maneuver is generally easier to perform, on occasion a larger loose body blocks visualization in either the medial or lateral compartment, which makes visualization for creation of an accessory PM or PL portal difficult.
- In general, transitioning into the posterior compartments may be necessary to access for meniscocapsular tears, meniscal root tear repairs, loose bodies, visualization of the posterior cruciate tibial footprint during PCL reconstruction, synovectomy, and in unusual situations, posterior capsular releases or Baker's cyst decompression.

BRIEF SUMMARY OF SURGICAL STEPS

- Suprapatellar pouch
- Patellofemoral joint
- Trochlear groove
- Medial gutter
- Lateral gutter
- Medial compartment
- Intercondylar notch
- Cruciate ligaments
- Lateral compartment
- Posterior compartments

REQUIRED EQUIPMENT

Tourniquet
30-Degree arthroscope
Arthroscopy tower, fluid system, pump, tubing
Arthroscopic graspers, scissors
Arthroscopic probe, Wissinger rod, switching sticks, knot tier
Cannulas
Spinal needle

TECHNICAL PEARLS

- Suprapatellar pouch → eyes at 12 o'clock to identify the proximal patellar pole when retracting
- Patellofemoral joint → eyes laterally with scope astride 30 degrees
- Trochlear groove → eyes at 6 o'clock
- Lateral gutter → eyes aimed medially, raising scope up when synovial folds visualized
- Medial gutter → eyes at 6 o'clock or aiming medially
- Medial compartment → eyes aimed laterally at the notch; in a tight knee, eyes may need to look up as well
- Placement of the scope on the anterior horn of the meniscus medially may provide a second way to visualize the posterior horn of the meniscus
- Intercondylar notch → the anterior cruciate ligament femoral insertion is best visualized with the eyes placed at 10 or 2 o'clock
- Lateral compartment → eyes at 12 o'clock to visualize the posterior horn of the meniscus, rotating laterally to inspect the midbody and anterior horn

COMMON PITFALLS

(When to call for the attending physician)

- Portals placed too inferiorly risk damage to the meniscus and prohibition of adequate visualization of the medial joint
- Aggressive débridement of fat pad may cause bleeding and an increase in postoperative pain
- Significant valgus stress to visualize the medial compartment may risk injury to the medial collateral ligament
- Aggressive insertion of trocar, scope, or probe may cause iatrogenic injury to articular cartilage
- A stiff knee may make entering the gutters difficult; starting in the patellofemoral joint and entering the compartments via the intercondylar notch is helpful in these cases
- Be careful with radiofrequency near the gutters; a blister can be caused by being too close to the skin

POSTOPERATIVE PROTOCOL

Weeks 1-2: Weight bearing as tolerated without assistance by 48 hours after surgery
Range of motion (ROM): Progress through passive, active, and resisted ROM as tolerated (goal: full extension by 2 weeks, 130 degrees of flexion by 6 weeks)
Patellar mobilization daily
Strengthening: Quad sets, straight leg raises (SLR), heel slides, etc.
No restrictions to ankle and hip strengthening
Modalities: Electric stimulation, ultrasound, heat before and after, ice before and after
Weeks 2-6: ROM: Continue with daily ROM exercises (goal: increase ROM as tolerated)
Strengthening: Increase closed chain activities to full motion arc; add pulley weights, theraband, etc.; progress strengthening activities (wall sits, lunges, balance ball, leg curls, leg press, plyometrics, squats, core strengthening)
Continue stationary bike and biking outdoors for ROM, strengthening, and cardiovascular
Modalities: Electric stimulation, ultrasound, heat before and after, ice before and after

POSTOPERATIVE CLINIC VISIT PROTOCOL

7-10 days: First postoperative visit for suture removal and ROM check
4-6 weeks: Second postoperative visit for gait, ROM, and strength check
8-10 weeks: Final postoperative visit

SUGGESTED READINGS

1. Frank RM, McCormick FM, Harris JD, et al. Diagnostic knee arthroscopy: surgical technique. <http://orthoportal.aaos.org/oko/article.aspx?article=OKO_SPO079#abstract>; 2014. Accessed 16.02.15.
2. Ward BD, Lubowitz JH. Basic knee arthroscopy part 1: patient positioning. *Arthrosc Tech*. 2013;2(4):e497-e499. doi:10.1016/j.eats.2013.07.010.
3. Ward BD, Lubowitz JH. Basic knee arthroscopy part 2: surface anatomy and portal placement. *Arthrosc Tech*. 2013;2(4):e501-e502. doi:10.1016/j.eats.2013.07.013.
4. Ward BD, Lubowitz JH. Basic knee arthroscopy part 3: diagnostic arthroscopy. *Arthrosc Tech*. 2013;2(4):e503-e505. doi:10.1016/j.eats.2013.07.012.
5. Ward BD, Lubowitz JH. Basic knee arthroscopy part 4: chondroplasty, meniscectomy, and cruciate ligament evaluation. *Arthrosc Tech*. 2013;2(4):e507-e508. doi:10.1016/j.eats.2013.07.011.
6. Jackson RW. Arthroscopic surgery. *J Bone Joint Surg Am*. 1983;65(3):416-420.
7. Kramer DE, Bahk MS, Cascio BM, Cosgarea AJ. Posterior knee arthroscopy: anatomy, technique, application. *J Bone Joint Surg Am*. 2006;88(suppl 4):110-121. doi:10.2106/JBJS.F.00607.
8. Morin WD, Steadman JR. Arthroscopic assessment of the posterior compartments of the knee via the intercondylar notch: the arthroscopist's field of view. *Arthroscopy*. 1993;9(3):284-290.

DIAGNOSTIC SHOULDER ARTHROSCOPY
SURGICAL TECHNIQUE

Rachel M. Frank | Brian J. Cole

CASE MINIMUM REQUIREMENTS

- N = 20 (shoulder arthroscopy)

COMMONLY USED CPT CODES

- CPT Code: 29805—Arthroscopy, shoulder, diagnostic, with or without synovial biopsy (separate procedure)
- CPT Code: 29806—Arthroscopy, shoulder, surgical; capsulorrhaphy
- CPT Code: 29819—Arthroscopy, shoulder, surgical; with removal of loose body or foreign body
- CPT Code: 29820—Arthroscopy, shoulder, surgical; synovectomy, partial
- CPT Code: 29821—Arthroscopy, shoulder, surgical; synovectomy, complete
- CPT Code: 29822—Arthroscopy, shoulder, surgical; débridement, limited
- CPT Code: 29823—Arthroscopy, shoulder, surgical; débridement, extensive
- CPT Code: 29825—Arthroscopy, shoulder, surgical; with lysis and resection of adhesions, with or without manipulation
- CPT Code: 29826—Arthroscopy, shoulder, surgical; decompression of subacromial space with partial acromioplasty, with or without coracoacromial release

The ability to perform a basic diagnostic shoulder arthroscopy is a critical skill for orthopaedic surgeons. With few exceptions, shoulder arthroscopy is likely to be performed multiple times per year, regardless of the field in which an orthopaedic surgeon ultimately decides to specialize. In many instances, especially for surgeons who specialize in shoulder and elbow surgery or sports medicine or practice general orthopaedic surgery, shoulder arthroscopy remains among the most common procedures performed. The surgical skills necessary for thorough, accurate, and efficient shoulder arthroscopy are typically developed early in residency training. With limitations in work hours, combined with the 2013 Accreditation Council for Graduate Medical Education (ACGME) implementation of skills training requirements for junior residents, development of excellent habits during initial training sessions is now, more than ever, imperative to build a foundation on which to expand one's ability to treat different shoulder pathologies arthroscopically. The purpose of this chapter is to provide up-to-date technical pearls for performing a thorough, accurate, and efficient diagnostic shoulder arthroscopy. In this chapter, the authors present the basic techniques for performing diagnostic shoulder arthroscopy in both the beach chair (BC) and lateral decubitus (LD) positions (Video 2-1). With appropriate set-up and positioning, both techniques are reliable with low complication rates. The BC position offers the advantage of easy conversion to open techniques, and the LD position may allow for lower suture anchor position on the glenoid. Of note, many different techniques are used to effectively navigate through the shoulder, and the technique presented here represents just one of these techniques. As such, the authors wish to emphasize that the reader understand the importance of learning and developing a specific routine for performing a diagnostic shoulder arthroscopy in order to perform the procedure in a routine fashion for every single shoulder.

SURGICAL TECHNIQUE

Room Set-Up

- Ensure that all appropriate equipment is in the room.
- Ensure that all implants and instruments are available and sterile.
- Confirm that the monitors are ergonomically positioned.
- Confirm that the video monitor, pump, and shaver systems are functional.
- The video monitor should be placed opposite the surgeon at head level.

Patient Positioning

Beach Chair

- A leg pad is placed securely against the patient's buttocks to ensure that the buttocks and back are firmly against the beach chair; this placement prevents sciatic, lower back, and pelvic injuries related to positioning.
- Place a facemask over the patient, with care taken to not obstruct the airway; protect the eyes, ears, and nose at all times.
  - If a facemask is not used, tape the patient's head into place in a neutral position with a towel over the forehead.
- A team effort then moves the patient from the supine to the beach chair position on the operating table (head of bed is elevated approximately 60 degrees). Confirm that the airway and facemask remain in a secured position, and confirm that the leg pad is firmly against the patient's buttocks and that the patient's back is firmly against the operating table.
- The upper portion of the operating table can then be adjusted to improve exposure of the posterior aspect of the shoulder, typically with sliding the back of the table toward the contralateral shoulder while shifting the patient's torso toward the operative side. Take care to confirm that the patient's head and neck remain in a neutral position.
- Folded towels can be placed behind the medial border of the ipsilateral scapula to stabilize it on the operating table.
- Take the shoulder through the range of motion (ROM) that is necessary for the intended operative procedure.
- Ensure that the patient's knees and elbows are appropriately padded.
- Turn the table 45 to 90 degrees to improve access to the patient for both the anesthesia team and the surgical team (Fig. 2-1).

Lateral Decubitus

- Ensure that the bean bag is on the operating table before attempting the transfer. A sheet should be under and on top of the bean bag.
- Transfer the patient to the operating table.
- A team effort is used to roll the patient into the lateral decubitus position on the bean bag, with the operative extremity up.
- Place the axillary roll under the patient, approximately 2 to 3 fingerbreadths distal to the axilla against the rib cage. This placement minimzes the pressure on the brachial plexus during the case.
- Position the bean bag as desired to ensure optimal exposure and access to the shoulder and all necessary portals.

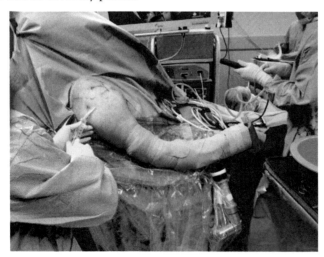

Figure 2-1 Intraoperative photograph shows final set-up for shoulder arthroscopy in the beach chair position.

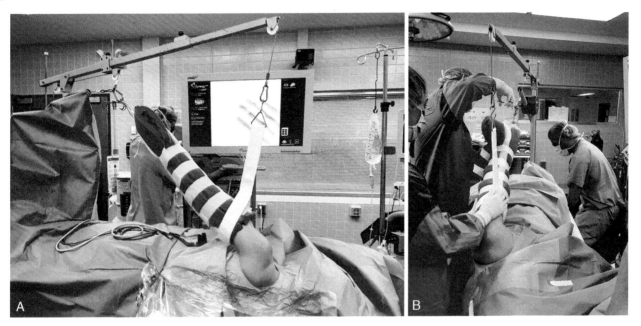

Figure 2-2 Intraoperative photograph shows traction set-up for shoulder arthroscopy in the lateral decubitus position (**A**, 30 to 40 degrees of abduction; **B**, 20 degrees of forward flexion).

- Inflate the bean bag.
- Secure the bean bag in place with heavy tape, with care taken to protect the skin of the patient.
- Ensure that bony prominences are well padded, especially the down arm and down leg at the ulnar nerve and peroneal nerve, respectively.
- Place a pillow between the legs to minimize pressure on the legs.
- Turn the table 45 to 90 degrees to improve access to the patient for both the anesthesia team and the surgical team (Fig. 2-2).

Prepping and Draping

- Two plastic drapes (sticky-u) are placed around the shoulder (one from proximal, one from distal) to create a barrier between the sterile preparation solution and the nonsterile portion of the patient.
- Skin preparation is performed per surgeon/institution preference. The authors typically use alcohol followed by a chlorhexidine preparation solution, with the arm suspended from a "candy cane" arm holder with Kerlix gauze (Covidien, Minneapolis) looped around the fingers
- The extremity is then draped in layers, as follows:
  - A down sheet is placed across the patient's body.
  - Two split drapes are placed above and below the shoulder, with the tails of the split drapes aimed toward the arm. The adhesive portions of the drapes should therefore create a barrier between the operative field and the plastic drapes that were placed before skin prepping. Be careful to maintain a generous working space so as to not "drape yourself out" of the operative field.
  - Use a sterile towel to grip the wrist as the circulating team removes the Kerlix from the fingers and removes the "candycane" holding the arm up.
  - Drape the hand, wrist, and forearm up to the elbow with an impervious stockinette followed by Coban wrapping (3M, Minneapolis, MN) around the stockinette.
  - Place the arthroscopy extremity drape over the arm as proximal as you can toward the barrier created by the split drapes, thus establishing the final sterile field. This drape typically has a hole in the center that creates a seal for the surgical field and plastic rectangular pouches that help to collect fluid during the

operative case, which should be aimed toward the floor such that they can be effective at collecting the fluid.

- The arthroscopy extremity drape is used by the anesthesia team to create a barrier to the surgical field.
- Ioban tape (3M) is then applied circumferentially around the extremity drape to create a barrier between the drape and the sterile field.

Beach Chair

- In the BC position, the arm can then either be (1) left free and held by an assistant or a mayo stand or (2) placed into an extremity holder.
- If the arm is left free, a draped mayo stand can be helpful at holding the arm in place during the operative procedure if no assistant is available.
- If an arm holder is to be used, the attachment for the support arm should be connected to the operating table via a standard table Clark rail and draped with the supplied sterile drape. The forearm should then be placed into the supplied foam-padded arm holder. The padded arm holder is then wrapped in Coban wrapping and attached to the arm support, which can be adjusted per the surgeon's preference with either the support arm itself or a foot pedal.

Lateral Decubitus

- In the LD position, the arm is then placed into the lateral decubitus traction device.
- Of note, before draping, the traction tower should be positioned appropriately (see Fig. 2-2). This system typically uses traction weights hung off of a pulley traction cable that is located away from the operative field, with several positioners located along the traction cable to allow for length, flexion, abduction, and traction adjustments as needed.
- The arm is placed into the supplied foam-padded arm sleeve, with care taken to protect the superficial radial nerve.

  • PEARL An extra abdominal pad (ABD pad) can be placed here for added protection.

- The sleeve is secured around the forearm with the supplied Velcro (Velcro USA Inc., Manchester, NH) straps, and then the pad is connected to the traction system with the supplied sterile S-hook with rope. An assistant (nonsterile) can then adjust the pulley system and weights to apply the appropriate traction and position. The goal is to maintain the arm in approximately 30 to 40 degrees of abduction and 20 degrees of forward flexion (see Fig. 2-2).
- Alternatively, a rolled towel can be placed in the axilla to provide joint distension without the need for a dual traction set-up.

  • PEARL Smaller degrees of flexion and abduction are needed for subacromial space access.

Landmarks and Portals

- Draw the following helpful landmarks with an indelible marking pen: acromion ("notch" and posterior+lateral borders), clavicle, coracoid process, AC joint.
- Standard portals for diagnostic arthroscopy are listed as follows (Figs. 2-3 and 2-4). These portals can be infiltrated with local anesthetic before incision.
  - Posterior portal: Standard viewing portal made 2 cm inferior and 1 cm medial to the posterolateral border of acromion in the "soft spot." In the LD position, this is typically located slightly more lateral than in the BD position. For palpation of the soft spot, it can be helpful to place the tip of the index finger in the "notch," the tip of the middle finger on the coracoid, and the thumb naturally in the position of the soft spot. Anatomically, this portal is located at the inferior edge of the infraspinatus (IS), or between the IS and teres minor. An 18-gauge spinal needle is inserted in the desired location, aiming toward the coracoid process, and the joint is insufflated with normal saline (Figs. 2-5 and 2-6). A skin incision is then made through only the skin and subcutaneous tissue, followed by insertion of the blunt trocar. When inserting the trocar and the scope, aim toward the coracoid process and attempt to palpate the junction between the glenoid rim and humeral head and then gently "push" through the posterior rotator cuff. Remember this same incision is used to access the subacromial space from the posterior (Fig. 2-7).

  • PEARL The axillary nerve typically lies 3 cm inferior to the posterior portal, and the suprascapular nerve lies 2 cm medial to the posterior portal.

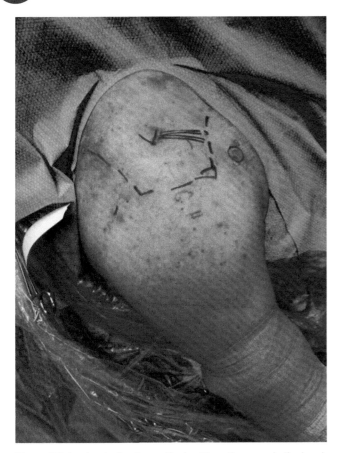

Figure 2-3 Landmarks for diagnostic shoulder arthroscopy in the beach chair position.

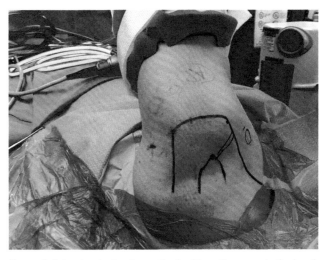

Figure 2-4 Landmarks for diagnostic shoulder arthroscopy in the beach chair position.

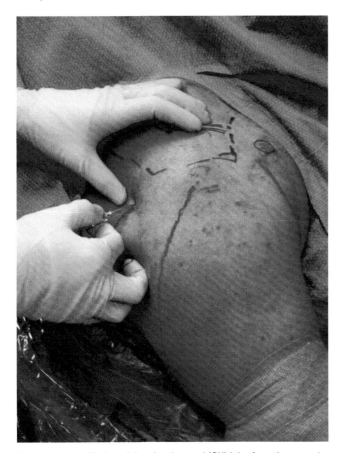

Figure 2-5 Insufflation of the glenohumeral (GH) joint from the posterior portal in the beach chair position.

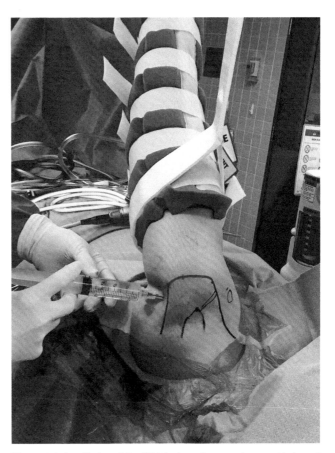

Figure 2-6 Insufflation of the GH joint from the posterior portal in lateral decubitus position.

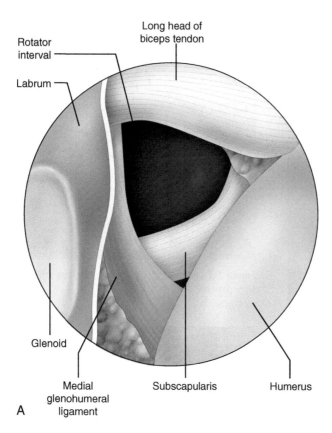

Rotator interval

Long head of biceps tendon

Labrum

Glenoid

Medial glenohumeral ligament

Subscapularis

Humerus

A

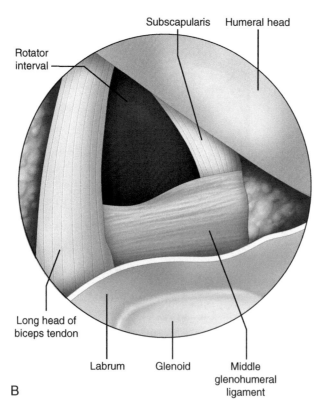

Subscapularis

Humeral head

Rotator interval

Long head of biceps tendon

Labrum

Glenoid

Middle glenohumeral ligament

B

Figure 2-7 Schematic of the appearance of the glenohumeral joint during diagnostic arthroscopy when viewing from the posterior, comparing (**A**) the beach chair position and (**B**) the lateral decubitus position. Structures visible include the glenoid, humeral head, labrum, long head of the biceps tendon, rotator interval, subscapularis tendon, and middle glenohumeral ligament.

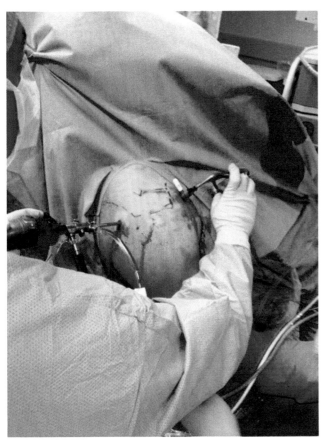

Figure 2-8 Intraoperative photograph shows anterior and posterior portals in the beach chair position.

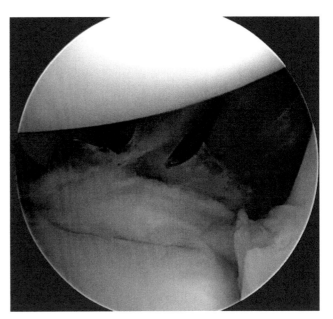

Figure 2-9 Intraoperative photograph shows anterior portal establishment (lateral decubitus position, left shoulder, viewing from posterior).

- Anterior portal (Figs. 2-8 and 2-9): Standard anterior working portal made approximately 1 cm inferior to the anterior margin of the acromion, between the anterolateral border of the acromion and the coracoid process; this portal position can be adjusted depending on the intended surgical procedure. This portal is established either via an inside-out (needle localization) technique or via an outside-in (advance posterior cannula into rotator interval, pass Wissinger rod through cannula and out through anterior soft tissues) technique. A skin incision is made only through the skin and subcutaneous tissue, and the trajectory for this portal goes through the deltoid, the pectoralis major, and ultimately the rotator interval (between the supraspinatus and the infraspinatus). This portal is lateral to the long head of the biceps tendon and just lateral to the middle glenohumeral ligament (MGHL).

> • PEARL Be sure to stay lateral to the coracoid to avoid damage to the neurovascular structures.

- Lateral portal: Typically used for subacromial space procedures, this portal is established with direct visualization with needle localization (viewing from posterior). A spinal needle is inserted 1 to 2 cm lateral to the lateral edge of the acromion in line with the posterior aspect of the AC joint. A skin incision is made only through the skin and subcutaneous tissue, and a blunt trocar is inserted through the deltoid and into the subacromial space.
- Several accessory portals can also be established, depending on the specific procedure to be performed:
  - Anterosuperior portal: This portal is helpful for Bankart repair, SLAP repair, and visualization during posterior labral repair. This portal is established via an outside-in technique, similar to that described previously for the standard anterior portal. This portal is established just inferior to the anterior border of the AC joint and enters the joint just anterior to the leading edge of the

supraspinatus. A threaded cannula is helpful to use after establishing this portal to prevent extravasation of fluid into the periarticular soft tissues.

- Anteroinferior (5 o'clock): This portal is also helpful for Bankart repair and is typically established percutaneously directly through the subscapularis muscle (transsubscapularis). This portal is typically established percutaneously with spinal needle localization; no cannula is used.

- Superior portal of Neviaser: This portal is helpful for rotator cuff repair, SLAP repair, and suprascapular nerve decompression and is typically made in the soft spot created by the clavicle (anteriorly), scapular spine (posteriorly), and acromion (laterally), also referred to as the "notch." This portal penetrates the trapezius muscle and should aim from medial to lateral in the supraspinatous fossa, with care taken to avoid injury to the suprascapular nerve by starting more medial.

- Port of Wilmington: This portal is helpful for SLAP repair and is made 1 cm lateral and 1 cm anterior to the posterolateral corner of acromion. This portal is typically established percutaneously with spinal needle localization; no cannula is used.

- Posterolateral portal (7 o'clock; Fig. 2-10): This portal is helpful for both anterior and posterior instability repair and is typically established percutaneously through or just inferior to the teres minor. Because of the proximity of the axillary nerve, one should always use dilators before placing a cannula in this portal.

- Typical diagnostic arthroscopy uses the standard posterior and standard anterior portal, which can be cheated superiorly or midglenoid, depending on the anticipated procedure.

Diagnostic Shoulder Arthroscopy

- A standard 30-degree arthroscope is adequate for diagnostic arthroscopy; however, a 70-degree arthroscope may be helpful to fully evaluate the anterior and inferior recesses.

- Regardless of the position of the patient, a routine diagnostic arthroscopy of the glenohumeral joint and the subacromial space should be performed in every patient. Several structures should be viewed from both the standard posterior viewing portal and the standard anterior working portal. Gaining different perspectives on the anatomy of the glenohumeral joint allows one to recognize all pathologies.

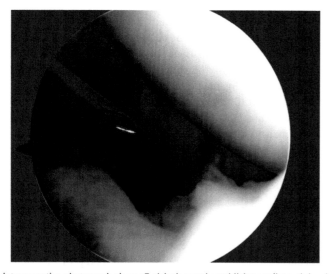

Figure 2-10 Intraoperative photograph shows 7 o'clock portal establishment (lateral decubitus position, left shoulder, viewing from posterior).

- In addition, several structures should be viewed from both the articular side (within the glenohumeral joint) and the bursal side (within the subacromial space).
- Once the standard posterior and anterior portals have been established as described previously, several structures should be viewed with the scope viewing from the posterior portal:
  - Rotator interval: Allows viewing of long head of the biceps tendon (LHBT), superior glenohumeral ligament (SGHL), MGHL, and subscapularis tendon.
  - Rotate the eyes of the camera inferiorly to fully view the subscapularis tendon and the anterior aspect of the glenohumeral joint inferior to the rotator interval.
  - Rotate the eyes superiorly to view the LHBT, superior labrum, and LHBT anchor. At this time, a probe can be inserted via the anterior portal and the LHBT can be "pulled" into the joint (pull from the superior aspect of the LHBT) to assess for LHBT pathology (i.e., lipstick lesion). The superior aspect of the labrum also can be probed to assess for a SLAP tear versus normal SLAP anatomic variants.
    - By moving the arm from adduction/neutral to 90 abduction–90 external rotation (ER), one may visualize a "peel back lesion" of the labral attachment of the LHBT at the superior aspect of the glenoid.
    - The SGHL is appreciated at the superior portion of the rotator interval, typically traveling with the LHBT.
    - The MGHL is variable in appearance, ranging from a well-defined structure to a cord-like structure (Buford complex, cord-like MGHL that inserts directly on the LHBT leaving a "bare" area of glenoid without labrum), to an attenuated nonsignificant structure.
  - Gently advance the scope into the joint and rotate the eyes inferiorly to allow for a better appreciation of the anterior and inferior structures of the joint, including the subscapularis tendon, MGHL, anterior inferior glenohumeral ligament (AIGHL), anterior-inferior labrum, and anterior-inferior joint capsule. The probe can be used to palpate these structures and assess for instability, with care taken not to violate the articular cartilage of the humeral head or glenoid.
    - The rolled upper border of the subscapularis defines the inferior border of the rotator interval.
    - Anterior labrum instability, and the possible presence of an anterior labrum periosteal sleeve avulsion (ALPSA) lesion, are indicative of anterior shoulder instability.
    - One should be sure to visualize the humeral attachments of the glenohumeral ligaments to rule out a humeral avulsion glenohumeral ligament (HAGL) or reverse-HAGL lesion.
  - Without pulling the scope out, rotate the eyes inferiorly and then posteriorly, which allows for evaluation of the AIGHL, inferior pouch, posterior recess (Fig. 2-11), and posterior inferior glenohumeral ligament (PIGHL).
  - Loose bodies are often present in the inferior pouch and posterior recess.
  - While withdrawing the scope slowly, but taking care not to withdraw from the joint, the eyes of the scope can be rotated superiorly, and the hand holding the scope can gently be lowered so that the camera is able to view the articular surface of the posterosuperior rotator cuff (supraspinatus and infraspinatus).
  - With the scope still in the posterior portal, rotate the eyes anteriorly to view the glenoid articular surface, including the bare spot, and the humeral head articular surface, including the bare area, which should not be confused for a Hill-Sachs lesion. The entirety of the humeral head can be visualized with gentle internal and external rotation of the humerus.
    - Document any articular cartilage softening, fissuring, or fragmentation (Fig. 2-12).
  - Next, gently withdraw the scope from the posterior portal and place it through the cannula in the anterior portal to allow a better appreciation of the posterior

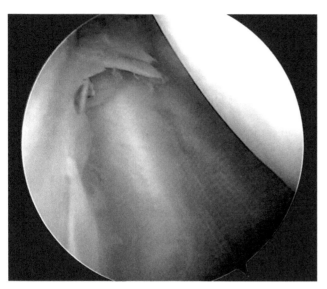

Figure 2-11 Arthroscopic photograph shows the posterior recess (beach chair position, right shoulder, viewing from posterior).

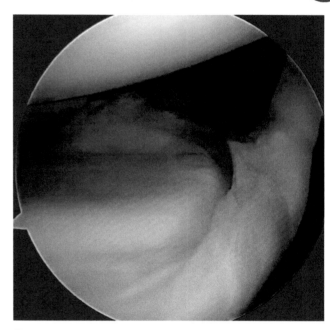

Figure 2-12 Arthroscopic photograph shows the glenohumeral joint (lateral decubitus position, left shoulder, viewing from posterior).

labrum, PIGHL, and posterior capsule. Once again, the probe can be used to palpate these structures and assess for instability, with care taken not to violate the articular cartilage of the humeral head or glenoid.

- With the scope still in the anterior portal, rotate the eyes anteriorly to view the glenoid articular surface, including the bare spot, and the humeral head articular surface, including the bare area, which should not be confused for a Hill-Sachs lesion.
- From this position, the eyes of the scope can be rotated superiorly, and the hand holding the scope can gently be lowered so that the camera is able to view the articular surface of the posterosuperior rotator cuff (supraspinatus and infraspinatus).
  - Document any cuff tissue fraying, calcification, or tearing (partial or full-thickness).
- Withdraw the scope and enter the subacromial space from the posterior portal. To do this, use the blunt trocar and aim the tip toward the anterolateral corner of the acromion, penetrating the deltoid muscle. Once the trocar has entered the subacromial space, you should be able to sweep your hand holding the trocar medially and laterally without any resistance. Insert the arthroscope, and the subacromial space should now be viewed as "a room with a view." Visualize the inferior acromion (by turning the eyes superior), subacromial bursa (by turning the eyes inferior), bursal side of the rotator cuff (eyes inferior), and undersurface of the coraco-acromial (CA) ligament (eyes superior). As discussed previously, the lateral portal can be established with direct visualization with spinal needle localization.
- While in the subacromial space, one can identify the bicipital groove, pectoralis major tendon insertion, and suprascapular nerve at the suprascapular notch and spinoglenoid notch.

Closure

- Portals are closed with 3-0 nylon sutures with mattress or figure-of-eight sutures.
- Dressings include gauze, ABD pads, and tape, with a sling.

BRIEF SUMMARY OF SURGICAL STEPS

Draw landmarks with an indelible marking pen: acromion ("notch" and posterior+lateral borders), clavicle, coracoid process, acromioclavicular joint

Establish posterior and standard anterior portals

Enter the GH joint through the posterior portal

View and probe the following structures:

- MGHL
- SGHL
- LHBT
- Biceps anchor
- Superior labrum
- Rolled edge of subscapularis
- Supraspinatus (articular side of rotator cuff)
- Infraspinatus (articular side of rotator cuff)
- Teres minor (articular side of rotator cuff)
- Articular surface of humeral head
- Bare spot of humerus
- Articular surface of glenoid
- Bare spot of glenoid
- Anterior labrum
- Posterior labrum
- Posterior capsular recess
- Axillary pouch and inferior labrum
- AIGHL

Switch scope to anterior portal and view the same structures

Switch scope to posterior portal and enter the subacromial space; visualize the following structures:

- Inferior acromion (by turning the eyes superior)
- Subacromial bursa (by turning the eyes inferior)
- Bursal side of the rotator cuff (eyes inferior)
- Undersurface of the CA ligament (eyes superior)

Establish the lateral portal can be established with direct visualization with spinal needle localization

TECHNICAL PEARLS

Beach Chair Advantages
- Ease of converting to open procedure
- More "natural" anatomy; easier for teaching
Arm free:
- Full rotational and abduction control
- Easy set-up; use a padded mayo stand
- Ease of performing open procedures
Arm holder:
- Commercially available positioners
- Helpful as a solo surgeon (no assistants needed)
- Hydraulic versus pneumatic versus mechanically controlled
- Allows for precise control of arm
- Allows for some degree of traction

Lateral Decubitus Advantages
- Less worry regarding cerebral hypoperfusion
- Improved ability to get access to inferior glenoid
- Improved access to posterior glenoid
- Improved visualization of subacromial space with 20 to 30 degrees of abduction
- Possibly decreased revision instability rates
- Possibly more ergonomic for the surgeon

REQUIRED EQUIPMENT

30-Degree arthroscope

Mayo stand or commercial arm holder (beach chair position)

Traction system with weights and pulleys, bean bag (lateral decubitus position)

Arthroscopy tower, fluid system, pump, tubing

Cannulas

Arthroscopic shaver, burr, radiofrequency device

Arthroscopic graspers, scissors

Arthroscopic elevator, probe, Wissinger rod, switching sticks, knot pusher

COMMON PITFALLS

(When to call for the attending physician)

Beach Chair Position
- Be aware of potential for cerebral hypotension
- Hypotensive anesthesia can be useful for the surgeon by reducing bleeding and therefore improving visualization
- Consider use of a beta-blocker (per anesthesia team)
- Consider location of blood pressure cuff placement
- Position buttocks up against bed to avoid pressure injury
- Avoid excessive ER to prevent brachial plexus strain
- Avoid contralateral elbow flexion more than 90 degrees to avoid an ulnar nerve injury
Be careful with head position
- Place head and neck in neutral to decrease risk of hypovascular incidents
- Ensure proper padding at the knees to avoid a peroneal nerve injury

Lateral Decubitus Position
- Ideal position: 15 degrees of forward flexion and 45 degrees of abduction
- Maximizes operative visibility, minimizes brachial plexus strain
Be aware of traction injuries
- Avoid extreme extension and abduction as a result of the musculocutaneous nerve
- Avoid use of more than 10 lb of traction
- Use additional padding for bony prominences
Greater trochanter
- Between body and bean-bag edges
- Be aware of head position; neutral neck position is critical
- Pay attention to the patient's normal cervical kyphosis
- Use head and ear donuts to avoid periauricular pressure injuries

General
- Draw landmarks and create portals before joint insufflation
- Use threaded cannulas when possible

POSTOPERATIVE PROTOCOL

Weeks 0-4: Passive ROM as tolerated with goals of 140 degrees forward flexion (FF)
and 40 degrees ER at the side
No abduction or 90-90 ER until at least 4 weeks
Sling for comfort for weeks 0-2
Grip strengthening allowed, but no resisted motions
Weeks 4-8: Increase passive and active ROM to tolerance without restrictions
Begin light isometric exercises with arm at side and advance with therabands as
tolerated
Weeks 8-12: Increase motion and strengthening as tolerated

POSTOPERATIVE CLINIC VISIT PROTOCOL

7-10 days: First postoperative visit for suture removal and ROM check
4-6 weeks: Second postoperative visit for gait, ROM, and strength check
8-10 weeks: Final postoperative visit

SUGGESTED READINGS

1. Frank RM, Saccomanno MF, McDonald LS, et al. Outcomes of arthroscopic anterior shoulder instability in the beach chair versus lateral decubitus position: a systematic review and meta-regression analysis. *Arthroscopy*. 2014;30(10):1349-1365. doi:10.1016/j.arthro.2014.05.008.
2. Skyhar MJ, Altchek DW, Warren RF, Wickiewicz TL, O'Brien SJ. Shoulder arthroscopy with the patient in the beach-chair position. *Arthroscopy*. 1988;4(4):256-259.
3. Paxton ES, Backus J, Keener J, Brophy RH. Shoulder arthroscopy: basic principles of positioning, anesthesia, and portal anatomy. *J Am Acad Orthop Surg*. 2013;21(6):332-342. doi:10.5435/JAAOS-21-06-332.
4. Neviaser TJ. Arthroscopy of the shoulder. *Orthop Clin North Am*. 1987;18(3):361-372.
5. Meyer M, Graveleau N, Hardy P, Landreau P. Anatomic risks of shoulder arthroscopy portals: anatomic cadaveric study of 12 portals. *Arthroscopy*. 2007;23(5):529-536. doi:10.1016/j.arthro.2006.12.022.
6. Lee JH, Min KT, Chun Y-M, Kim EJ, Choi SH. Effects of beach-chair position and induced hypotension on cerebral oxygen saturation in patients undergoing arthroscopic shoulder surgery. *Arthroscopy*. 2011;27(7):889-894. doi:10.1016/j.arthro.2011.02.027.
7. Peruto CM, Ciccotti MG, Cohen SB. Shoulder arthroscopy positioning: lateral decubitus versus beach chair. *Arthroscopy*. 2009;25(8):891-896. doi:10.1016/j.arthro.2008.10.003.
8. Chalmers PN, Sherman S. Patient positioning, portal placement, normal arthroscopic anatomy, and diagnostic arthroscopy. In: Cole BJ, Sekiya JK, eds. *Surgical Techniques of the Shoulder, Elbow, and Knee*. 2nd ed. Philadelphia: Elsevier; 2014:3-12.

ANTERIOR CRUCIATE LIGAMENT RECONSTRUCTION WITH PATELLAR TENDON AUTOGRAFT OR ALLOGRAFT

Andrew Joseph Riff | Michael Collins | Brian Forsythe

CASE MINIMUM REQUIREMENTS

- ACL tear in a young patient who is returning to sports
- Symptomatic knee instability in a patient with ACL insufficiency
- Multiligamentous knee injury

COMMONLY USED CPT CODES

- CPT Code: 29888—Arthroscopically aided ACL repair/augmentation or reconstruction
- CPT Code: 29888-22—Commonly used modifier for revision ACL reconstruction
- CPT Code: 29882—Arthroscopy, knee, surgical; with meniscus repair (medial or lateral)
- CPT Code: 29883—Arthroscopy, knee, surgical; with meniscus repair (medial and lateral)

COMMONLY USED ICD9 CODES

- 844.2—Tear of cruciate ligament injury of the knee
- 836.0—Tear of medial cartilage or meniscus
- 836.1—Tear of lateral cartilage or meniscus

Anterior cruciate ligament (ACL) reconstruction is one of the most common orthopaedic procedures, with an estimated incidence between 100,000 and 250,000 cases annually in the United States. Approximately 70% of ACL injuries are noncontact injuries; the remaining 30% are contact injuries. The most common mechanism is a noncontact deceleration event with a sudden change in direction against a planted foot (i.e., cutting). Injuries occur most commonly in the late teens and early twenties and, according to a recent metaanalysis, are roughly three times more common in females than in males in soccer and basketball. After ACL rupture, reconstruction is recommended for young athletes who hope to return to sports and for less active patients with symptomatic instability (i.e., recurrent "giving way"). Some literature suggests that ACL reconstruction helps prevent meniscus tears and chondral injury; however, high-quality evidence that it prevents osteoarthritis is lacking. O'Connor, Laughlin, and Woods showed that delay of ACL reconstruction beyond 6 months from injury resulted in a 1.5-fold increased risk of meniscal injury in men and a 3.4-fold increased risk in women when compared with reconstruction within 2 weeks of injury.

The most controversial topics in ACL reconstruction include technique used to establish the femoral tunnel (anteromedial portal versus transtibial), graft selection (patellar tendon versus hamstring), and indication for use of allograft versus autograft. Although transtibial ACL reconstruction has rendered favorable outcomes since the early 1990s, the proportion of surgeons who use an independent drilling technique has increased dramatically in recent years (from 10% in 2006 to 68% in 2013). Advocates of the anteromedial portal technique contend that independent drilling permits more anatomic placement of the femoral footprint and improved rotator stability; however, this technique comes with a risk of shorter tunnels and an increased risk of posterior cortical blowout. Central-third patellar tendon (BTB) is considered by many surgeons to be the gold standard graft because it is associated with lower rates of failure when compared with hamstring autograft in a large volume registry and systematic review studies. However, this technique comes with the drawbacks of fixed graft length (risk of graft-construct mismatch), higher risk of donor site morbidity (anterior knee pain and patellar fracture), and risk of physeal closure in the pediatric population. Allograft ACL reconstruction witnessed a dramatic rise in popularity in the late 1990s because of reduced donor site morbidity, motion loss, and operative time; however, its popularity was tempered in the early 2000s because of a few highly publicized cases of graft-associated infection. Improved techniques of secondary sterilization seem to have minimized the risk of infection but have also imparted deleterious biomechanical effects to the graft, which have resulted to an alarmingly high failure rate in young patients (2.6 to 4.2 times that of BTB autograft in one study). According to the current literature, allografts should be used sparingly in patients under the age of 30 years. The senior author favors a technique that uses flexible reaming from the anteromedial portal to establish the femoral tunnel. With regard to graft choice, BTB autograft is preferred in young contact athletes and in younger females with ligamentous laxity, as long as the physes are closed. The authors' allograft of choice is also BTB, treated with low-dose irradiation.

SURGICAL TECHNIQUE

Room Set-Up

The following steps are shown in an instructional video (Video 3-1)
- The operating table is positioned in the typical location within the operating room.
- A second sterile back table should be established by the surgical technician and should have sufficient workspace with the instruments needed for graft preparation.

Patient Positioning

- Surgery is performed with the patient supine and after administration of prophylactic antibiotics and general anesthetic.
- Before final positioning, examination of the injured knee with anesthesia is conducted. This examination should include pivot shift and Lachman testing to confirm the diagnosis of ACL insufficiency and grade of ACL insufficiency, respectively. The collateral ligaments should also be evaluated at full extension and at 30 degrees. A dial test at 30 and 90 degrees of knee flexion and a check for anteromedial and posterolateral rotary instability at 90 degrees of knee flexion should also be performed.
- A padded tourniquet is placed high on the operative thigh.
- Most surgeons place the thigh in a leg holder with the operative leg hanging off the end of the table and the contralateral leg in a lithotomy leg holder. The senior surgeon prefers to drape the leg free with a lateral post along the proximal thigh (Fig. 3-1). A bump is taped to the table just distal to the contralateral knee to permit easy flexion of the operative knee to 90 degrees during graft harvest (Fig. 3-2). Draping the leg free improves the ease of hyperflexion for passing the femoral guidepin and for femoral bone plug fixation.
- If the pivot shift is positive, the authors proceed with graft harvest before diagnostic arthroscopy.
- If the pivot shift is equivocal, diagnostic arthroscopy is performed before harvesting of the graft (or thawing of the allograft).

Prepping and Draping

- A nonsterile U-drape is placed around the tourniquet.
- The knee is preliminarily scrubbed with alcohol to reduce bioburden.
- Final preparation is performed with chlorhexidine gluconate.
- The knee is draped with a sterile U-drape and then with an extremity drape.

Patellar Tendon Harvest

- In the setting of definitively positive pivot shift test results, patellar tendon autograft harvest can be performed before diagnostic arthroscopy to permit placement of arthroscopic portals within the harvest wound and to allow for graft preparation during diagnostic arthroscopy.
- An 8-cm incision is made from the inferior order of the patella to the medial aspect of the tibial tubercle (Fig. 3-3). The incision is carried down sharply until the transverse fibers of the paratenon are encountered.
- Skin flaps are raised, and the paratenon is divided longitudinally and preserved.

COMMONLY USED ICD10 CODES

- M23.61—Other spontaneous disruption of anterior cruciate ligament of knee
- M23.20—Derangement of unspecified meniscus due to old tear or injury
- M23.21—Derangement of anterior horn of medial meniscus due to old tear or injury
- M23.22—Derangement of posterior horn of medial meniscus due to old tear or injury
- M23.23—Derangement of other medial meniscus due to old tear or injury
- M23.24—Derangement of anterior horn of lateral meniscus due to old tear or injury
- M23.25—Derangement of posterior horn of lateral meniscus due to old tear or injury
- M23.26—Derangement of other lateral meniscus due to old tear or injury

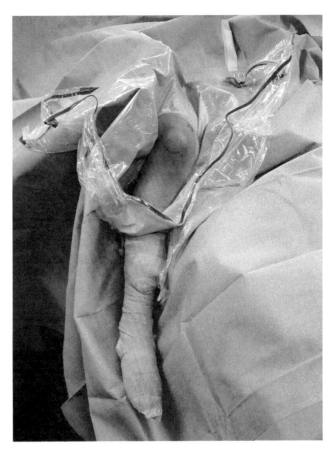

Figure 3-1 The leg is draped free with a lateral post in place to permit a resting position in 90 degrees of flexion but also allow improved ease of hyperflexion compared with a leg holder. Furthermore, leg positioning and surgery are more easily performed if a skilled assistant is not available.

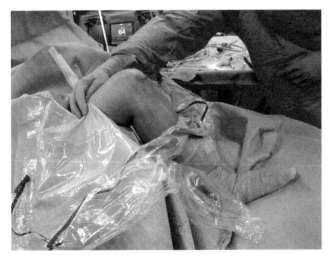

Figure 3-2 A bump taped to the table just distal to the contralateral knee allows the knee to be brought to 90 degrees of flexion for graft harvest and prevents the leg from sliding down the bed.

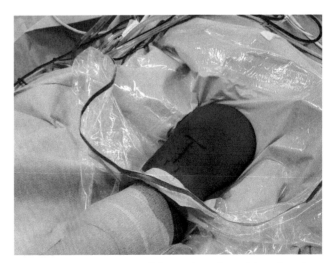

Figure 3-3 Patellar tendon graft harvest is performed through an 8-cm incision from the inferior pole of the patella to the proximal aspect of the tibial tubercle.

- Electrocautery is used to score the periosteum that surrounds the patellar and tibial bone plugs, with measurements of 10×20 mm and 10×30 mm on the patellar and tibial sides, respectively.
- The corners of the patella and tibia harvest sites are drilled with a 2-mm drill bit to a depth of 8 mm to facilitate graft liberation (Fig. 3-4).
- An oscillating saw is used, at an angle toward midline, to harvest equilateral triangular plugs from the patella and tibia.
- When the proximal patella and distal tibia crosscuts are made, the saw blade is angled 45 degrees relative to the cortex to avoid creation of an additional stress riser medial or lateral to the longitudinal cuts (Fig. 3-5).
- Once the cuts are complete, the bone plugs are gently levered from the patellar and tibial beds with a $\frac{1}{4}$-in osteotome. The authors refrain from striking the osteotome with a mallet on the patellar side to protect the cartilage surfaces.
- The patellar tendon is marked with pen to define the medial and lateral margins of the graft, 10 mm apart (Fig. 3-6).
- A #11 blade is used to harvest the patellar tendon medially and laterally in line with the longitudinal orientation of its fibers (Fig. 3-7) and in line with the patellar and tibial bone plugs.

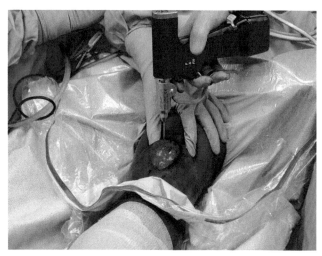

Figure 3-4 A 2-mm drill bit is used to penetrate the cortex and the corners of the graft to improve the ease of liberation of the bone plugs from their osseous beds.

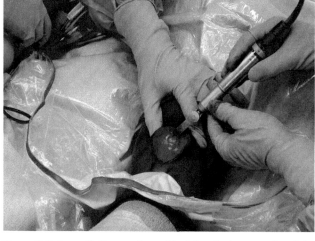

Figure 3-5 An oscillating saw is used to define the bony margins of the patellar and tibial bone plugs. When the proximal and distal crosscuts are made, the blade is held at a 45-degree angle relative to the cortex to avoid extending beyond the medial and lateral longitudinal cuts.

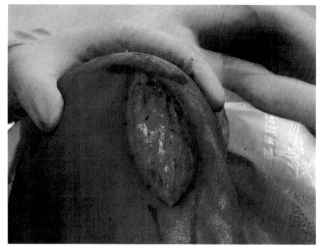

Figure 3-6 After the paratenon is incised and the medial and lateral flaps are elevated, the tendon is marked with a marking pen to define the medial and lateral margins of the graft 10 mm apart.

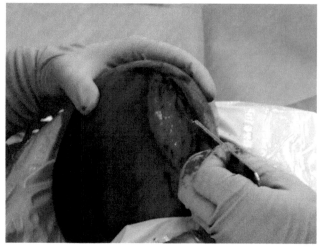

Figure 3-7 A #11 blade is used to cut the patellar tendon medially and laterally in line with the longitudinal fibers of the tendon.

- Note that the authors typically begin with the patellar bone cut, followed by the patellar tendon cut and ending with the tibial bone cut.

Graft Preparation

- On the back table, the first assistant measures and records the total graft length, the length of the bone plugs, and the length of the tendinous portion.
- With a sagittal saw, bone plugs are tubularized to easily pass through a 10-mm sizing tube.
- A 0.062-in K-wire is used to place a drill hole through the tibial and femoral bone plugs, respectively. No. 2 FiberWire (Arthrex, Naples, FL) sutures are placed through these drill holes for assistance with graft passage and tensioning.
- A marking pen is used to mark the tenoosseous junctions of both plugs and the cortical surface at the end of the tibial bone plug (Fig. 3-8).
- The graft is placed in a moist lap sponge, marked, and put in a safe location.
- The graft location should be communicated to every member of the surgical team.

Hamstring Harvest

- The pes anserinus is composed of the sartorius, semitendinosus, and gracilis tendons. These three tendons have a common attachment roughly 2 cm distal and 2 cm medial to the tibial tubercle.
- A 1-inch incision is made 2 cm distal and 2 cm medial to the tibial tubercle.
- Dissection is taken down to sartorial fascia, and the fascia is incised in an inverted "L" fashion, with a transverse limb along the superior border of the gracilis and a longitudinal limb along the attachment at the tibia (Fig. 3-9).
- The gracilis and semitendinosus tendons are dissected free from the posterior aspect of the sartorial fascia and whip-stitched with #2 Ethibond (Ethicon, Somerville, NJ).
- After control is established with the Ethibond suture, care is taken to completely release tethering to extratendinous bands, specifically the two large bands often found from the semitendinosus to the medial head of the gastrocnemius. If these are not thoroughly released, the risk of premature amputation of the tendon is increased.
- The tendons are then harvested with a close-ended, blunt-tipped tendon stripper.

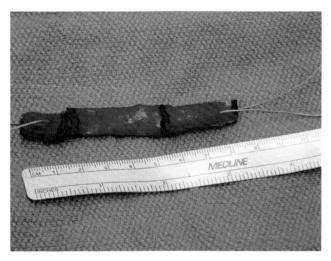

Figure 3-8 After the bone plugs have been appropriately sized, no. 2 FiberWire sutures are placed through the bone plugs for graft passage and the graft is marked along both tenoosseous junctions and at the end of the tibial bone plug.

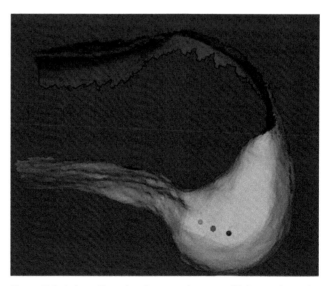

Figure 3-9 A three-dimensional computed tomographic image shows the location of the native footprint of the anteromedial bundle *(green dot),* the posterolateral bundle *(blue dot),* and a central location *(red dot),* which is used as the center point for graft placement.

- The harvested tendons are then taken to the back table and placed on a tensioning board with 15 lbs for 15 minutes to minimize creep.
- The grafts are then placed through a 10-mm EndoLoop with an EndoButton (Smith & Nephew, Andover, MA).

Diagnostic Arthroscopy

- When the diagnosis is clear and graft harvest precedes diagnostic arthroscopy, the arthroscopic portals and instrumentation are placed through the harvest wound (Fig. 3-10).
- Arthroscopy is performed before graft harvest in the event of equivocal pivot shift test results or with plans to use an allograft. In this case, athroscopic portals are established, including standard anterolateral, anteromedial, and accessory transpatellar tendon portals (Fig. 3-11).
- The anterolateral portal is established with the knee in 90 degrees flexion and placed just lateral to the patellar tendon at the level of the inferior border of the patella. This relatively "high" position affords an excellent view of the tibia ACL footprint.
- The anteromedial portal is established with direct visualization. Care must be taken when this portal is established because it will be used for femoral tunnel reaming. A spinal needle is used to localize this portal. The needle should enter the joint directly above the anterior horn of the medial meniscus. Its trajectory must allow unencumbered access to the femoral ACL footprint and should be as perpendicular to the lateral wall as possible. Nevertheless, the needle must be sufficiently far from the medial femoral condyle to prevent iatrogenic injury during reaming.

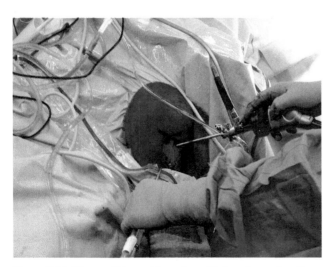

Figure 3-10 When graft harvest is performed before diagnostic arthroscopy, arthroscopic portals and instrumentation can be placed through the harvest wound.

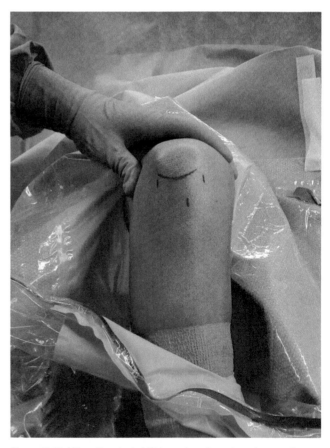

Figure 3-11 When the pivot shift is equivocal or when plans are for use of an allograft, diagnostic arthroscopy is performed with anterolateral, anteromedial, and accessory transpatellar tendon portals.

■ Diagnostic arthroscopy is performed in a systematic fashion to (1) assess the patellar and trochlear cartilage; (2) evaluate for loose bodies in the suprapatellar pouch, lateral gutter, and medial gutter; (3) assess the chondral and meniscal integrity in the medial and lateral compartments (Fig. 3-12); (4) verify the presence of an ACL tear (Fig. 3-13); and (5) ensure posterior cruciate ligament (PCL) integrity.

Anatomic Dissection and Preparation

■ The wall of the lateral femoral condyle is visualized through the transpatellar or parapatellar portal, and the dissecting instruments are passed through the anteromedial portal.

■ The ACL stump is débrided with a combination of arthroscopic biter, full-radius shaver, and radiofrequency probe (Figs. 3-13 and 3-14). The center points of the anteromedial (AM) and posterolateral (PL) bundles are identified and marked on the femoral wall. Care is taken to outline the the lateral intercondylar ridge ("resident's ridge") and the lateral bifurcate ridge on the femoral wall (Fig. 3-15).

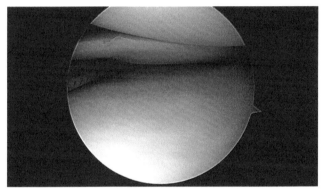

Figure 3-12 Diagnostic arthroscopy should include careful inspection of the chondral surfaces and both menisci as success of meniscal repair is improved in the setting of anterior cruciate ligament reconstruction.

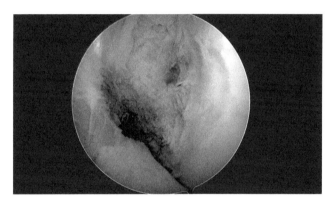

Figure 3-13 After débridement of the anterior cruciate ligament stump, residual soft tissue on the lateral wall of the intercondylar notch is used to identify bony topographic landmarks of the native femoral anterior cruciate ligament footprint.

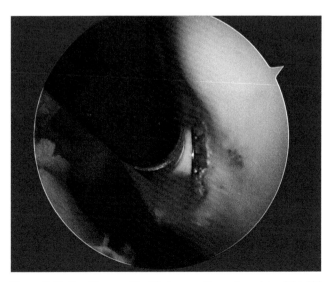

Figure 3-14 The ridges are identified, as are the center points of the AM and PL bundles, with a radiofrequency wand.

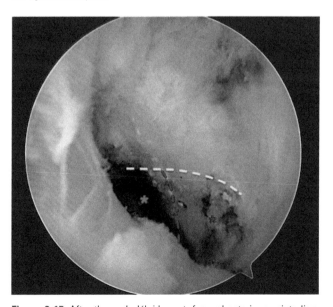

Figure 3-15 After thorough débridement, femoral anterior cruciate ligament footprint anatomy can be easily visualized. The *green asterisk* represents the origin of the anteromedial bundle, the *blue asterisk* represents the origin of the posterolateral bundle, the *red line* represents the bifurcate ridge, and the *yellow line* represents the lateral intercondylar ridge. The *red asterisk* represents the ideal location for femoral guide pin placement.

- The tibial footprint is carefully dissected with radiofrequency. The center points of the AM and PL bundles are identified and marked, along with the anterior intertubercular ridge (Fig. 3-16).
- Note: The senior author rarely performs a notchplasty, unless overgrowth has occurred from previous notchplasty (in revision cases.) If the surgeon feels that the notch is stenotic, a ¼-in curved osteotome may be placed through the inferomedial portal to excise bone anterior to the footprint. Free fragments are removed with a grasper. The notchplasty may then be fine tuned with a spherical or cylindrical burr.

Femoral Tunnel

- With the femoral footprint visualized through the transpatellar portal, a curved guide is advanced through the anteromedial portal and positioned 1 mm posterior to the bifurcate ridge, approximately 1 to 2 mm below the intercondylar ridge. The guide is rotated 10 degrees below the horizontal plane, slightly superolateral. A flexible guidewire is then advanced through the lateral femoral cortex and thigh, with the knee at 120 degrees of flexion (Figs. 3-17 and 3-18).
- The location where the pin exits the skin can be used to confirm appropriate pin position. A pin that exits the anterior thigh suggests an overly vertical trajectory, whereas a pin that exits directly laterally suggests an overly horizontal trajectory and risk of a shorter femoral tunnel.
- The guide is removed, and a 10-mm flexible cannulated reamer is advanced over the wire, with care taken to avoid injuring the chondral surface of the medial femoral condyle.

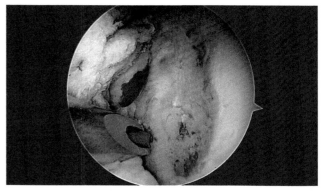

Figure 3-17 The flexible femoral aiming guide is advanced to the femoral anterior cruciate ligament footprint and held with an orientation roughly 10 degrees cephalad relative to the tibial plateau.

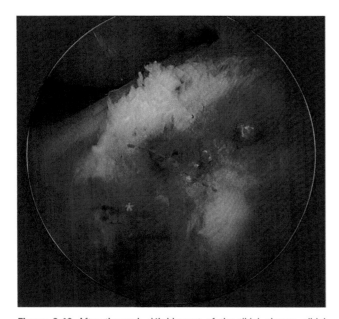

Figure 3-16 After thorough débridement of the tibial plateau, tibial anterior cruciate ligament footprint anatomy can be easily visualized. The *green asterisk* represents the insertion of the anteromedial bundle, the *blue asterisk* represents the insertion of the posterolateral bundle, and the *red line* represents the anterior intertubercular ridge. The *red asterisk* represents the ideal location for tibial guide pin entry.

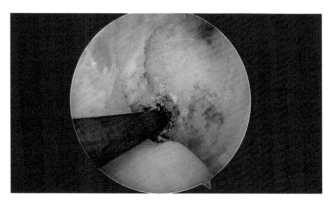

Figure 3-18 The guide is withdrawn, and the location of the guide pin is inspected.

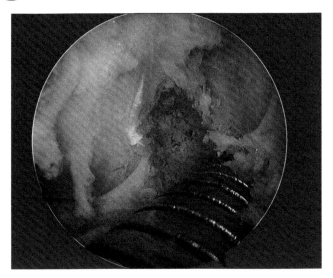

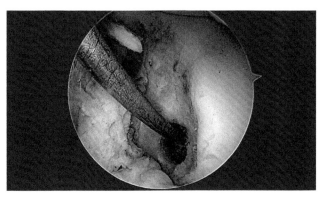

Figure 3-20 After reaming of the initial 10 mm of the femoral tunnel, the reamer is withdrawn and the preliminary tunnel is inspected to ensure integrity of the posterior cortex.

Figure 3-19 The reamer is then advanced over the guide pin. The knee is flexed to 120 degrees, and the tunnel is initially reamed to a depth of 10 mm.

- With direct visualization, the reamer is advanced over the pin to an initial depth of 10 mm (Fig. 3-19). At this point, the reamer is retracted and the preliminary tunnel is inspected to ensure integrity of the posterior wall (Fig. 3-20).
- The reamer then is readvanced and reamed to a depth of 25 to 30 mm.
- Flexible reaming should be performed with the knee still at 120 degrees of flexion to prevent kinking of the flexible guidewire.
- The reamer then is removed, and bony debris is cleared from the socket with a shaver.
- The arthroscope then is switched to the anterolateral portal, and the socket is carefully inspected to ensure circumferential integrity (Fig. 3-21).
- The flexible guide pin is left in place for later graft passage.
- The superior aspect of the tunnel is notched with a hexagonal screwdriver, or notching device, to facilitate interference screw placement for BTB autografts/allografts. This pilot hole is placed at roughly the 10 o'clock position in right knees and the 1 o'clock position in left knees.

Tibial Tunnel

- A variable angle tibial aiming guide is used to create an appropriately positioned tibial tunnel.
- Either a point-to-point or a point-to-elbow aiming guide may be used. One should be aware of which type of guide is used to ensure that the guide pin enters at the appropriate position intraarticularly.
- The angle of the guide is determined based on the length of the soft tissue portion of the graft, with the N+10 rule, to minimize graft tunnel mismatch (e.g., 45-mm soft tissue graft = 55-degree angle). For most grafts, the aimer is set to 65 degrees.
- The aiming tip of the guide is placed through the accessory transpatellar tendon portal (Fig. 3-22).
- The guide should be placed so that the pin enters the joint between the intercondylar spines on the anterior intertubercular ridge, the midpoint between the AM and PL bundle origins (see Fig. 3-16).
- If an autograft is used, the tibial aiming guide can be placed through the harvest wound. However, if an allograft is used, a 3-cm incision is established over the anteromedial tibia at the midpoint between the posterior tibia cortex and tibia tubercle, along the superior border of the pes tendons.
- The skin is retracted, and the cannulated guide arm is advanced onto the anteromedial tibia. It should contact the tibia roughly 1.5 cm medial to the tibial tubercle

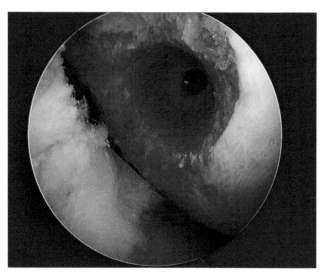

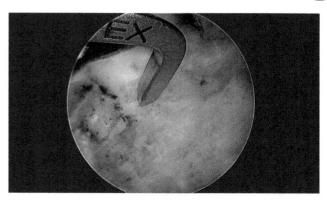

Figure 3-22 The point of the tibial aiming guide is advanced through the accessory transpatellar tendon portal and onto the tibial footprint.

Figure 3-21 After the femoral tunnel has been reamed, the scope is placed through the anteromedial portal and advanced up the tunnel to ensure circumferential integrity of the tunnel.

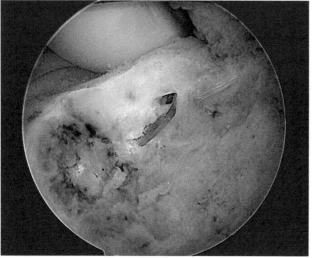

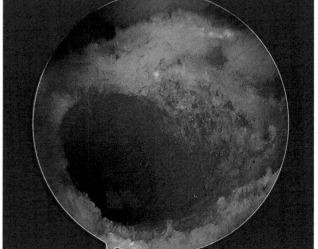

Figure 3-23 The tibial guide pin is drilled with direct visualization. It should enter the joint on the anterior intertubercular ridge, at the midpoint between the AM and PL bundle origins.

and 1 cm proximal to the pes tendon insertion. This area is the transition between the vertically oriented medial collateral ligament (MCL) fibers and the obliquely oriented pes fibers.

- The guide pin is advanced with direct visualization to confirm appropriate position in the center of the tibial footprint (Fig. 3-23).
- The guide pin is then overreamed with a 10-mm straight reamer.
- After reaming, a rongeur and shaver are used to remove any loose bone and periosteum around the periphery of the tibial orifice. A shaver is also used to remove loose bony debris within the tunnel and to smooth the posterior aspect of the intra-articular tunnel aperture to ensure easy graft passage.

Graft Passage

- The free ends of a looped #2 Ethibond then are placed through the eyelet of the flexible passing pin, and the pin is pulled through the anterolateral thigh so that the free ends exit the thigh and the looped end is left within the notch.

- A grasper is placed up the tibial tunnel and used to retrieve the looped end of the passing stitch.
- The graft is retrieved from the back table by the surgeon who will be passing the graft.
- The suture passed through the femoral bone plug is passed through the loop of the passing stitch, and the passing stitch is pulled out through the thigh.
- The leg is extended while the graft is pulled through the tibial tunnel to align the vector of pull with the tibial tunnel (Fig. 3-24).
- With the assistance of a curved hemostat or arthroscopic probe, the femoral bone plug is oriented and seated into the femoral tunnel.

Graft Fixation

- A 1.2-mm nitinol guidewire is placed through the anteromedial portal into the pilot hole, the site of the previously established femoral tunnel notch.
- An 8 × 20–mm PEEK BioInterference (Arthrex, Naples, FL) screw is advanced over the wire, after tapping with an 8-mm instrument.
- The knee should be flexed to 120 degrees during screw insertion to increase the distance between the screw and the graft and to minimize graft damage. Flexion of the knee also allows the screw to be inserted collinear with the graft and minimizes divergence.
- Care should be taken during insertion of the graft that the screw does not appear to be lacerating the graft.
- Once the screw is half-seated, the guidewire can be removed and the screw advanced until it is flush with the base of the femoral bone plug.
- Once the femoral bone plug has been fixated, tension is applied to the tibial sutures and the graft is cycled about 10 times to diminish graft creep.
- The graft is also examined arthroscopically during range of motion to ensure that it is not impinging in the notch in full extension (Fig. 3-25).
- Tibial fixation is then performed with the knee in 10 degrees of flexion to ensure that fixation does not "capture" the knee and result in a postoperative flexion contracture.
- The tibial bone plug is rotated 180 degrees to orient the cortex facing anteriorly. This orientation allows the cancellous surface of the bone plug to heal to cancellous bone on the posterior aspect of the tibial tunnel.
- With the knee in 10 degrees of flexion, tension is applied on the tibial suture and a gentle posterior drawer is applied to reduce the knee (Fig. 3-26). A nitinol wire

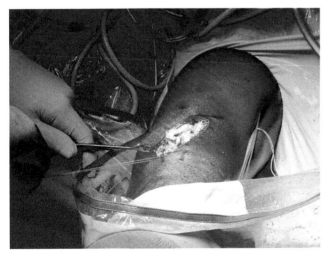

Figure 3-24 The graft is passed with the knee in full extension so that the trajectory of graft pull is parallel to the tibial tunnel.

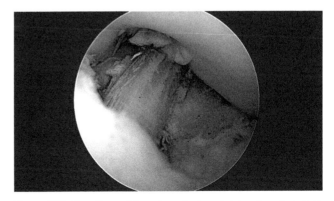

Figure 3-25 Once the graft is in place, the knee is taken through a range of motion to ensure that there is no graft impingement on the roof of the intercondylar notch.

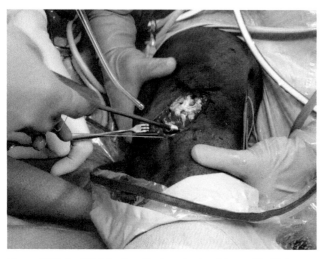

Figure 3-26 For tibial fixation, the knee is placed in roughly 10 degrees of flexion and a gentle posterior drawer is applied to reduce the tibia on the femur. The graft may be rotated 180 degrees externally to reproduce the ribbon-like morphology of the anterior cruciate ligament (and its two functional AM and PL bundles.)

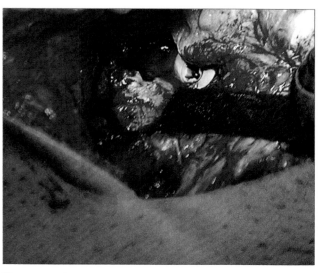

Figure 3-27 Once fully seated, the BioInterference screw should ideally be flush with the anterior tibial cortex and at roughly the same level as the distal extent of the tibial bone plug.

is placed along the graft on the lateral and anterior aspect of the tibial socket to medialize the graft in its tunnel.

- A 10 × 20–mm PEEK BioInterference screw is advanced over the guidewire after tapping with a 9-mm instrument, just deep to the anterior tibial cortex to prevent painful hardware (Fig. 3-27).
- In the event of graft-tunnel mismatch, a variety of strategies may be used.
  - In the event of subtle mismatch, the graft can be rotated up to 540 degrees to shorten the construct roughly 10% without significantly altering the construct's biomechanical properties.
  - Some authors propose redrilling the femoral socket to further recess the graft.
  - For more significant mismatch, some authors advocate flipping the bone plug 180 degrees onto the soft tissue portion of the graft (shortening the construct by the length of the tibial bone plug).
  - Alternatively, one can use a free-bone-block modification where the tibial bone plug is transected at the tenoosseous junction to create a pseudo-quad tendon graft. In this case, a grasping stitch is placed in the soft tissue, the bone plug is placed anterior to the soft tissue in the tunnel, and the construct is secured with an interference screw.
- Finally the graft is inspected and probed to ensure appropriate graft orientation and tension (Fig. 3-28).
- The knee is ranged to ensure full range of motion, and gentle Lachman testing is performed to ensure appropriate graft tension.

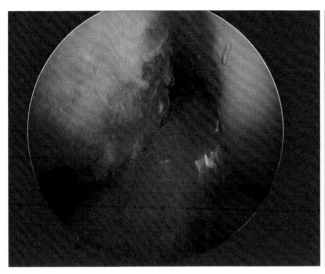 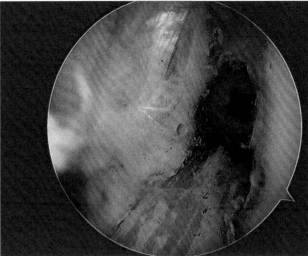

Figure 3-28 Once fixated, the graft is inspected and probed to ensure appropriate trajectory and tension.

BRIEF SUMMARY OF SURGICAL STEPS

- Patient positioning and examination with anesthesia
- Graft harvest (if diagnosis is clear)
- Graft preparation
- Diagnostic arthroscopy
- Topographic anatomic dissection and preparation
- Femoral tunnel reaming
- Tibial tunnel reaming
- Graft passage
- Graft fixation

TECHNICAL PEARLS

- Before the anteromedial portal is established, care should be taken to localize the portal with the spinal needle so that the trajectory permits access to the femoral ACL footprint but avoids the medial femoral condyle.
- Flexible reaming should be performed through the AM portal and visualized through the transpatellar portal for improved visualization and reduced risk of iatrogenic injury to the fat pad and medial femoral condyle. The posterior wall may be simultaneously observed.
- If passing the graft into the femoral tunnel is difficult, ensure that the tibial plug is not caught on the anterior tibial orifice.
- When the nitinol wire is placed for femoral fixation, ensure that it is parallel to the bone plug to minimize divergence, which may result in graft fracture, fixation failure, or tunnel blowout.
- Tibial fixation should be done in full extension or 10 degrees of flexion to ensure that fixation does not "capture" the knee and limit knee extension.

REQUIRED EQUIPMENT

Arthroscope (4.0-mm)

No. 2 FiberWire × 2 (graft preparation)

Femoral aiming guide

Flexible guide pin (femoral tunnel reaming)

Clancy flexible drill bits (femoral tunnel reaming)

#2 Ethibond (looped, for graft passage)

"Tip" or "elbow" tibial aiming guide

Tibial guide pin

10-mm full fluted reamer (tibial tunnel reaming)

Nitinol guidewire

8 × 20–mm PEEK BioInterference screw (femoral fixation, patellar tendon grafts)

10 × 20–mm PEEK BioInterference screw (tibia fixation, patellar tendon grafts)

COMMON PITFALLS

(When to call for the attending physician)

- Error in tunnel positioning is the most common technical cause of ACL reconstruction failure.
- Insufficient ACL stump débridement from the femoral and tibial footprints increases the likelihood of nonanatomic tunnel placement and predisposes to "Cyclops" lesions.
- Horizontal femoral guide pin placement increases the likelihood of a shortened femoral tunnel.
- Inadequate clearance of soft tissue debris from the tibial orifice and interarticular aperture can make graft passage very challenging.
- Placement of the femoral interference screw with the knee in resting position (instead of 120 degrees flexion) increases the likelihood of graft laceration or divergent screw placement.
- Placement of the tibial interference screw in flexion increases the likelihood of postoperative flexion contracture.

POSTOPERATIVE PROTOCOL

Phase IA: Early mobilization (0 to 2 weeks)

Goals: Decrease pain and swelling, achieve full extension, attain voluntary quad contraction

Treatment recommendations: Ice, active range of motion, passive range of motion, quad sets, patellar mobilization, straight leg raises, full arc quads (without weight), prone knee flexion, calf and hamstring stretching, locking knee brace at all times (locked at 0 degrees for first 7 days, except during exercise)

Phase IB: Late mobilization (2 to 6 weeks)

Goals: Full flexion, good quad control, normal gait

Treatment recommendations: Phase IA + mini squats, partial quad arcs (weight as tolerated), toe raises (weigh as tolerated), step ups (locking brace during ambulating; brace unlocked when there is no lag with the straight leg raise)

Phase IIA: Early strengthening (6 weeks to 3 months)

Goals: Strength 60% of the opposite limb

Treatment recommendations: Phase IB + increased closed chain activities (mini squats, bike riding, StairMaster [StairMaster, Vancouver, WA]), gait training, proprioceptive training, supervised jogging, discontinuation of knee brace

Phase IIB: Late strengthening (3 to 5 months)

Goals: Strength 80% of the opposite limb

Treatment recommendations: Phase IB + increased intensity of plyometrics, increased jogging/running intensity, jump rope; jogging begins at 3.5 months for autograft and 4 months for allograft

Phase III: Functional (5 months and beyond)

Goals: Return to full activity, work, and sport

Treatment recommendations: Progressive plyometrics, incline plyometrics, jogging, running, bounding, skipping, hopping, sport simulation

Criteria for return to sport: One leg hop test (90% of contralateral leg), jog without limp, full-speed run without limp, shuttle run without limp, figure 8 running without limp, single-leg vertical jump (90% of contralateral leg), squat and rise from squat

POSTOPERATIVE CLINIC VISIT PROTOCOL

Patients are typically seen in the office at 1 to 2 weeks, 6 to 8 weeks, 3 months, and 6 months after surgery.

SUGGESTED READINGS

1. Barrett GR, Luber K, Replogle WH, Manley JL. Allograft anterior cruciate ligament reconstruction in the young, active patient: Tegner activity level and failure rate. *Arthroscopy*. 2010;26(12):1593-1601. doi:10.1016/j.arthro.2010.05.014.
2. Duquin T, Wind W, Fineberg M, Smolinski R, Buyea C. Current trends in anterior cruciate ligament reconstruction. *J Knee Surg*. 2010;22(01):7-12. doi:10.1055/s-0030-1247719.
3. Forsythe B, Kopf S, Wong AK, et al. The location of femoral and tibial tunnels in anatomic double-bundle anterior cruciate ligament reconstruction analyzed by three-dimensional computed tomography models. *J Bone Joint Surg Am*. 2010;92(6):1418-1426.
4. Hewett TE, Myer GD, Ford KR. Anterior cruciate ligament injuries in female athletes: part 1, mechanisms and risk factors. *Am J Sports Med*. 2006;34(2):299-311. doi:10.1177/0363546505284183.
5. McAllister DR, Joyce MJ, Mann BJ, Vangsness CT. Allograft update: the current status of tissue regulation, procurement, processing, and sterilization. *Am J Sports Med*. 2007;35(12):2148-2158. doi:10.1177/0363546507308936.
6. O'Connor DP, Laughlin MS, Woods GW. Factors related to additional knee injuries after anterior cruciate ligament injury. *Arthroscopy*. 2005;21(4):431-438. doi:10.1016/j.arthro.2004.12.004.
7. Persson A, Fjeldsgaard K, Gjertsen JE, et al. Increased risk of revision with hamstring tendon grafts compared with patellar tendon grafts after anterior cruciate ligament reconstruction: a study of 12,643

patients from the Norwegian Cruciate Ligament Registry, 2004-2012. *Am J Sports Med*. 2014;42(2):285-291. doi:10.1177/0363546513511419.

8. Prodromos CC, Han Y, Rogowski J, Joyce B, Shi K. A meta-analysis of the incidence of anterior cruciate ligament tears as a function of gender, sport, and a knee injury-reduction regimen. *Arthroscopy*. 2007;23(12):1320-1325.e6. doi:10.1016/j.arthro.2007.07.003.

9. Reinhardt KR, Hetsroni I, Marx RG. Graft selection for anterior cruciate ligament reconstruction: a level I systematic review comparing failure rates and functional outcomes. *Orthop Clin North Am*. 2010;41(2):249-262. doi:10.1016/j.ocl.2009.12.009.

10. Sutton KM, Bullock JM. Anterior cruciate ligament rupture: differences between males and females. *J Am Acad Orthop Surg*. 2013;21(1):41-50. doi:10.5435/JAAOS-21-01-41.

CHAPTER 4

TOTAL HIP ARTHROPLASTY

Bryan D. Haughom | Aaron G. Rosenberg

Hip arthritis is commonly encountered in the practice of orthopaedic surgery and can result from a multitude of etiologies (osteoarthritis, inflammatory arthritis, posttraumatic arthritis, sequelae of childhood hip disease, postseptic arthritis, etc). Nonoperative management strategies include weight loss, mechanical aids, nonsteroidal antiinflamatory agents, and intrarticular injection. Other operative treatments for hip arthritis include arthroscopy, periarticular osteotomy, joint resurfacing procedures, and arthrodesis, but this chapter focuses on the most commonly performed procedure for arthritis of the hip, the total hip arthroplasty (THA).

Related to the increasingly successful outcomes after THA and the evidence of improved longevity of modern constructs, the indications for THA in the management of hip arthritis have increased to include younger patients. THA is one of the most commonly performed hip procedures in the United States, with 284,000 primary THAs performed in 2009 and current estimates indicating a projected increase of 174% by the year 2030. From the original cemented design of Sir John Charnley, the modern THA includes use of components cemented in place or, as is more commonly performed in the United States, use of components implanted in cementless fashion.

Although the outcomes are typically excellent, with improvements in function and pain, the procedure is not without its risks. Patients should be counseled with regards to the potential risks of the periopertiave period (e.g., anesthetic risks, deep venous thrombosis, intraoperative fracture) and the long-term risks (e.g., periprosthetic infection, dislocation, aseptic loosening, corrosion). Furthermore, treating physicians should consider the patient's underlying medical comorbidities when discussing these risks and when determining the optimal implants or surgical approach. For example, anterior or lateral surgical approaches, larger femoral head articulations, constrained implants, and possibly dual-mobility articulations may be more appropriate for patients at high risk for dislocation, including patients with neurologic disorders (e.g., Parkinson's disease, seizure disorders, spasticity), and those patients with cognitive dysfunction or substance abuse problems.

A variety of surgical approaches to THA are available, including anterior, anterolateral, direct lateral, and posterior. The bulk of this chapter focuses on the posterior approach because this is the most commonly used approach in the United States. However, each of the approaches has advantages, and ultimately the approach is determined by the treating surgeon.

Preoperative evaluation requires assessment of hip range of motion, the presence of contracture(s), and leg length discrepancies and adequate radiographs. Radiographs should include an anteroposterior view of the pelvis and an anteroposterior and lateral view of the affected hip. The use of a sizing marker to determine magnification may allow for more accurate preoperative templating to estimate the planned position and size of the components.

CASE MINIMUM REQUIREMENTS

- 30 Total hip arthroplasties are required by the Accreditation Council for Graduate Medical Education (ACGME) for graduation

COMMONLY USED CPT CODES

- CPT Code: 27130—Arthroplasty, acetabular and proximal femoral prosthetic replacement (total hip arthroplasty), with or without autograft or allograft
- CPT Code: 27132—Conversion of previous hip surgery to total hip arthroplasty, with or without autograft or allograft
- CPT Code: 27236—Open treatment of femoral fracture, proximal end, neck, internal fixation, or prosthetic replacement

COMMONLY USED ICD9 CODES

- 715.15—Osteoarthritis of the hip
- 714.0—Rheumatoid arthritis

COMMONLY USED ICD10 CODES

- M16—Osteoarthritis of hip
- M05—Rheumatoid arthritis with rheumatoid factor

SURGICAL TECHNIQUE

Room Set-Up

- A standard operating room table is used, centered under the operative room lights, with sufficient room for the anesthesia team to have access to the head of the bed (Fig. 4-1).
- The operating room should employ laminar flow type ventilation and many surgeons wear body exhaust suits, both of which are thought to decrease the risk of infection.

Patient Positioning

- Patients are initially positioned supine on the operating room table, and a Foley catheter is frequently placed.
- After administration of a general or neuraxial anesthetic, the patient is placed in either a lateral decubitus position with the operative hip facing the ceiling or the supine position, depending on the surgical approach.
- Care is taken to pad bony prominences (e.g., ankles, fibular head; Fig. 4-2).

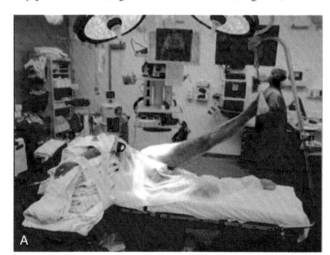

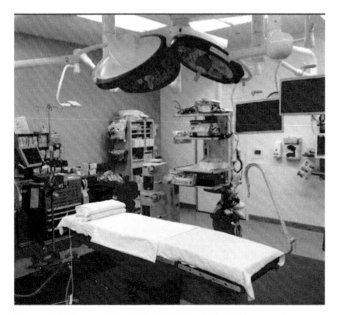

Figure 4-1 The operating table is in the middle of the operating room, centered beneath the lights.

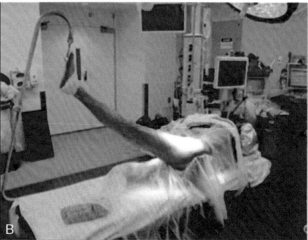

Figure 4-2 For the posterior approach to the hip, the patient is positioned in the lateral position. Hip positioners are used to keep the pelvis stationary. **A,** All bony prominences are well padded, and the arms are held in a forward flexed position. **B,** For the surgical preparation, the leg is held in a leg holder in an externally rotated position, which helps lock the knee in extension.

- Devices designed to secure the patient in the lateral position are used to prevent pelvic motion during acetabular preparation. Ranging from pegboards to bean bags, hip positioners require two points of contact. The anterior positioner has two points of contact with the patient: the pubis and the anterior superior iliac spine. The posterior positioner is placed at the level of the sacrum.
- In the lateral position, an axillary roll is placed to minimize pressure on the neurovascular structures of the upper extremity.
- In the lateral position, blankets or an arm holder are used to position the arms so that the top arm remains in neutral adduction. The patient's torso then is secured to the bed with heavy tape; a towel is used to protect the skin from the adhesive (see Fig. 4-2).
- In the supine position, the patient's arms are extended to approximately 90 degrees, on arm boards, with the lower arm palm up.
- Lateral and anterior approaches may use the supine position.

Prepping and Draping

- The operative hip is shaved in an atraumatic fashion with electric clippers.
- The operative leg is held in a leg holder with the leg abducted and externally rotated (see Fig. 4-2). An impermeable plastic drape is the applied to the operative leg, shielding the perineum.
- Standard preparation is undertaken with an alcohol-, chlorhexidine-, or iodine-based product.
- Surgical towels are placed circumferentially around the hip, and a sterile impermeable U-drape is applied to the perinium (Fig. 4-3).
- The operative leg is taken out of the leg holder at this time, and an impermeable stockinette is applied to the foot and overwrapped with Coban (3M, St. Paul, MN).
- A lower extremity drape then is applied.
- Two Ioban dressings (3M) then are applied to the hip to complete the draping. The first (smaller) Ioban dressing is applied longitudinally to the medial aspect of the leg, and the second (larger) Ioban dressing is applied transversely over the posterior, lateral, and anterior aspects of the hip. Marking of the skin with lines orthogonal to the incision before application of the Ioban dressing is useful to facilitate later closure (Fig. 4-4).

Surgical Approaches

- A number of surgical approaches have been described for THA, including the direct anterior, anterolateral, direct lateral, and posterior approaches. Each of these approaches takes advantage of a different internervous or intermuscular plane. They are all viable options for the placement of a THA, and use of any is largely dictated by surgeon preference and patient factors.
- The anterior (Smith-Peterson) approach to the hip takes advantage of the internervous plane between the sartorius (femoral nerve) and tensor fasciae latae (superior gluteal nerve) superficially and the rectus femoris (femoral nerve) and gluteus medius (superior gluteal nerve) deep. Care must be taken to avoid the lateral femoral cutaneous nerve during the superficial dissection. This approach is performed with the patient in a supine position.
- The anterolateral (Watson-Jones) approach to the hip uses the muscular interval between the tensor fascia latae and the gluteus medius. There is no internervous plane in this approach because both muscles are innervated by the superior gluteal nerve.
- The direct lateral (Harding) approach is a muscle splitting approach with no true internervous plane. In this approach, the gluteus medius and the vastus lateralis are split to gain access to the hip joint. Note that both muscles are split distant from their respective sites of innervation. However, care should be taken not to extend

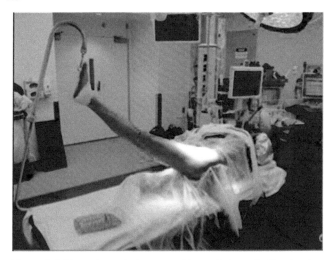

Figure 4-3 The perineum is first covered in surgical towels. Care is taken to keep the towels as posterior as possible. Also note the use of body exhaust suits in this image.

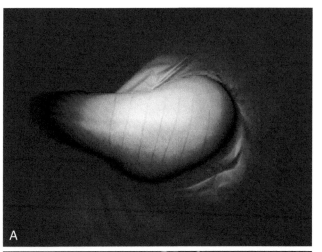

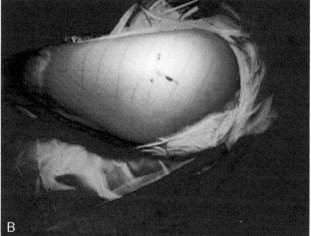

Figure 4-4 **A,** Before application of the Ioban dressing (3M, St. Paul, MN), marks are made on the skin to facilitate skin closure. **B,** The greater trochanter is palpated and drawn, and the surgical incision is marked on the skin.

the incision too far proximally because the superior gluteal nerve is encountered approximately 5 cm proximal to the greater trochanter.

- The posterior (Southern) approach to the hip is the most extensile of the hip approaches. It uses a muscle splitting approach through the gluteus maximus (Figs. 4-5 and 4-6). To complete the approach to the hip, the hip external rotators must be removed from the greater trochanter (Fig. 4-7). Although these are later repaired to bone, patients are at a slightly increased risk of dislocation through this approach. This risk can be mitigated with meticulous repair of the short external rotator muscles. At the time of muscular detachment, tag sutures should be placed in the capsule and short external rotators to facilitate later repair. Repair may be performed with a strong nonabsorbable suture from tendon to periosteum or through bone tunnels made with a 2.0-mm drill. Because the posterior approach is the most commonly used approach in modern orthopaedics, this approach is described in greater detail.
- Before the posterior approach to the hip is started, the greater trochanter is palpated and marked out. The incision is roughly 10 cm long, starting posterior and proximal to the greater trochanter and traveling distally and inferiorly. The incision should cross the greater trochanter at the juncture of the anterior one third and posterior two thirds of the trochanter (see Fig. 4-4).

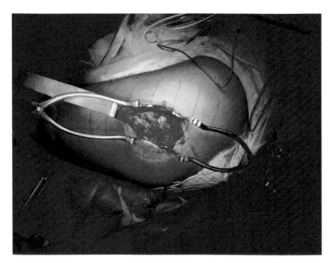

Figure 4-5 After the skin is incised, electrocautery is used to establish hemostasis. The dissection is carried down to the level of the fascia, pictured here, and a Cobb elevator is used to clear off the fascia. Self-retaining retractors are useful during this portion of the approach.

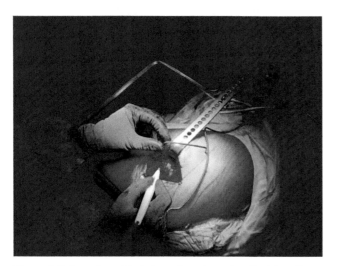

Figure 4-6 A number of techniques have been described to estimate changes in leg length and offset. A simple technique is depicted in which a pin is placed in the ilium, bent, and used as simple measuring implement. The site where the pin hits the greater trochanter is marked with electrocautery and is used at the end of the case to compare leg length and offset.

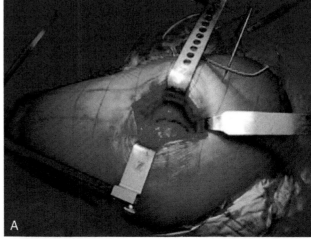

A

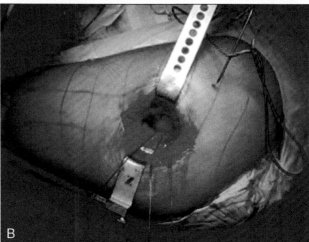

B

Figure 4-7 After the fascia is incised, and the bursa is removed, the short external rotators become visible. **A,** These are removed near their insertion. **B,** Once they are removed, they are tagged for later closure.

- Self-retaining retractors are used in this superficial layer as hemostasis is established, and electrocautery is used to the level of the deep fascia (see Fig. 4-5). A Cobb elevator is used to clear a plane to facilitate closure.
- The deep fascia is incised in line with the gluteus maximus fibers and a Charnley retractor is placed deep to this fascia, exposing the gluteal musculature and the external rotators.
- After removal of the bursa overlying these muscles, the external rotators are removed as one sleeve and the capsulotomy is performed. Alternatively this can be done in layers. Tag stitches are placed to facilitate later closure. Once this step has been accomplished, dislocation can be undertaken (see Fig. 4-7).

Dislocation and Neck Osteotomy

- Before hip dislocation is attempted, the surgeon should adequately débride adherent capsular tissue and osteophytes about the acetabular rim. Protrusio of the femoral head may increase the difficulty of dislocation and require more extensive soft tissue dissection and in situ osteotomy of the femoral neck or head to allow removal of the head from the acetabulum in fragments.
- Dislocation requires a combination of traction (to break any vacuum phenomenon) and rotation. Anterior dislocation requires placement of the limb in a figure 4 position, and posterior dislocation requires flexion, adduction, and external rotation.
- Once dislocated, osteotomy of the neck is a critical part of both femoral component placement and acetabular exposure. Preoperative templating is needed to accurately assess the level of the neck osteotomy and must be made in reference to a reproducible landmark that can be accessed after dislocation (Figs. 4-8 and 4-9).
  - From the posterior approach, this is usually the superior aspect of the lesser trochanter.
  - From the anterior, the saddle point (junction of the superolateral neck and a point just anterior to the piriformis fossa) is more accessible.
- Care must be taken during osteotomy of the neck to avoid extension into the greater trochanter, which may promote trochanteric fracture. Homan retractors can be placed on the inferior and superior femoral neck to protect surrounding structures.

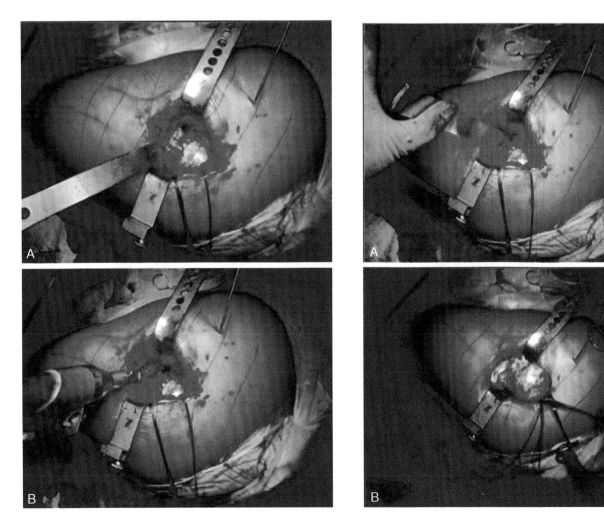

Figure 4-8 A, Retractors are placed under the femoral neck; and **B,** an oscillating saw is used to perform the neck cut.

Figure 4-9 A, A straight osteotome and **B,** point clamp are used to remove the femoral head.

Making an excessively vertical osteotomy results in excessive shortening of the remaining neck in comparison with the expected, template position.

Acetabular Preparation

- After resection of the femoral head, the acetabulum must be exposed. Adequate débridement of extraneous capsular tissue at the periphery such as the labrum is necessary so that the entirety of the acetabulum can be visualized for adequate positioning of the reamer and the implant.
- Additional débridement of the anterior capsule can be entertained at this step, depending on the degree of preoperative flexion contracture. Care should be taken, however, to avoid overzealous capsular resection because this can lead to postoperative instability.
- Retractors are sequentially placed about the periphery of the acetabulum to adequately retract the femur and soft tissue (Fig. 4-10). Specifically, an anterior acetabular retractor is placed over the anterior rim of the acetabulum and a posterior acetabular retractor is placed.
- Reaming begins with a hemispherical reamer several sizes smaller than the templated size of the final implant, with débridement first of remaining cartilage and pulvinar. Once the cartilage and soft tissue have been débrided, larger reamers are used to remove any medial osteophyte and subchondral bone for eventual impaction of the acetabular component. The surgeon must ream in the position the cup will ultimately be placed in because this restricts the eventual position of cup impaction (Fig. 4-11).
- Optimal positioning of the acetabular component is in 45 ± 10 degrees of abduction and 20 ± 10 degrees of anteversion. Cup position can be determined during surgery with bony and soft tissue landmarks. Computer navigation also has been described as a means of appropriate positioning.
- Consideration should be given to supplementary screw fixation in the acetabular shell (as long as the selected design allows for this). Screws ideally should be placed in the posterior superior quadrant of the acetabulum, followed by the anterior

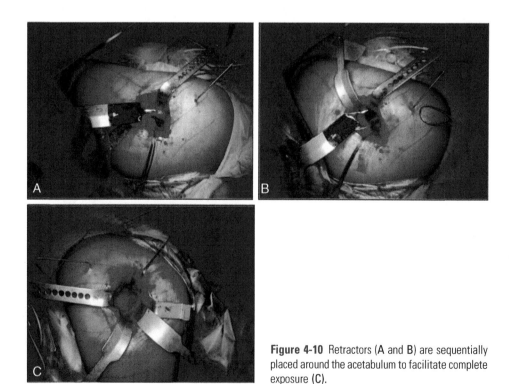

Figure 4-10 Retractors (A and B) are sequentially placed around the acetabulum to facilitate complete exposure (C).

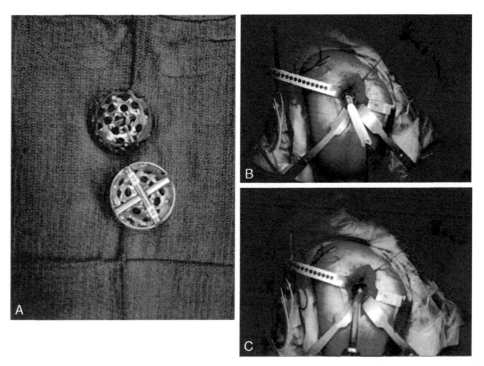

Figure 4-11 **A,** Hemispherical reamers are used to remove soft tissue and cartilage from the acetabulum. Care is taken to ream in the direction **(B)** of eventual implantation **(C).**

superior quadrant in the event that inadequate bone is present in the posterior superior quadrant.

■ After impact of the acetabular shell, an osteotome or rongeur can be used to remove any impinging osteophytes that might lead to postoperative instability.

■ Once the acetabular shell is firmly in place, a trial or the actual liner is then impacted in place (Fig. 4-12).

Femoral Preparation

■ Preparation of the femoral canal varies by stem fixation type and geometric characteristics.

■ Cemented components require avoidance of component varus and maintenance of a rough endosteal interface to permit cement interdigitation and appropriate use as a grout rather than a glue.

■ For femoral preparation, the proximal femur must be adequately visualized. This is accomplished with a proximal femoral elevator, placed under the proximal femoral metaphysis. The assistant facilitates this maneuver by placing the leg in a position of internal rotation and flexion.

■ After a lateral box-cutting osteotome is used to lateralize the rasp's starting point in the piriformis fossa, a starting awl can be used to centralize the rasp in the canal (Fig. 4-13).

■ After this, the surgeon uses sequentially larger broaches to prepare the metaphysis and proximal diaphysis for implantation. The broaches should be placed as laterally as possible in the canal, and care should be taken to impact the broaches in the appropriate amount of anteversion to avoid intraoperative fracture and varus implantation (Fig. 4-14).

■ Sequentially larger rasps are used until the cortical bone is encountered and the rasp no longer advances readily or the anticipated template size is reached. This is best accomplished by matching the patient's natural anteversion (Fig. 4-15). Even, gentle mallet blows are used to impact the broaches into the canal.

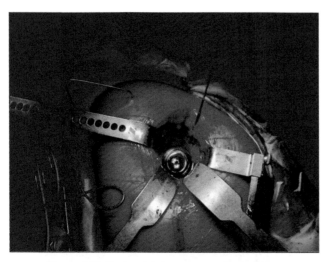

Figure 4-12 Final acetabular component implantation.

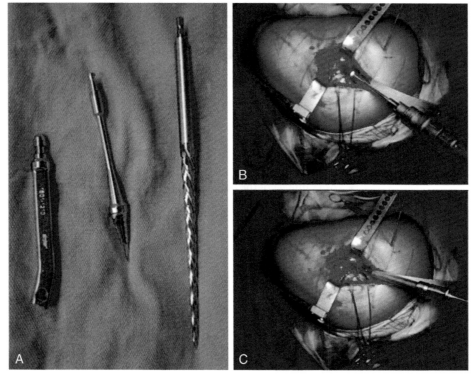

Figure 4-13 **A,** A box chisel, entry reamer, and canal finder (from *left* to *right*). **B** and **C,** A starting awl can be used to centralize the rasp in the canal.

- Cementless implants may require rasping only or a combination of reaming and rasping.
- Metaphyseal filling implants (usually anatomic or tapered designs) require rasping only, and sequentially larger rasps are used until the cortical bone is encountered and the rasp no longer advances readily or the anticipated template size is reached. In these stems, the initial fixation depends on an interference fit of the implant in the proximal femur.
- Stems designed for more distal fixation via ingrowth and press fit into a machined cylindrical segment of the diaphysis require reaming of the intramedullary canal until reasonably solid endosteal bone is reached.
- After reaming, broaches are used to prepare the metaphysis. Broaching should begin before the final anticipated size is reached with reamers to ensure that there is no significant mismatch between distal and proximal segment sizing.

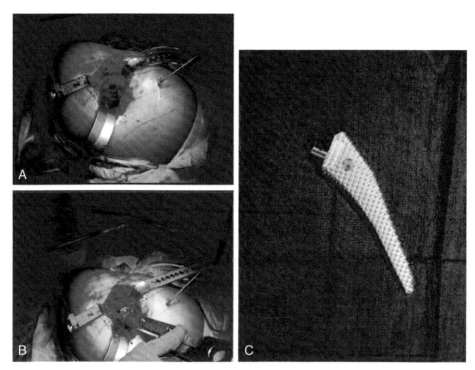

Figure 4-14 **A,** An entry reamer and canal finder are used before broaching with sequentially larger femoral broaches (**B** and **C**).

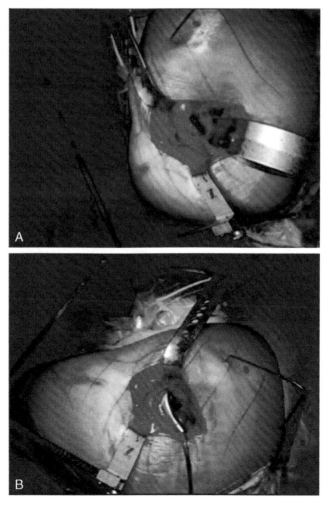

Figure 4-15 Broaching is facilitated with a proximal femoral elevator, which brings the femur out of the wound. **A,** Note that the femoral broaches were inserted in a direction that matched the patient's native anteversion. **B,** After broaching, the final implant is placed; care is taken to ensure the final implant sits at the same level as the largest broach.

- Once the final size broach has been impacted, trial femoral neck and head sizes are implanted based on preoperative templating and intraoperative assessment of appropriate implant size by the criteria noted previously, and the construct is assessed.

Construct Assessment

- *Stability.* The operative hip is taken through the extremes of motion. In the event of instability, the surgeon must determine whether additional femoral offset, larger head size, or a lipped acetabular liner is necessary. Furthermore, reevaluation of the acetabular component position may be necessary because component malposition has been shown to be a common source of early postoperative instability (Fig. 4-16).
- *Leg length.* Leg length discrepancies after THA are a common source of patient dissatisfaction, although the functional implications are unknown. Evaluation of leg lengths are performed in several ways (Fig. 4-17). Preoperative radiographs are used to determine the degree to which any length discrepancies have developed, in an effort to guide any corrective lengthening that may be performed. During surgery, a number of measuring devices have been used to estimate the amount of lengthening based on fixed bony landmarks. Fixed anatomic structures, such as the patella, may be compared between both legs as a rough estimate as well. And finally, the soft tissue tension may be assessed with application of a traction force with the leg in extension for evaluation of the degree of distraction at the level of the joint as a surrogate for the degree of lengthening. Note that component stability trumps leg length discrepancy.

Final Component Insertion

- After femoral preparation has been performed, the trial components have been inserted, and the final construct has been evaluated, the final femoral component

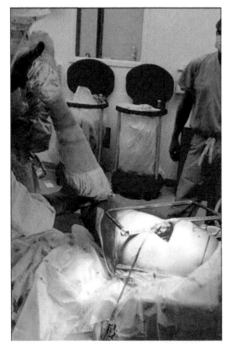

Figure 4-16 The stability of the construct is assessed by taking the patient through a range of motion.

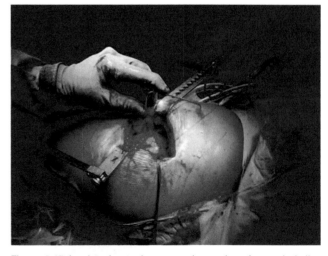

Figure 4-17 Leg lengths can be assessed a number of ways, including here with the use of the previously inserted wire. The position of the wire relative to the mark made at the beginning of the case is compared to determine any changes in leg length.

size is noted. The component is then impacted into the femoral canal with careful attention noted to the final component position. Final component position should mirror that of the trial components. Impaction beyond the level of the trial components may suggest the presence of an intraoperative fracture.

- Once the final component is in place, and the construct has been deemed stable, attention is turned to a meticulous closure.

Closure

- After final implantation of components, particularly in the case of a lateral or posterior approach to the hip, with disruption of either the gluteus medius or short external rotators, a meticulous closure is necessary. Before this, a providone-iodine bath is performed, according to Brown and colleagues (Fig. 4-18). Capsular closure is performed, and as previously stated, large nonabsorbable suture is used to repair the short external rotators (in the posterior approach) or the gluteus medius (in the case of a lateral approach). These may be anchored with either suture to the periosteum or through bone tunnels. This has been shown to decrease the rate of postoperative instability (Fig. 4-19).
- The fascia, subcutaneous tissues, and skin then are closed in a layered fashion, and an impermeable dressing is applied (Fig. 4-20).

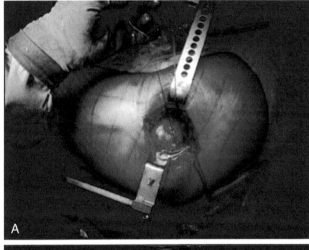

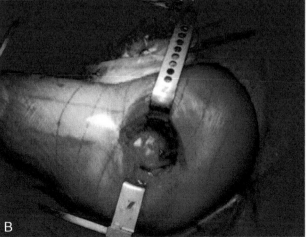

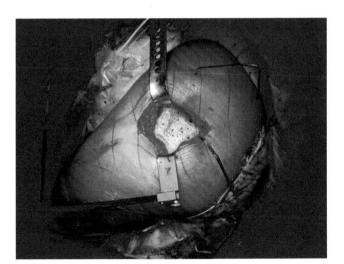

Figure 4-18 The wound is copiously irrigated, and a providone-iodine soak is performed as described by Brown and colleagues.

Figure 4-19 Care is taken to repair the capsule **(A)** and external rotators **(B)**; this has been shown to decrease the rate of dislocation after a posterior approach.

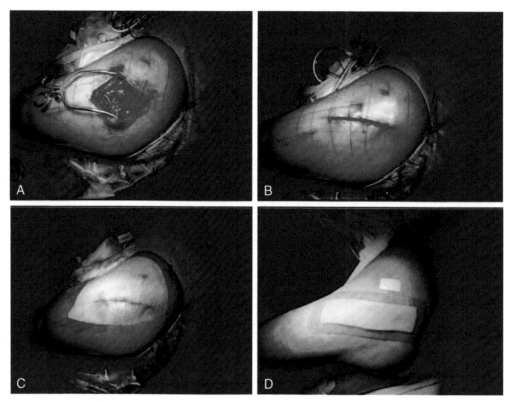

Figure 4-20 The wound is closed in layers, first with **A,** the fascia; **B,** subcutaneous fat; and **C,** skin. **D,** Finally, an impermeable dressing is applied to the hip.

BRIEF SUMMARY OF SURGICAL STEPS

- Superficial dissection
- Capsule management
- Dislocation
- Neck osteotomy
- Acetabular and femoral preparation
- Trialing
- Implantation
- Closure

TECHNICAL PEARLS

- Preoperative templating helps avoid mistakes and prevent malpositioning of components during surgery.
- Adequate visualization of the acetabulum helps ensure proper component position.
- Acetabular component position should be 45 ± 10 degrees of abduction and 20 ± 10 degrees of anteversion.
- Supplementary acetabular screws should be placed in the posterior superior quadrant of the acetabulum.
- Femoral positioning should match the patient's natural anteversion.
- When the femoral broaches are impacted, size mismatch with preoperative templates may be a clue that the component is in a varus position.
- A final femoral component position that is more distally seated than trials may suggest an intraoperative fracture.
- If intraoperative instability persists despite increased offset, increased head size, and elevated liners, the acetabular component may be malpositioned.

REQUIRED EQUIPMENT

Preoperative templated radiographs

Laminar flow/body exhaust suits

Self-retaining hip retractors (e.g., Charnley retractor) and manual hip retractors (e.g., large Homan, acetabular retractors)

Large oscillating saw/osteotomes

Long-handled electrocautery/knife handles

Acetabular reamers

Femoral reamers/broaches

Trial implants

COMMON PITFALLS

(When to call for the attending physician)

- In the case of intraoperative fracture
- In the case of component mismatch with preoperative templated sizes
- In the event that screws are to be placed in any quadrant outside of the posterior superior quadrant or if screw lengths are greater than 25 mm
- In the case of significant intraoperative bleeding
- During assessment of component stability
- During the final component impaction

POSTOPERATIVE PROTOCOL

The primary objectives of the acute postoperative period are prevention of infection and medical complications, pain control, and early mobilization. Three doses of perioperative antibiotics and anticoagulation therapy are started on the night of surgery. A number of anticoagulant agents have been deemed appropriate by the American Academy of Orthopaedic Surgery. At the authors' institution, Warfarin is used unless a contraindication is noted. Deep venous thrombosis prophylaxis is continued for 3 weeks after surgery. In addition, sequential compression devices (SCDs) are used during surgery and throughout the postoperative admission.

Pain control is started during surgery with the use of neuraxial anesthesia. If an epidural catheter is left in place, an epidural PCA (patient controlled analgesia) is utilized for 1 to 2 days after surgery. Alternatively, patients can undergo transition to an intravenous PCA with supplemental long-acting oral opiates. Oral analgesia is started on postoperative day 1 regardless.

Patients are ideally mobilized on the night of surgery, not only to hasten their recovery but also to minimize the risk of blood clot formation. Physical therapists and occupational therapists work closely with patients during the postoperative period to educate them regarding new activity restrictions. Activity restrictions are particularly necessary when a posterior approach is used; patients are instructed to avoid deep hip flexion, hip abduction, and excessive internal rotation. In the case of a lateral approach, active abduction is limited for the first 3 weeks after surgery to maximize the healing at the site of abductor repair.

POSTOPERATIVE CLINIC VISIT PROTOCOL

Patients are seen in the office at 2 to 3 weeks, 6 weeks, 3 months, 6 months, and 1 year and annually thereafter. At the first visit, the wounds are inspected (and if used, sutures or staples are removed). Patients again are counseled as to activity restrictions, and in the case of the lateral approach, active abduction is initiated. Anticoagulation therapy is stopped. Radiographs are taken and compared with films taken in the postoperative recovery unit. Care is taken to evaluate for any evidence of component migration or fracture. At subsequent visitis, radiographs are scrutinized for evidence of osteointegration and any component wear or aseptic loosening. In addition, at each postoperative visit, patients are queried regarding potentially worrisome signs of infection or loosening (e.g., new pains).

SUGGESTED READINGS

1. Barrack RL. Dislocation after total hip arthroplasty: implant design and orientation. *J Am Acad Orthop Surg*. 2003;11:89-99.
2. Brooks PJ. Dislocation following total hip replacement: causes and cures. *Bone Joint J*. 2013; 95-B:67-69.
3. Brown NM, Cipriano CA, Moric M, Sporer SM, Della Valle CJ. Dilute betadine lavage before closure for the prevention of acute postoperative deep periprosthetic joint infection. *J Arthroplasty*. 2012;27:27-30.
4. Kurtz S, Ong K, Lau E, Mowat F, Halpern M. Projections of primary and revision hip and knee arthroplasty in the United States from 2005 to 2030. *J Bone Joint Surg Am*. 2007;89:780-785.
5. Kwon MS, Kuskowski M, Mulhall KJ, Macaulay W, Brown TE, Saleh KJ. Does surgical approach affect total hip arthroplasty dislocation rates? *Clin Orthop Relat Res*. 2006;447:34-38.
6. *American Academy of Orthopaedic Surgeons*. Preventing venous thromboembolic disease in patients undergoing elective hip and knee arthroplasty. <http://www.aaos.org/Research/guidelines/VTE/VTE_full_guideline.pdf>; 2011. Accessed 01.11.14.
7. Wasielewski RC, Cooperstein LA, Kruger MP, Rubash HE. Acetabular anatomy and the transacetabular fixation of screws in total hip arthroplasty. *J Bone Joint Surg Am*. 1990;72:501-508.

5

TOTAL KNEE ARTHROPLASTY

Michael D. Hellman | Tad Gerlinger

Total knee arthroplasty is the gold standard for degenerative conditions about the knee. The goals of surgery include pain relief, restoration of functional range of motion, and restoration of alignment. The two classic philosophies for performing total knee arthroplasty are measured resection and gap balancing.

The measured resection technique was developed for cruciate-retaining (CR) total knee arthroplasty. A strict adherence to maintaining the joint line position is critical to ensure proper posterior cruciate ligament (PCL) tensioning and overall implant survival. If the PCL is too tight, excessive tibiofemoral rollback occurs, which risks posterior wear. If the PCL is too loose, excessive femoral anterior translation occurs, which risks anterior wear. Measured resection relies on anatomic landmarks for determination of femoral component rotation.

The gap balancing technique was developed for cruciate-substituting (also known as posterior stabilized [PS]) total knee arthroplasty. The goal of gap balancing is to achieve even rectangular gaps both in extension and in flexion. Typically the tibial and distal femoral cuts are made first, followed by ligament releases to correct any deformity. Once a balanced extension gap has been created, the knee is flexed and the posterior femoral cut is determined based on the balanced ligament tension. Gap balancing relies on the tension of the soft tissues in flexion for determination of femoral component rotation.

This chapter describes a measured resection technique for implanting a cemented cruciate-retaining total knee arthroplasty.

SURGICAL TECHNIQUE

Room Set-Up

- Preoperative radiographs should be displayed in the room (weight-bearing anteroposterior [AP], lateral, sunrise, skier, and mechanical axis views).
- Preoperative templating (either acetate or digital) should be displayed in the room.
- The device company representative should have components available either inside the room or just outside of the room.

Patient Positioning

- Anesthesia can consist of general, spinal, or combined spinal-epidural.
- The patient should be supine; take care to pad all bony prominences.
- Apply a sequential compression device to the contralateral leg.
- Insert a Foley catheter.
- Bump the patient's pelvis so that the knee is neutral with the patella pointing toward the ceiling. Rolled blankets or sheets are often used as the bump.
- Shave the patient's leg that is overlying the operative field.
- Apply a nonsterile tourniquet to the proximal thigh.
- Lift the leg with a candy cane lithotomy leg holder and an ankle support strap (Fig. 5-1).

CASE MINIMUM REQUIREMENTS

- 30 total knee arthroplasties required

COMMONLY USED CPT CODES

- CPT Code: 27447—Arthroplasty, knee, condyle and plateau; medial *and* lateral compartments with or without patella resurfacing (total knee arthroplasty)
- CPT Code: 27487—Revision of total knee arthroplasty, with or without allograft; femoral and entire tibial component
- CPT Code: 27442—Arthroplasty, femoral condyles or tibial plateau(s), knee
- CPT Code: 27443—Arthroplasty, femoral condyles or tibial plateau(s), knee; with débridement and partial synovectomy
- CPT Code: 27445—Arthroplasty, knee, hinge prosthesis (e.g., Walldius type)
- CPT Code: 27446—Arthroplasty, knee, condyle and plateau; medial *or* lateral compartment

COMMONLY USED ICD9 CODES

- 715.16—Primary osteoarthritis of lower leg
- 715.26—Secondary osteoarthritis of lower leg
- 714.0—Rheumatoid arthritis
- 714.30—Juvenile rheumatoid arthritis
- 905.4—Late effect of injury/fracture

- Apply a nonsterile U-drape just distal to the tourniquet.
- Apply an electrocautery grounding pad on either the patient's belly or the contralateral thigh.
- If a leg holder device will be used (i.e., Alvarado Knee Holder [Zimmer, Warsaw, IN]), install the initial bar and support plate assembly on the bed.

Prepping and Draping

- Provisionally prepare the operative leg with rubbing alcohol–soaked 4 × 4–in gauze pads.
- Prepare the operative leg with a preferred surgical solution (i.e., chlordexidine gluconate+isopropyl alcohol, providone-iodine scrub with povidone-iodine prep).
- Wear a helmet and battery pack ("space-suit").
- Proceed with scrubbing, gowning, and gloving; wear one additional pair of gloves for draping.
- Apply a sterile half-sheet drape over the distal end of the table.
- Apply a sterile blue towel around the proximal thigh just distal to the nonsterile U-drape; secure it with a towel clip.
- Apply a sterile half-sheet drape over each arm board.
- Apply an impervious sterile U-drape around the thigh at the level of the blue towel from proximal to distal.
- Apply another impervious sterile U-drape around the thigh at the level of the blue towel from distal to proximal (Fig. 5-2).
- Hold the leg at the calf with a blue towel and have the circulating nurse remove the candy cane lithotomy leg holder and ankle support strap from the operative field.
- Place an impervious stockinette from the foot to the midcalf.
- Wrap the leg with a self-adherent wrap from the foot to just proximal to the end of the stockinette (i.e., Coban [3M, St. Paul, MN]; Fig. 5-3).
- With a surgical marking pen, mark multiple horizontal lines across the knee, perpendicular to the anticipated incision, to later aid in skin closure.
- Flex the knee to 90 degrees and carefully apply an antimicrobial incise drape (i.e., Ioban [3M]) circumferentially around the distal operative field.
- Extend the knee and apply the antimicrobial incise drape to the proximal operative field; no skin should be uncovered.
- Remove top gloves.
- Apply an extremity drape; the leg can now be set down onto the operative field.
- If a leg holder device will be utilized, apply the sterile portion.

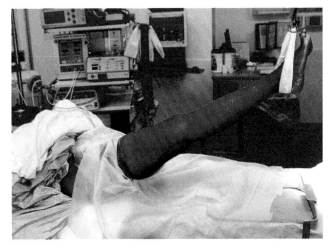

Figure 5-1 The patient's leg is properly positioned and ready for prepping and draping.

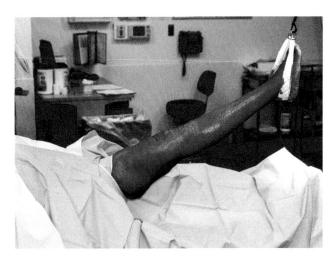

Figure 5-2 The patient's leg is prepped, and draping is underway.

- If a tourniquet will be used for the entire procedure, apply an esmarch wrap from foot to proximal thigh, bend the knee to 90 degrees, and inflate.

Exposure

- Flex the knee and identify and mark the patella and the tibial tubercle.
- Make a longitudinal incision just medial to the tibial tubercle; the incision is made long enough to avoid excessive traction to skin edges, usually about 12 cm in length (Fig. 5-4).
- Sharply dissect through subcutaneous tissue down to layer 1 fascia/retinaculum; use rakes on each side of the skin incision to provide uniform tension.
- A sponge or lap can be used to bluntly clear off subcutaneous tissue until the joint capsule is visualized; proximally the muscle fibers of the vastus medialis obliquus (VMO) should also be visible.
- Make a medial parapatellar arthrotomy either with an electrocautery or sharply with a knife.
- Have an assistant ready with the suction to remove synovial fluid from the operative field as the arthrotomy is made.
- Retract the patella laterally with a double Hohmann retractor and sharply remove the anterior cruciate ligament and the anterior horn of the medial meniscus.
- Elevate the deep fibers of the medial collateral ligament (MCL) and the medial capsule just distal to the tibial articular surface around to the posteromedial corner; use a single-prong Hohmann retractor at the medial joint line.
- With the medial retractor in place, extend the knee, identify excess medial synovium under the joint capsule, and excise; an army-navy retractor medially can be helpful (Fig. 5-5).
- With the knee extended, remove the patella fat pad with care; be careful not to cut the patella tendon or avulse it with excessive retraction.
- Remove the anterior horn of the lateral meniscus and then use an osteotome to release the lateral structures just distal to the tibial articular surface; use a double Hohmann retractor at the lateral femoral condyle.
- Use a rongeur to remove any osteophytes that reside along the medial joint line and lateral joint line and along the contour of the femoral condyles.
- Use electrocautery to remove the suprapatella fat pad and anterior synovium from the femur.
- Note that once the femur or tibia has been cut, removal of the menisci from their capsular attachments is much easier.
- Use a laminar spreader on the medial side when excising the lateral meniscus and on the lateral side when excising the medial meniscus (Fig. 5-6).

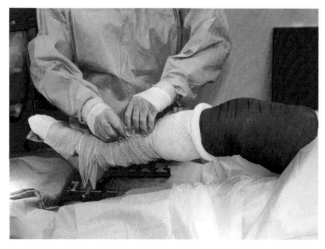

Figure 5-3 The patient's leg is fully prepped and draped.

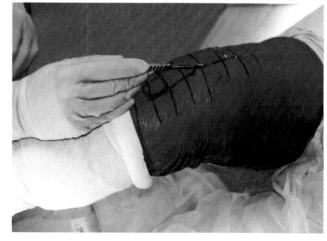

Figure 5-4 A skin incision is made for a medial parapatellar approach.

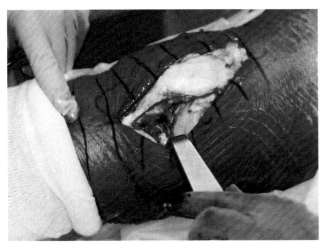

Figure 5-5 A medial-sided release of the tibia is performed. A Hohmann retractor is used deep to the superficial medial collateral ligament.

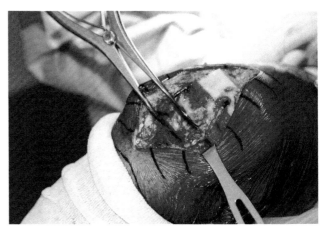

Figure 5-6 A laminar spreader is used to expose the menisci. Note how the medial and lateral space is even.

Bone Preparation and Component Sizing

Femur

- Femoral cuts should be performed with the knee in flexion.
- Typically, knee joint retractors are used to expose the more proximal aspects of the femur, a double Hohmann retractor hinged on the lateral femoral condyle is used to evert the patella, and a single Hohmann retractor at the medial joint line is used to protect the MCL.
- Intramedullary alignment instrumentation is typically used for the femoral bone resection (Fig. 5-7).
- Make an entry portal into the femoral intramedullary canal with an entry reamer just medial to Whiteside's line and about 1 cm anterior to the origin of the PCL.
- Place the distal femoral resection guide into the femoral canal (typically in 5 degrees of valgus), secure the cutting block with pins (mallet or power driver), and remove the intramedullary guide from the cutting block.
- Perform the distal femoral cut; consider the optional cut for a knee with significant flexion contracture.
- Remove the pins and the distal femoral cutting block.
- Place the anterior/posterior sizer against the resected distal femur by sliding it underneath the posterior femoral condyles (typically in 3 degrees of external rotation or parallel to the epicondylar axis).
- Measure the AP size of the femur from the central scale with the sizing tip touching the anterior femur; consider using the medial-lateral (M/L) sizer at this time as well (Fig. 5-8).
- Drill two location holes for the four-in-one cutting block into the distal femur through the sizing guide and then remove the guide.
- Place the appropriately sized four-in-one cutting block into the two location holes (Fig. 5-9).
- Tap the block with a mallet to ensure it is sitting flush against the resected distal femur and secure the cutting block with pins.
- Perform the anterior, posterior, and chamfer femoral cuts.
- Remove the four-in-one cutting block.
- Finish the cuts with a reciprocating saw.
- Remove posterior femoral osteophytes with a curved osteotome and mallet.

Tibia

- Extramedullary alignment instrumentation is typically used for tibial bone resection (Figs. 5-10 and 5-11).

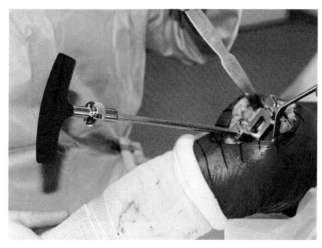

Figure 5-7 An intramedullary guide is used to cut the distal femur. Two Hohmann retractors are used to expose the femoral condyles.

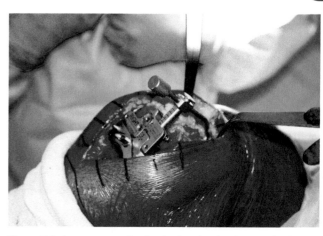

Figure 5-8 An anteroposterior sizer is placed under the posterior femoral condyles, and the central scale sizing tip is positioned over the anterior femur.

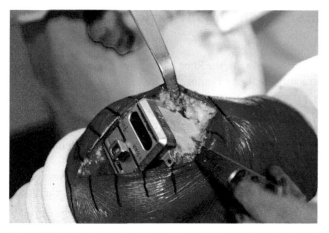

Figure 5-9 A four-in-one block is used to cut the femur. Note the "grand piano" sign of the anterior femur after a cut was made with the correct external rotation.

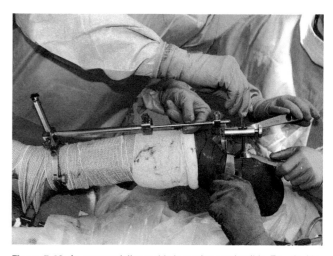

Figure 5-10 An extramedullary guide is used to cut the tibia. Two double-prong Hohmann retractors and a single-prong Hohmann retractor are used to expose the proximal tibia.

- Typically the tibia is subluxated for better exposure with a double-prong Hohmann retractor at the PCL, a double-prong Hohmann retractor at the lateral tibial plateau, and a single-prong Hohmann retractor at the medial tibial plateau.
- Apply the tibial extramedullary alignment guide to the patient's leg.
- Adjust the tibial extramedullary guide so that it is in neutral varus/valgus alignment; typically the proximal end is centered over the tibial tubercle, and the distal end is centered over the second metatarsal or the center of the ankle joint (Fig. 5-12).
- Adjust the alignment guide's distance from the leg to ensure that the appropriate tibial slope will be cut (based on the design of the prosthesis being used).
- Dial the alignment guide proximal or distal so that 2 mm of bone will be resected from the plateau side with more cartilage/bone loss.
- Alternatively, dial the alignment guide proximal and distal so that 10 mm of bone will be resected from the plateau side with less cartilage/bone loss.
- Perform the medial and lateral tibial cuts, leaving a central bone island to not cut the PCL.
- Remove the pins and the extramedullary tibial cutting guide.
- With a reciprocating saw, cut just medial and lateral to the PCL attachment.

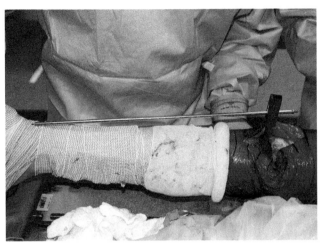

Figure 5-11 A spacer block and an alignment rod are used to check the alignment of the tibia.

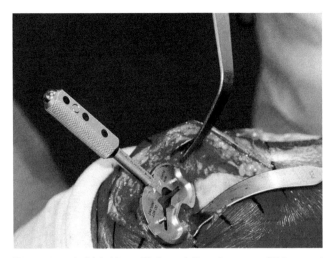

Figure 5-12 A tibial sizing guide is used. Note the correct tibial external rotation.

- Remove each tibial plateau with a rongeur, osteotome, and electrocautery.
- Remove excessive PCL bone island with a double-action rongeur.
- Find a tibial sizer tray that fits both medial to lateral and anterior to posterior with the trial in slight external rotation, aligning near the junction of the middle and medial thirds of the tibial tubercle.
- With the knee in extension, insert a spacer block with an alignment drop rod to ensure the tibial cut was neutral.

Patella
- The patella cut should be done with the knee in extension (Fig. 5-13).
- Place a towel clip just distal to the patella through the patella tendon and just proximal to the patella through the quadriceps tendon; apply tension through the towel clips to stabilize the patella.
- A patella clamp surface cutting guide can be used to accurately cut the patella.
- The patella is cut with a measured resection technique with the exception that at least 12 mm of patella should remain after the cut to decrease the likelihood of patella fracture.
- Patella sizers are used to select the correct patella size, and drill holes are made for the patella pegs with the sizer's guide holes.

Trialing and Balancing
- The knee should be in flexion.
- Place a femoral trial onto the resected femur by lifting up on the femur and striking in place with a mallet.
- Change the knee position to extension (Fig. 5-14).
- Place a tibial trial onto the tibia and insert a 10-mm poly trial.
- Test the knee's range of motion (goal is 0 to 130 degrees).
- Test the tightness of the trial components in both extension and flexion.
- Test for anterior liftoff of the components (PCL is too tight) and excessive femoral anterior translation (PCL is too loose).
- Test the knee for valgus and varus stability in extension and flexion.
- Place an alignment drop rod through the trial components to test for valgus and varus malalignment.
- If the knee is too loose in both flexion and extension, increase the poly trial.
- If the knee has a persistent flexion contracture, first reassess that all posterior femoral osteophytes have been removed; a posterior capsular release may be performed as needed.

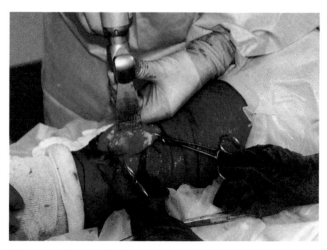

Figure 5-13 Two towel clips are used to stabilize the patella as it is cut with a saw.

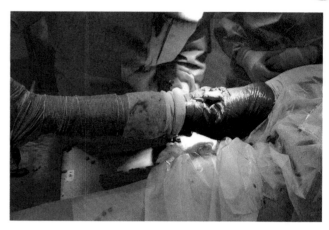

Figure 5-14 The knee is tested for medial and lateral stability with the knee trial components in place.

- If the knee has a persistent varus malalignment (the spacer block is tight medially), first reassess that all the medial tibial plateau and medial femoral condyle osteophytes have been removed.
- If the knee has persistent varus malalignment, perform a more in-depth subperiosteal dissection of the superficial MCL without disrupting the insertion, which is 6 to 8 cm distal to the joint line.
- If the knee has persistent valgus malalignment (spacer block is tight laterally), ensure osteophytes are removed and perform a lateral release as needed to balance the knee.

Cementing and Closure

- If a tourniquet is only being used for cementing, cover the wound with a dry lap sponge, apply an esmarch wrap, bend the knee to 90 degrees, and inflate the tourniquet.
- Have the scrub technician begin mixing the cement and start a cement timer (Fig. 5-15).
- Use a pulsatile lavage to clean the femur, tibia, and patella of any debris and marrow from the exposed bony surfaces (Fig. 5-16).
- Dry the bone with a clean lap sponge.
- Take the cement gun and fill the tibial metaphysis with cement; press the cement into the metaphysis with your finger.
- Additional cement should be applied to the bottom of the tibial component.
- Press the tibial component onto the tibia and use an impactor and mallet to fully seat.
- Use a freer-elevator and toothless pickup instrument to clean any extravasated cement out of the knee.
- Apply cement to the femur by pressing the cement into the femoral condyles with your finger.
- Additional cement should be applied to the posterior condyles of the femoral component.
- Press the femoral component onto the femur and use an impactor and mallet to fully seat the component (Figs. 5-17 and 5-18).
- Use a freer-elevator and toothless pickup instrument to clean any extravasated cement out of the knee.
- Place the trial poly between the femoral and tibial components and fully extend the knee.

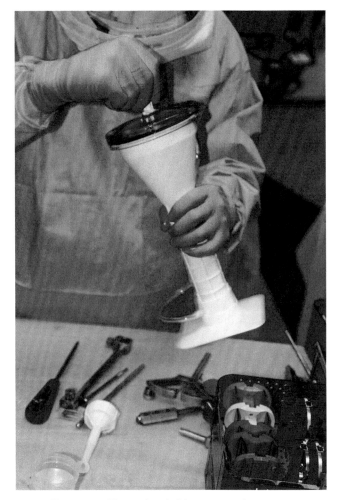

Figure 5-15 The scrub technician prepares the cement.

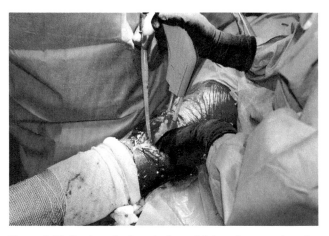

Figure 5-16 The knee is cleared of any debris and marrow from the exposed bony surfaces.

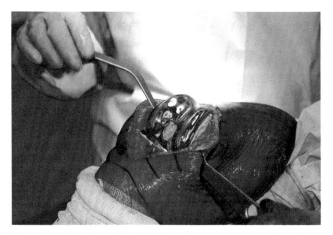

Figure 5-18 The femoral and tibial prostheses are cemented into place.

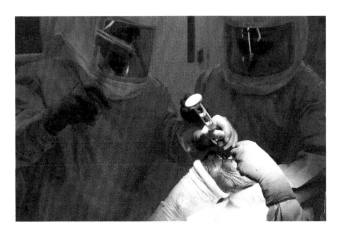

Figure 5-17 A secondary impactor and mallet are used to seat the femoral prosthesis.

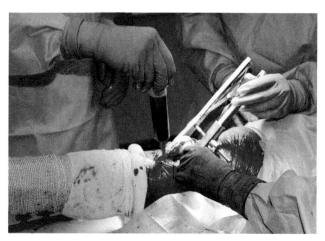

Figure 5-19 A dilute providone-iodine lavage is poured into the joint after the components are cemented in place.

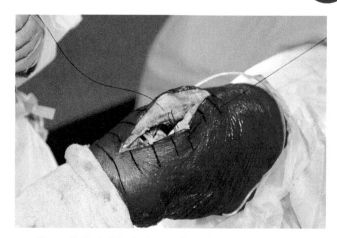

Figure 5-20 A #2 barbed suture is used to close the capsule.

- Apply cement to the patella by pressing the cement onto the cut bone surface with your finger.
- Additional cement should be applied to the back of the patella button.
- Press the patella component onto the patella with a patella clamp.
- Use a freer-elevator and toothless pickup instrument to clean any extravasated cement out of the knee.
- Mix a dilute providone-iodine lavage (0.35%) and pour into the knee joint (Fig. 5-19).
- Allow the lavage to sit for 3 minutes before irrigating the knee with saline solution.
- Allow the cement to fully dry, remove the trial tibial component, and search for any loose cement fragments.
- Insert the tibial polyethylene liner and be sure it locks into position.
- Insert a Hemovac drain that exits the knee superolaterally.
- Close the capsule with either a #1 Vicryl (Ethicon, Somerville, NJ) suture (figure-of-eight stitching) or a #2 barbed suture (running baseball stitching; Fig. 5-20).
- Close the subdermal layer with either a 2-0 Monocryl (Ethicon, Somerville, NJ) suture (simple stitching) or a 0 barbed suture (running baseball stitching).
- Close the skin with a stapler.
- Apply a nonadherent dressing of your choice (i.e., petrolatum gauze dressing).
- Wrap the leg with a bulky cotton padding and an elastic bandage wrap.

BRIEF SUMMARY OF SURGICAL STEPS
• Prep and drape
• Expose the femur and tibia
• Cut the distal femur
• Cut the tibia
• Cut the posterior and anterior femur
• Trial components
• Cement components
• Close

REQUIRED EQUIPMENT
Lower extremity draping pack
Company specific prosthesis system tray
Company specific implants
Powered instrumentation tray

TECHNICAL PEARLS

- If the knee has a significant valgus deformity, perform a very small medial release at the beginning of the case.
- If the knee has a significant varus deformity, perform a large medial release at the beginning of the case.
- If the knee has a significant flexion contracture, perform the optional cut at the beginning of the case.
- If the knee is not balancing correctly after the measured resection cuts are performed, always consider soft tissue releases before removing more bone.

COMMON PITFALLS

(When to call for the attending physician)

- If the medial collateral ligament is incompetent
- If the posterior cruciate ligament is incompetent
- If significant deformity is present, making it difficult to expose the knee
- If you have trouble balancing the knee
- If you think you need to remove more bone than the cuts described in this chapter

POSTOPERATIVE PROTOCOL

The patient should have both mechanical and chemoprophylaxis therapy prescribed immediately after surgery. Twenty-three hours of perioperative intravenous antibiotics should also be prescribed (usually cefazolin or clindamycin if the patient is penicillin allergic). A multimodal pain management strategy should be initiated. Physical therapy should begin as soon as the patient can tolerate, usually on postoperative day 0 or day 1. If a drain was used, it should be removed on postoperative day 1. Patients usually go home, but some need additional care at a rehabilitation center. If a patient does go home, home physical therapy should be prescribed. If a patient goes to a rehabilitation center, inpatient therapy should be continued. Usually patients need some type of assist device for the first 3 weeks after surgery. At 3 weeks, the wound is checked, range of motion is assessed, and deep venous thrombosis (DVT) prophylactic medication is discontinued. At 6 weeks, a patient's range of motion should be approximately 0 to 100 degrees. If the patient does not have this motion, aggressive physical therapy should be prescribed with the understanding that a knee manipulation with anesthesia may be necessary. Zero to 110 to 115 degrees of motion is considered a successful outcome.

POSTOPERATIVE CLINIC VISIT PROTOCOL

Patients are usually seen back in the office at 3 weeks, 6 weeks, and 6 months and for annual follow-up visits. Postoperative radiographs should be obtained at 6 weeks and 6 months and at annual follow-up visits.

SUGGESTED READINGS

1. American Academy of Orthopaedic Surgeons. *AAOS guideline on preventing venous thromboembolic disease in patients undergoing elective hip and knee arthroplasty.* <http://www.aaos.org/Research/guidelines/VTE/VTE_guideline.asp>. Accessed 14.12.14.
2. Berger RA, Crossett LS, Jacobs JJ, Rubash HE. Malrotation causing patellofemoral complications after total knee arthroplasty. *Clin Orthop Relat Res.* 1998;356:144-153.
3. Brown NM, Cipriano CA, Moric M, Sporer SM, Della Valle CJ. Dilute betadine lavage before closure for the prevention of acute postoperative deep periprosthetic joint infection. *J Arthroplasty.* 2012; 27(1):27-30.
4. Gililland JM, Anderson LA, Sun G, Erickson JA, Peters CL. Perioperative closure-related complication rates and cost analysis of barbed suture for closure in TKA. *Clin Orthop Relat Res.* 2012;470(1): 125-129.

CHAPTER 6

OPEN REDUCTION AND INTERNAL FIXATION OF FEMORAL NECK FRACTURES

Daniel J. Stinner

Hip fractures occur in a bimodal distribution with the vast majority in the elderly population as the incidence rate increases with age. Hip fractures in the elderly patient population commonly occur after low-energy trauma (e.g., fall from standing) and more commonly present as a subcapital femoral neck fracture. As the aging population continues to increase, the rate of hip fractures is expected to grow with it, which poses a significant healthcare problem as the 1-year mortality rate for hip fractures ranges from 14% to 36%. Femoral neck fractures in younger patients are much less common and are typically caused by high-energy trauma (e.g., motor vehicle collision). These fractures present more commonly as basicervical or more vertically oriented femoral neck fractures, which is important to recognize during preoperative planning because it can affect implant selection and placement.

Patients typically present with the injured limb shortened and externally rotated as the fracture deformity results in femoral shortening, varus, and anterior angulation. An anteroposterior (AP) pelvis radiograph should be obtained, in addition to AP and lateral radiographs of the injured hip and femur. The AP pelvis radiograph can be used to assist in preoperative templating if an arthroplasty is performed, or it can be used to allow assessment of the neck-shaft angle of the uninjured side for comparison and assessment of quality of reduction when open reduction and internal fixation is planned. The surgeon should be aware that the mean femoral neck-shaft angle is 130 $\pm$ 7 degrees, with femoral anteversion approximately 10 $\pm$ 7 degrees, in both preoperative planning and assessment of fracture reduction.

Two fracture classifications are commonly used for femoral neck fractures. The first is the Garden classification: I, incomplete, valgus impacted; II, complete, nondisplaced; III, complete, partially displaced; and IV, complete, totally displaced. Garden I and II femoral neck fractures are considered stable, and patients commonly undergo operative fixation without open reduction and visualization of the fracture site. Garden III and IV femoral neck fractures, on the other hand, are considered unstable, and patients subsequently should undergo open reduction and internal fixation. The other fracture classification, perhaps less commonly used but equally important in that different fixation constructs might be used based on the classification, is the Pauwels classification. This system groups femoral neck fractures into three categories based on the orientation of the fracture pattern measured from the horizontal: Pauwels I, less than 30 degrees; Pauwels II, 30 to 50 degrees; and Pauwels III, more than 50 degrees.

A femoral neck fracture should always be ruled out when a patient presents with a femoral shaft fracture after high-energy trauma (Fig. 6-1). In this scenario, the author prefers to obtain, in addition to dedicated views of the ipsilateral hip, including an AP internal rotation view, a computed tomographic (CT) scan of the pelvis that includes fine cuts through the femoral neck to ensure that the diagnosis is not missed, which occurs in up to 9% patients with femoral shaft fractures.

The patient's actual and physiologic age, functional status, bone quality, fracture comminution, and fracture displacement are important in consideration between open reduction and internal fixation or arthroplasty in patients with displaced femoral neck fractures. A young patient (<65 years old) with a displaced femoral neck fracture

CASE MINIMUM REQUIREMENTS

- N = 30 Hip fractures (includes femoral neck and inter/per/subtrochanteric femur fractures)

COMMONLY USED CPT CODES

- CPT Code: 27235—Percutaneous fixation of femoral neck, fracture not visualized
- CPT Code: 27236—Open treatment of femoral neck fracture with internal fixation or hemiarthroplasty

COMMONLY USED ICD9 CODES

- 820—Femoral neck fracture
- 820.0—Transcervical fracture (closed)
- 820.02—Closed fracture of midcervical section of neck of femur
- 820.03—Closed fracture of base of neck of femur
- 820.08—Closed fracture of unspecified part of neck of femur

COMMONLY USED ICD10 CODES

- S72.00—Fracture of unspecified part of neck of femur
- S72.01—Unspecified intracapsular fracture of femur
- S72.02—Fracture of epiphysis (separation) (upper) of femur
- S72.03—Midcervical fracture of femur
- S72.04—Fracture of base of neck of femur
- S72.05—Unspecified fracture of head of femur
- S72.06—Articular fracture of head of femur
- S72.09—Other fracture of head and neck of femur

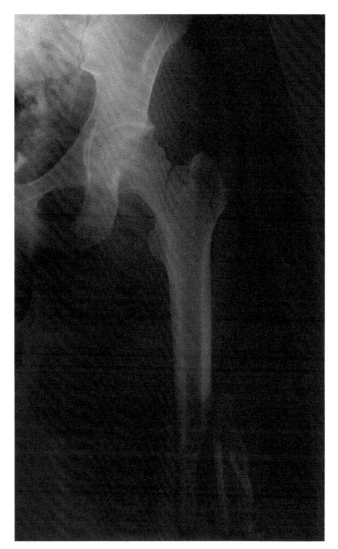

Figure 6-1 A radiograph shows ipsilateral femoral neck and shaft fractures.

(Garden III or IV) should undergo open reduction and internal fixation. In patients older than 65 years, prosthetic replacement is typically preferred because of the higher rate of failure with open reduction and internal fixation and the good results that can be obtained with arthroplasty. Patients with Garden I and II fractures can commonly undergo screw fixation alone (without an open reduction), but the author cautions that nondisplaced femoral neck fractures are not common in younger patients.

The femoral head receives most of its blood supply from the medial branch of the deep circumflex artery, which enters the femoral neck posteriorly. This vessel can be damaged or kinked with a femoral neck fracture, which has led many to advocate urgent open reduction and internal fixation in an effort to minimize the risk of avascular necrosis; however, the data remain inconclusive regarding the need for urgent management. Despite this, the author's preference is to perform open reduction and internal fixation within 24 hours of presentation when possible.

Complications specifically associated with femoral neck fractures include avascular necrosis of the femoral head and femoral neck nonunion. Avascular necrosis occurs in 10% to 40% of patients, and a higher risk is associated with greater initial displacement and poor reduction. There is a potential decreased risk with reduced time to reduction and decompression of the intracapsular hematoma, but the literature supporting this is inconclusive. Nonunion occurs in 10% to 30% of displaced fractures and is higher with malreduction, which is commonly varus or anterior angulation, so the surgeon should make every attempt to obtain an anatomic reduction. Several

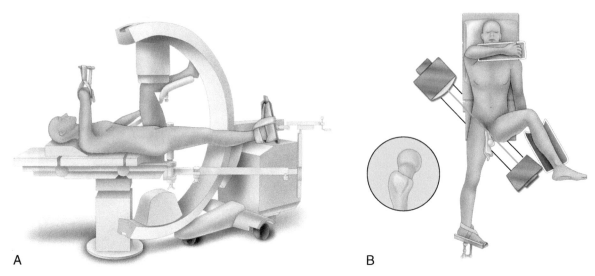

A   B

Figure 6-2 A, Schematic shows patient and image intensifier positioning to allow for adequate fluoroscopic images during open reduction internal fixation of femoral neck fractures. **B,** Note the image intensifier coming from the opposite side of the patient at an angle of approximately 45 degrees.

options are available for the treatment of a femoral neck nonunion, but treatment commonly includes a valgus intertrochanteric osteotomy in the younger patient or consideration for conversion to total hip arthroplasty in the older patient.

SURGICAL TECHNIQUE

Room Set-Up (Fig. 6-2)

- A radiolucent table with an unobstructed view of the hip must be used. This can be either a radiolucent flat top table or a fracture table, based on surgeon preference.
  - If the radiolucent flat top table is used, the entire operative extremity can be draped into the operative field to allow manipulation by the surgeon. Alternatively, skeletal traction can be applied.
  - If a fracture table is used, the distal segment can be manipulated and traction applied through the table.
- The author prefers the use of the radiolucent flat top table when open reduction and internal fixation is planned.
- For intraoperative imaging, a large C-arm, coming in from opposite side of the table, is used.
- The view box should be positioned at the foot of the bed.
- The author prefers to ensure appropriate imaging can be obtained before the start of the case once the patient is positioned to include an AP and lateral view of the hip.
  - Taping the floor can speed the process of moving between images when the C-arm is coming in and out.
    - Tape an "L" around the front wheel and around a rear wheel.
- Surgical scrub technician and table are on the same side as the surgeon.

Patient Positioning

- The patient is positioned supine with a bump under the operative hip.
- Secure the ipsilateral arm across the chest so it does not interefer with the C-arm when a lateral view of the hip is obtained.
- With free leg or skeletal traction, use an elevated leg ramp to minimize the deforming forces (relaxing the hip flexors).

Prepping and Draping

- Prepare the entire exposed extremity all the way up to the most inferior rib across to midline whenever possible.
- Sterile towels are placed around the extremity and operative limb and secured with staples.
- Two split impervious drapes are used when prepping in the entire extremity.
  - When the fracture table is used, an additional split drape is placed around leg just proximal to the fracture boot.
- Use two split drapes or a split (around the leg) and bar drape (head side of the exposed field).
  - When the fracture table is used, an addition split or bar drape is placed around the leg just proximal to the fracture boot.
- Appropriate preoperative antibiotics should be administered (author's usual preference is a first generation cephalosporin, i.e., cephazolin 2 g, given intravenously [IV]).
- Final time-out is performed before skin incision.

Closed Reduction

- A closed reduction can be attempted before prepping when a fracture table is used or after the prepping and draping if the operative extremity is draped into the surgical field, which allows gross manipulation of the limb.
- The most common maneuver for reduction is the Ledbetter maneuver: hip flexion, external rotation, and abduction and gentle traction, followed by hip extension and internal rotation.
- Imaging may grossly underestimate the amount of true displacement, so confirmation with multiple fluoroscopic views is necessary.

Surgical Approaches

- Watson-Jones (anterolateral) approach (see Video 6-1):
  - Advantages: Single approach for fracture exposure, reduction, and implant placement.
  - Disadvantages: Visualization of the femoral neck can be more difficult in obese patients.
  - Incision: Curvilinear incision that begins approximately 2 to 4 cm posterior and distal to the anterosuperior iliac spine (ASIS) and extends toward the tip of the greater trochanter and then curves distally and slightly medially for approximately 10 cm along the anterior portion of the proximal femur (Fig. 6-3).
  - Exposure: The interval between the tensor fascia lata and gluteus medius is developed. Typically, a fat stripe can be found in this interval, which facilitates identification of the interval (Fig. 6-4). The anterior border of the gluteus medius and minimus is retracted posteriorly, and the tensor fascia lata is retracted anteriorly to expose the anterior capsule. Capsulotomy is then performed (Fig. 6-5). After reduction, implants can be placed without the need for an additional skin incision (Fig. 6-6).
- Modified Smith-Petersen approach:
  - Advantages: Excellent exposure of the anterior femoral neck.
  - Disadvantages: Requires separate incision for implant placement.
  - Incision: Starts just distal to ASIS and extends distally approximately 10 cm (Figs. 6-7 and 6-8).
  - Exposure: The interval between the sartorius and the tensor fascia lata is identified and developed. Once the appropriate plane is identified, the author prefers to use either army-navy or Sofield retractors to develop the interval through blunt dissection, taking the tensor fascia lata laterally and the sartorius medially (Fig. 6-9). The lateral femoral cutaneous nerve is frequently encountered and

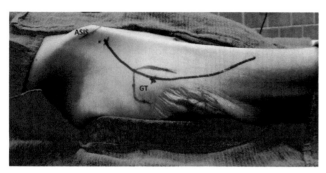

Figure 6-3 The skin incision for the Watson-Jones approach begins 2 to 4 cm posterior and distal to the anterosuperior iliac spine *(ASIS)* and is curvilinear, centered over the greater trochanter *(GS)*.

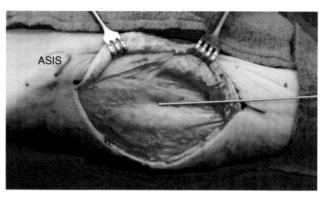

Figure 6-4 Superficial dissection down to fascia with the Watson-Jones approach to the hip. The fat strip that can be seen deliniating the interval between the tensor fascia lata and the gluteus medius is shown by the pointer. *ASIS,* Anterosuperior iliac spine.

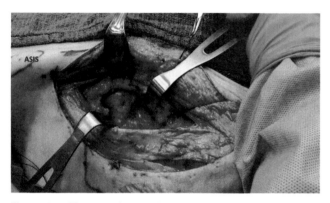

Figure 6-5 After capsulotomy, the surgeon can easily visualize the femoral neck *(*)* and has access within the wound for implant placement *(+)* without having to make an additional incision. *ASIS,* Anterosuperior iliac spine; *GT,* greater trochanter.

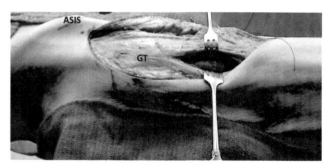

Figure 6-6 A view from the lateral side of the patient with the leg slightly internally rotated shows the deep dissection for implant placement on the lateral border of the proximal femur during the Watson-Jones approach. *ASIS,* Anterosuperior iliac spine; *GT,* greater trochanter.

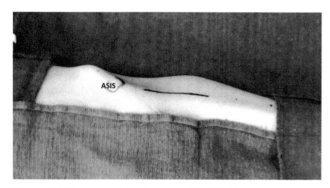

Figure 6-7 The skin incision for the modified Smith-Petersen approach begins two fingerbreadths distal to the anterosuperior iliac spine *(ASIS)* and extends toward the lateral border of the patella for approximately 10 cm.

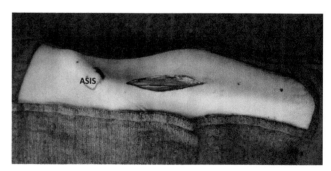

Figure 6-8 The skin incision for the modified Smith-Petersen approach is then carried down to the fascia and the interval between the Sartorius and the tensor fascia lata is developed.

should be retracted medially with the sartorius. To avoid damage to the nerve, the skin incision can be made 1 to 2 cm posterior to the ASIS and the fascial incision made over the tensor fascia lata. The tendonous portion of the rectus is found overlying the capsule and should be elevated off of the hip capsule.

- Additional exposure can be gained by detaching the direct head of rectus femoris tendon origin. When doing so, the author prefers to place a heavy braided suture within the tendon to allow for easy retraction and repair at the end of the case. Ensure that a cuff of tendon is left attached to the ASIS to allow repair during closure. Slight flexion of the hip also releases the rectus, psoas, and sartorius muscles.

Capsulotomy

- The iliocapsularis muscle is elevated sharply from the anterior capsule, and either a Z-shaped, an inverted T-shaped (as shown in Video 6-1), or a T-shaped capsulotomy is performed based on surgeon preference. When performing a T-shaped capulotomy, the capsule is typically elevated off the intertrochanteric line for adequate visualization (Fig. 6-10).
- Be careful not to damage the labrum with the proximal aspect of the transverse limb of the capsulotomy if performing a T-shaped capsulotomy or the limb extending closest to the acetabulum if performing a Z-shaped capsulotomy.
- An intraoperative image with the use of a radiodense object can be used to localize the optimal site for the capsulotomy dependent on the particular fracture.
- Heavy, nonabsorbable sutures are placed in each corner of the capsulotomy to aid in retraction and can be used or replaced during closure of the capsulotomy (Fig. 6-11).
- Avoid the use of Hohmann retractors or retractors that, when placed, hinge on the posterior aspect of the femoral neck because they may damage the blood supply to the femoral head.
  - Ideal retractors include Sofield or Hibbs retractors.

Reduction Techniques

- The proximal fragment is commonly posterior to the distal fragment. In addition, femoral shortening commonly is seen.
- Lateral traction combined with axial traction, with either a bone hook or a Schanz pin placed in the distal segment, can provide enough room to disimpact and bring

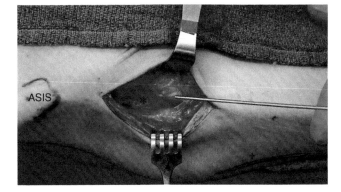

Figure 6-9 After the use of army-navy retractors to bluntly dissect through the superficial and deep intervals of the modified Smith-Petersen approach, the capsule is identified *(*)*. The straight head of the rectus is overlying the medial aspect of the capsule (shown here with the *pointer*) and can either be retracted medially (author's preference) or released from its origin with repair done at the conclusion of the case. Use of this approach requires a second incision for the placement of implants, which is shown by the *+*. *ASIS,* Anterosuperior iliac spine.

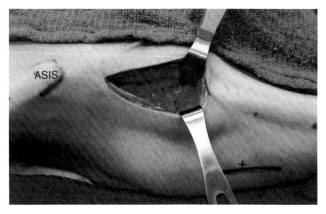

Figure 6-10 The proposed T-shaped capsulotomy is shown deep within the wound for the modified Smith-Petersen approach. Again, use of this approach requires a second incision for the placement of implants, which is shown by the *+*. *ASIS,* Anterosuperior iliac spine.

the proximal fragment into an appropriate position to allow for fine tuning of the fracture reduction.

- A ball-spike placed on the anterior femoral neck and applying a posterior directed force can aid in reducing the sagittal plane deformity.
- A 2.5-mm drill hole can be placed at the femoral head neck junction.
  - With use of a modified large Weber clamp, one tine can be placed in the drill hole and the other either over the lateral aspect of the greater trochanter or through a second drill hole in the distal fragment (Fig. 6-12).
  - Similarly, a Jungbluth reduction clamp can be used if modified Weber clamps are not available (Figs. 6-13 and 6-14).
- With this technique, it is important to ensure that the posterior aspect of the fracture is not gapping open as anterior compression is obtained.
- A Schanz pin can be placed in the femoral head or neck to use to manipulate or rotate the proximal fragment.
  - When placing the Schanz pin, anticipation of the reduction maneuver is important to ensure that the Schanz pin will not be impeded by soft tissues or the acetabulum (4.0-mm to 5.0-mm Schanz pin in the femoral head/neck; 5.0-mm can be used in the greater trochanter/proximal femur; Fig. 6-15 and Video 6-1).
- Ensure that an anatomic reduction has been obtained both with direct visualization of cortical surfaces exposed (ideal locations to visualize include the anterior cortex and the inferior cortex) and through the use of intraoperative fluoroscopy on both AP and lateral views.
- Once the fracture is reduced, it is held in place with either modified Weber clamps or multiple 2.0-mm K-wires.
  - When placing these K-wires, avoid placement where the planned hardware will go.
- If comminution is present anteriorly and inferiorly and precludes obtaining and maintaining an anatomic reduction, a 2.4-mm or 2.7-mm staight or reconstruction plate can be contoured and temporarily secured to maintain the reduction until the definitive fixation is applied.

Fixation Constructs

- The most common method of fixation includes 6.5-mm or 7.3-mm cannulated screws, with washers.

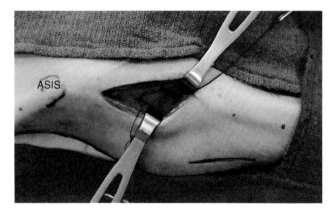

Figure 6-11 After capsulotomy, the femoral neck *(*)* is well visualized with the modified Smith-Petersen approach. Sutures were placed in the ends of the joint capsule to aid in retraction. *ASIS,* Anterosuperior iliac spine.

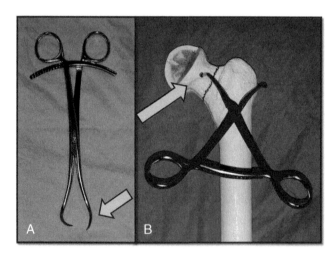

Figure 6-12 A Weber clamp can be modified, where one tine is straightened (**A**, *green arrow*), which allows it to be easily placed into a 2.5-mm drill hole in the femoral neck (**B**, *green arrow*). The fracture can then be compressed when the other tine from the Weber clamp is placed over the greater trochanter as shown in **B**.

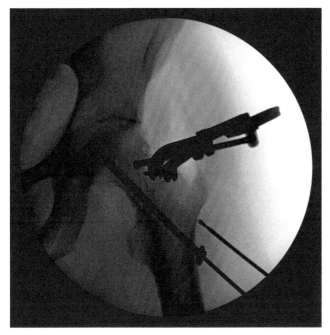

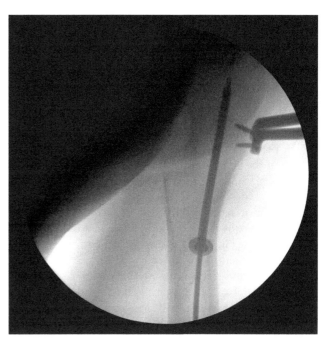

Figure 6-13 An anteroposterior fluoroscopic view of the hip shows the use of a Jungbluth clamp to provide compression across the superior aspect of the femoral neck, which was the site of maximal displacement as the fracture hinged inferomedially. The author typically places all three guidewires before placement of cannulated screws; however, in this case, the inferior screw was placed first to obtain more balanced compression across the fracture site because the Jungbluth clamp was placed superiorly.

Figure 6-14 A lateral fluoroscopic view of the hip shows the use of a Jungbluth clamp with unicortical screws, which does not interfere with intended fixation.

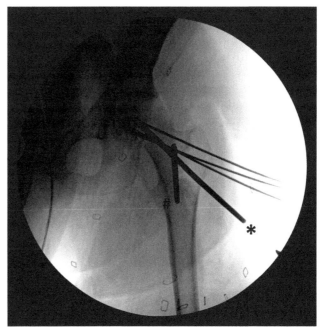

Figure 6-15 A femoral neck fracture is reduced with the aid of two Schanz pins, one placed in the femoral head (*) and one placed in the femoral neck (#). The reduced fracture can then be temporarily held with K-wires placed in a position that does not interfere with intended fixation.

- Three screws are placed in an inverted triangle arrangement; additional screws do not appear to offer any mechanical advantage.
- The starting point for all screws should be above the level of the lesser trochanter to minimize the risk of an iatrogentic subtrochanteric femur fracture.
- Screws should be placed to optimize compression across the fracture site (i.e., perpendicular to the fracture site).
- Screw spread is also important to minimize postoperative fracture displacement; place at the periphery.
- The posterior superior quadrant should be avoided to minimize the risk of disruption of the blood flow to the femoral head.
- When placing a screw to obtain compression, place the screw furthest from any potential comminution, which is most commonly posterior and inferior (i.e., place the anterior-superior screw first), to avoid creating a deformity.
  - If this is not a concern, ideal placement is the inferior screw first along the inferior cortex in the AP and centrally on the lateral. This screw helps resist inferior displacement.
  - The second screw is a posterior-superior screw along the posterior cortex on the lateral and central in the head on the AP. This screw resists posterior displacement and anterior angulation when the patient is rising from a seated position.
  - The final screw is an anterior screw, anterior on lateral and central on the AP.
- Avoid a superior screw because of risk of damage to the lateral epiphyseal artery branches.
- It is always important to range the hip after surgery with fluoroscopy to ensure no in-out-in.
- Reasons to consider other implant and fixation constructs:
  - Pauwels III and basicervical femoral neck fractures: Because of increased shear forces across a vertically oriented fracture (Pauwels III), several alternative fixation constructs have been used successfully.
    - These constructs most commonly include either the use of an additional horizontally placed screw (i.e., perpendicular to the fracture line) or the use of a dynamic hip screw (DHS) with an antirotation screw.
    - For these fractures, the author prefers to use a low-angle sliding hip screw, placed in a similar location to the inferior screw in a three-screw construct, with two cannulated screws placed proximally, making the base of the inverted triangle when able.
  - Because of the limited purchase in the proximal fragment of basicervical fractures, a DHS with antirotation screw should be considered for this fracture pattern.

BRIEF SUMMARY OF SURGICAL STEPS

- Ensure appropriate fluoroscopic images can be obtained once patient is positioned
- Use Watson-Jones or modified Smith-Petersen approach
- Correct location for capsulotomy can be confirmed with a radiodense instrument as a marker while an anteroposterior view of the hip is obtained if the surgeon is unsure
- Expose the fracture
- Reduce the fracture and hold in place with the use of reduction aids
- Ensure that varus and anterior angulation have been corrected by obtaining both anteroposterior and lateral views of the hip
- Stabilize the fracture with the three cannulated screws or dynamic hip screw and antirotation screw construct, dependent on type of femoral neck fracture
- Obtain multiple fluoroscopic images at varying angles to ensure all hardware is in an appropriate position and anatomic reduction has been obtained
- Close capsule with a heavy, nonabsorbable suture, followed by closure of fascial layer and skin (use of drain dependent on surgeon preference)

TECHNICAL PEARLS

- Obtain images before the start of the case and mark the C-arm and the location of the base to make intraoperative images easier to obtain
- Use a radiodense instrument and an anteroposterior view of the hip to plan the ideal location for the capsulotomy if unsure
- Schanz pins placed in the femoral neck and greater trochanter are ideal for gaining control of the fragments (see Fig. 6-15)
- With use of a Weber clamp, it is easier to place one end on the femoral neck if it is modified (i.e., straighter rather than curved) and the other end on the greater trochanter (see Fig. 6-12)
- A ball-spike applied to the anterior femoral neck with a downward force can be used to correct the apex anterior angulation
- With a dynamic hip screw, use an antirotation screw to prevent twisting at the fracture site when placing the dynamic hip screw

REQUIRED EQUIPMENT

Major orthopaedic set
Additional retractors: Hibbs or Sofield
Large Weber clamp, modified ideal with one tip straighter rather than curved (see Fig. 6-12)
Ball-spike
Schanz pins (4-mm to 5-mm for the femoral head/neck and 5-mm for the greater trochanter)
Minifragment plates available
6.5-mm/7.3-mm or 7.0-mm cannulated screw set
Dynamic hip screw implant set (if use of dynamic hip screw is anticipated) Handheld power/drill

COMMON PITFALLS

(When to call for the attending physician)

- Inability to obtain a good lateral view of the femoral neck; spend time before prepping the patient to ensure the view can be obtained and mark the C-arm to make it easy to obtain during surgery
- Poorly placed capsulotomy; check with a fluoroscopic image and a radiodense instrument to identify the ideal location if unsure
- Failure to correct varus; ensure an appropriate amount of traction and abduction of the leg
- Failure to correct anterior angulation; use a ball-spike on the anterior cortex of the femoral neck with a posterior directed force to correct
- Overcompression of screws can lead to loss of reduction if comminution is present or eccentric compression is applied (Figs. 6-16 and 6-17)
- Twisting at the fracture site when tightening the dynamic hip screw (when used) can be avoided with placement of an antirotation screw
- Screws that are too long or in-out-in can be avoided by taking fluoroscopic views at multiple angles, not just the anteroposterior and lateral

POSTOPERATIVE PROTOCOL

Postoperative antibiotics are not required but, if given, should not be given beyond 24 hours from surgery. Because of the high risk of deep venous thrombosis associated with hip fractures, all patients should receive a minimum of 3 weeks of systemic chemoprophylaxis. The author's preference is to use low-molecular-weight heparin for 3 weeks followed by transition to aspirin 325 mg twice a day for an additional 3 weeks. Sequential compression devices are used until discharge but must not inhibit postoperative mobilization.

For patients with stable fracture patterns (Garden I and II) who undergo operative stabilization with cannulated screws without requiring an open reduction, immediate full weight-bearing is allowed. For patients with unstable fracture patterns (Garden III and IV) requiring open reduction and internal fixation, touch-down weight-bearing

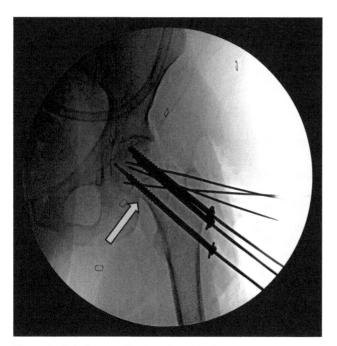

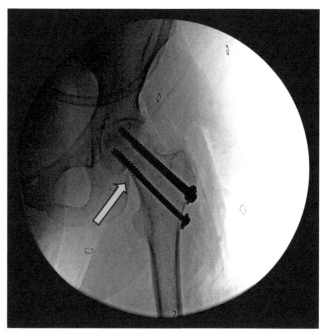

Figure 6-16 A fluoroscopic view of the hip shows anatomic reduction *(green arrow)* before final tightening of all cannulated screws.

Figure 6-17 A fluoroscopic view of the hip shown in Figure 6-16 shows slight loss of reduction *(green arrow)* because of overcompression of the inferior screw.

with an assistive device is allowed immediately with transition to full weight-bearing at 10 to 12 weeks.

Physical therapy is not routinely ordered but is allowed for patients who need assistance with mobilization. Progression of weight-bearing after 10 to 12 weeks involves the the demonstration of safe mobilization with the current assistive device. When patients are able to fully bear weight and are mobilizing well with crutches or a walker, they can progress to the use of a cane carried in the opposite hand and then wean from all assistive devices. When radiographs show bony union and the patient is able to be fully weight-bearing without discomfort, gradual return to strenuous activity/running/sports is allowed.

POSTOPERATIVE CLINIC VISIT PROTOCOL

All patients are seen at 2 to 3 weeks after surgery for a wound check and suture and staple removal. Confirmation that the patient is taking deep venous thrombsis medication is performed, in addition to an assessment of the patient's mobilization. If the patient is having difficulties mobilizing with the assistive device, physical therapy is initiated. No radiographs are obtained unless concern exists for possible loss of reduction.

The patient returns for follow-up at 6 weeks with radiographs taken to include low AP pelvis and radiographs of the operative hip (AP and lateral). Mobilization with the patient's assistive device again is assessed.

At 12 weeks, radiographs again are obtained to include low AP pelvis and radiographs of the operative hip (AP and lateral). Unless there are radiographic or clinical concerns for a nonunion, progression to full weight-bearing is initiated.

Radiographs and clinical assessment again are performed at 6 months and 1 year after surgery. If there are concerns for delayed union, nonunion, or the development of avascular necrosis, more frequent follow-up is allowed and progression of weight-bearing can be slowed.

SUGGESTED READINGS

1. Aharonoff GB, Koval KJ, Skovron ML, Zuckerman JD. Hip fractures in the elderly: predictors of one year mortality. *J Orthop Trauma*. 1997;11(3):162-165.
2. Bhandari M, Tornetta P 3rd, Hanson B, Swiontkowski MF. Optimal internal fixation for femoral neck fractures: multiple screws or sliding hip screws? *J Orthop Trauma*. 2009;23(6):403-407.
3. Fisher MA, Matthei JD, Obirieze A, et al. Open reduction internal fixation versus hemiarthroplasty versus total hip arthroplasty in the elderly: a review of the National Surgical Quality Improvement Program database. *J Surg Res*. 2013;181(2):193-198.
4. Iorio R, Schwartz B, Macaulay W, Teeney SM, Healy WL, York S. Surgical treatment of displaced femoral neck fractures in the elderly: a survey of the American Association of Hip and Knee Surgeons. *J Arthroplasty*. 2006;21(8):1124-1133.
5. Kyle RF, Cabanela ME, Russell TA, et al. Fractures of the proximal part of the femur. *Instr Course Lect*. 1995;44:227-253.
6. Macaulay W, Nellans KW, Garvin KL, Iorio R, Healy WL, Rosenwasser MP. Prospective randomized clinical trial comparing hemiarthroplasty to total hip arthroplasty in the treatment of displaced femoral neck fractures: winner of the Dorr Award. *J Arthroplasty*. 2008;23(6 suppl 1):2-8.
7. Schmidt AH, Leighton R, Parvizi J, Sems A, Berry DJ. Optimal arthroplasty for femoral neck fractures: is total hip arthroplasty the answer? *J Orthop Trauma*. 2009;23(6):428-433.
8. Zuckerman JD, Skovron ML, Koval KJ, Aharonoff G, Frankel VH. Postoperative complications and mortality associated with operative delay in older patients who have a fracture of the hip. *J Bone Joint Surg Am*. 1995;77(10):1551-1556.

CHAPTER 7

INTERTROCHANTERIC FEMUR FRACTURES

INTRAMEDULLARY HIP SCREW

Nicole A. Friel | Ivan S. Tarkin

Intertrochanteric hip fractures encompass fractures in the area of the proximal femur from the extracapsular femoral neck to the area just distal to lesser trochanter. The incidence of hip fractures in the United States is 250,000, and the rate continues to increase. Fractures usually occur in the elderly with osteoporotic bone as a result of low-energy falls; high-energy trauma is typically causative for the younger patient with intertrochanteric hip fracture. Fractures are generally classified as stable or unstable, based on the involvement of the posteromedial buttress. When the posteromedial cortex is intact, the bone is able to resist medial compressive loads once reduced. Unstable fractures, in which the posteromedial cortex is comminuted, collapse into varus and retroversion when loaded. Unstable fractures include reverse obliquity fractures and fractures with subtrochanteric extension.

The goal of treatment is to safely and efficiently restore mobility while minimizing the risk of medical complications and technical failure. Nonoperative management is reserved for patients with multiple medical comorbidities that put them at unacceptable risk of anesthesia or surgery. Medical evaluation and optimization should occur before surgery, and transient medical imbalances, such as electrolyte and fluid imbalance, are addressed before surgery. Studies reveal increased morbidity when surgery is delayed in a geriatric population more than 48 to 72 hours, so prompt attention and teamwork by all involved teams is crucial.

Two implants are widely used to treat intertrochanteric hip fractures: the dynamic hip screw (DHS) and the intramedullary hip screw (IMHS; Fig. 7-1). The intramedullary hip screw combines the sliding compression screw with an intramedullary nail. It has gained significant popularity for the effective treatment of both stable and unstable intertrochanteric fracture variants.

Intramedullary hip screws are most suitable for unstable fractures, including reverse obliquity patterns, fractures with subtrochanteric extension, and fractures with a compromised integrity of the lateral femoral wall because of their superior biomechanics. The intramedullary hip screw acts as a buttress to prevent excessive shaft medialization (Video 7-1). Further, an intramedullary hip screw has the advantage of a closed, percutaneous insertion, which preserves the biology at the fracture site. The use of cephalomedullary nails for intertrochanteric fractures has dramatically risen in the last decade, with an increase from 3% in 1999 to 67% in 2006.

SURGICAL TECHNIQUE

Room Set-Up

- A radiolucent fracture table is positioned in the center of the room.
- Fluoroscopy is brought in from the well leg side with monitor placement at the bottom of the table in the sight line of the surgeon.

CASE MINIMUM REQUIREMENTS

- N = 30 (hip fractures)

COMMONLY USED CPT CODES

- CPT Code: 27244—Treatment of intertrochanteric, peritrochanteric, or subtrochanteric femoral fracture; with plate/screw type implant, with or without cerclage
- CPT Code: 27245—Treatment of intertrochanteric, peritrochanteric, or subtrochanteric femoral fracture; with intramedullary implant, with or without interlocking screws or cerclage
- CPT Code: 27236—Open treatment of femoral fracture, proximal end, neck, internal fixation or prosthetic replacement

COMMONLY USED ICD9 CODES

- 820.21—Closed
- 820.31—Open

COMMONLY USED ICD10 CODES

- S72.14—Intertrochanteric fracture of femur
- S72.10—Unspecified trochanteric fracture of femur
- S72.11—Fracture of greater trochanter of femur
- S72.12—Fracture of lesser trochanter of femur

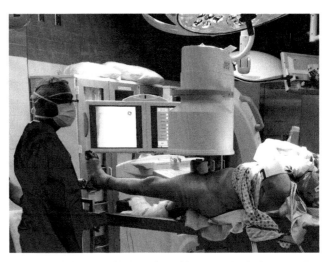

Figure 7-2 A fracture table is used to achieve reduction in the vast majority of geriatric hip fractures via ligamentotaxis. The scissored position is the preferred posture with the affected leg in slight adduction. The ipsilateral arm is adducted across the chest with padding and secured with a wrist restraint. The fluoroscopy screen is in line with the operator sight line.

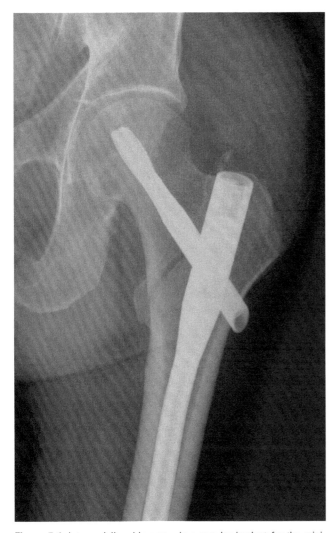

Figure 7-1 Intramedullary hip screw is a popular implant for the minimally invasive management of an intertrochanteric fracture.

Patient Positioning

- With use of multiple assistants, the patient is transferred from the ward bed onto the fracture table.
- A well-padded perineal post is used.
- The affected lower extremity is secured to the fracture table with a well-padded foot holder (Fig. 7-2).
- Based on equipment availability, surgeon preference, and the patient's body habitus, the contralateral (well) leg can be postured in a scissored or hemilithotomy position and secured to the fracture table with the appropriate attachment.
- To facilitate lateral fluoroscopy, the arm on the affected side is adducted across the chest.
- Usage of a wrist restraint is commonplace to secure the limb over padding.
- The contralateral arm is extended over an arm board.
- Adequate anteroposterior (AP) and lateral fluoroscopic images should be obtained before draping.

Fracture Manipulation of Fracture Table

- Perform fracture reduction with fluoroscopic visualization.
- Longitudinal traction can reduce the fracture by ligamentotaxis.

- Intertrochanteric fractures are usually reduced with traction of the leg. Reduction should be confirmed in both AP and lateral views.
- If unable to achieve adequate reduction, plan to perform a percutaneous or open reduction.

Prepping and Draping

- Prepare the operative field in the usual manner per surgeon preference.
- Extend the sterile field from just above the iliac crest to just beyond the knee and from the midline anteriorly to the midline posteriorly.
- Block draping can be performed, or alternatively, specialty drapes such as a vertical isolation drape (shower curtain) can be used (Fig. 7-3).

Reduction

- If inadequate reduction was obtained, percutaneous reduction techniques can aid in reduction.
    - A ball-spike pusher may be used.
    - Alternatively, eccentrically placed Schanz pins can serve as joysticks to achieve reduction (Fig. 7-4).
- If reduction cannot be achieved percutaneously, a limited or formal open reduction can be used.
    - A direct lateral approach to the femur is used.
    - A collinear clamp is popular for holding reduction during nail instrumentation when open reduction is necessary (Fig. 7-5).
- Most low-energy geriatric fractures reduce with closed manipulation with or without percutaneous applied reduction aids.
- Typically, high-energy intertrochanteric fractures in the young patient require an open reduction strategy because the adjacent soft tissue sleeve is severely disrupted and reduction via ligamentotaxis is ineffective.

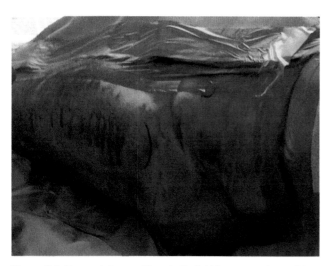

Figure 7-3 Prep and drape with a sterile field large enough to achieve the appropriate trajectory for a percutaneous starting portal.

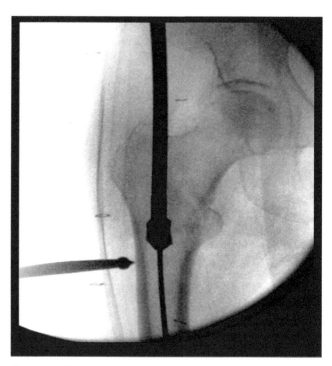

Figure 7-4 Reduction of intertrochanteric fractures can be refined with percutaneous strategies with a ball-spike pusher or Schanz pins as joysticks.

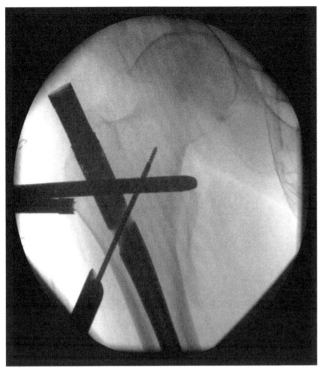

Figure 7-5 Open reduction is seldom necessary for low-energy intertrochanteric fractures. In contrast, high-energy intertrochanteric fractures in younger patients almost always require an open reduction. A collinear clamp is a useful reduction tool.

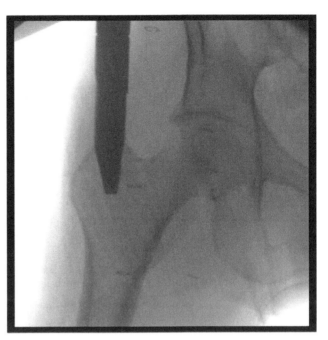

Figure 7-6 The ideal starting point for an intramedullary hip screw is just medial to the tip of the greater trochanter at the junction of the anterior third/posterior two thirds.

Start Point

- The ideal starting point is on the medial edge of the greater trochanter at the junction of the anterior third/posterior two thirds.
  - Because the greater trochanter is a posterolateral structure, this location aligns the nail with the intramedullary canal of the femur (Fig. 7-6).
- Cannulated technique is exercised to achieve a precise starting point that can be performed purely percutaneously.
- A percutaneously placed K-wire on the lateral aspect of the femoral shaft can serve as a guide for the appropriate starting point trajectory (Fig. 7-7).
- Alternatively, a strategic limited incision can be made cephalad to the greater trochanter in line with the femur, and then one can proceed with achieving a starting point (Fig. 7-8).
- Biplanar fluoroscopy is used to determine accurate guidewire position.
- A cannulated drill or awl can be used to create the proximal entry portal in the greater trochanter.

Femoral Preparation

- A ball-tip guidewire is inserted through the established greater trochanteric entry portal across the reduced fracture and then advanced into the distal femur.
  - For long nails, ensure that the guidewire stays in the center-center position distally by checking the position radiographically in the AP and lateral planes.
- Reaming is performed to achieve a path for intramedullary hip screw.
- Avoid "wedging" the fracture open with the reamers (Fig. 7-9).
- Use of a reamer medializing tool and ball-spike pusher on femoral shaft can avoid the wedge effect (Fig. 7-10).

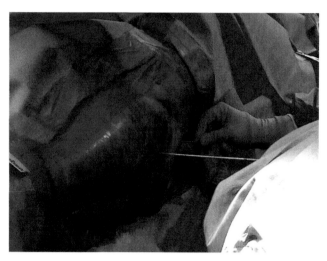

Figure 7-7 The starting point can be achieved percutaneously with cannulated technique. A second K-wire can be placed on the lateral aspect of the femur as a reference.

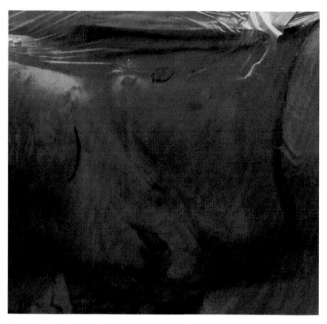

Figure 7-8 A limited incision can be made centered over the percutaneously placed starting point guidewire. Dissection is carried through skin, subcutaneous tissue, and investing gluteal fascia.

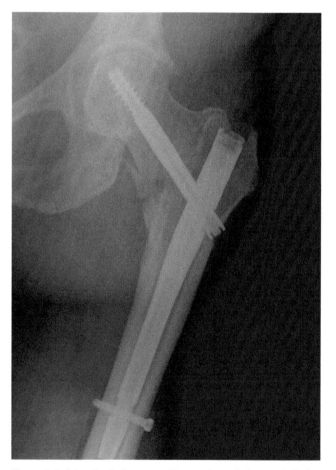

Figure 7-9 Suboptimal alignment of intertrochanteric fracture including shaft lateralization/varus from wedging of the fracture by the nail.

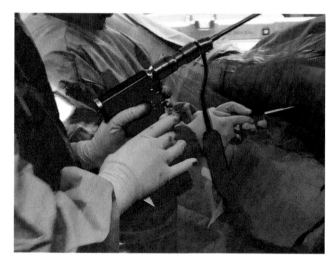

Figure 7-10 Maintaining fracture reduction/manicuring an adequate path for the nail with reaming can avoid the wedge effect. The ball-spike pusher and reamer medializing tool are helpful for avoiding this phenomenon.

- Ream at least 1 mm larger than the diameter of the nail.
  - Note that a typical IMHS has a larger proximal diameter and a larger reamer needs to be used in the peritrochanteric region versus in the diaphysis and distal femur.
- Reaming is slow yet deliberate.

Nail Insertion

- Assemble the nail and guide system on the back table so that the Herzog curve and anterior bow of nail are oriented correctly.
- Check the reliability of the guide by passing a drill bit through the cannula then nail.
- Insert the tip of the nail, with its associated nail assembly, into the prepared proximal femur.
- For long nails, begin the insertion of the nail with the guide handle in the anterior position to negotiate the proximal femur and then slowly rotate the nail into the lateral position with version that matches the individual patient.
- Insertion of the nail can be completed with lightly striking the nail down the shaft with a mallet.
- The final position of the nail is determined by the position of the barrel in relation to the head/neck segment.
  - Ideal positioning directs the lag screw into the center-center position.

Proximal Targeting

- Correct positioning of the nail is crucial to ensure that the lag screw is placed in the center of the femoral head in the AP and lateral planes (Fig. 7-11).
- Cannulated technique is used.
  - Verify the position of the guide pin on AP and lateral radiographic views.
  - The pin should lie within the central third of the femoral neck and head on both radiographic views.
  - When the correct position of the guide pin is achieved in both planes, advance it to within 5 to 10 mm of the articular surface of the femoral head.

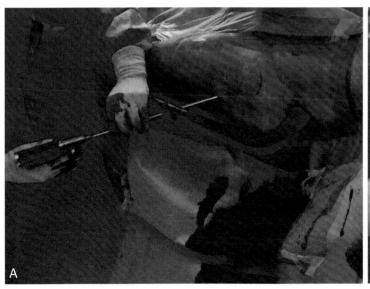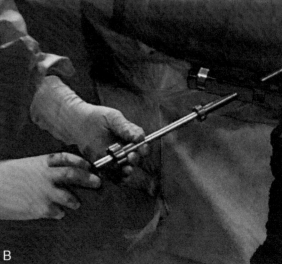

Figure 7-11 A, Cannulated tecthnique is necessary for precise positioning of intramedullary hip screw lag in the center-center position with optimal tip to apex distance (TAD). **B,** Tapping for the screw is only necessary when good bone stock is evident.

- The sum of the distance from the tip of the lag screw to the apex, less correction for magnification, should be 25 mm or less for optimal screw purchase in the head.

Lag Screw Insertion

- The guidewire is measured, and the triple reamer is set to manicure an appropriate path for the screw.
- Use radiographs while reaming to ensure that the guide pin is not being pushed through the femoral head into the joint.
- Use a tap for the lag screw in young patients with strong bone.
- Tapping is unnecessary in patients with osteoporotic bone.
- Insert the lag screw into the proximal femur to the desired level with radiographic control.
- Apply set screw.
  - Typically after seating the set screw, the screw is loosened a half turn to allow for sliding of the screw within the barrel.
  - This process achieves dynamic compression of the fracture with weight-bearing.
- With most systems, compression can be achieved during surgery with the guide and accessories.
- Alternatively, in selected cases, fully seat the set screw to achieve a fixed angle device.

Distal Locking

- Unstable fracture patterns require distal locking; stable fracture patterns do not require distal locking (Fig. 7-12).
- Lock the distal end of a short nail with the guide.
- Lock the distal end of a long intramedullary hip screw with standard freehand techniques.

Closure

- Close the proximal operative wound in layered fashion over a suction drain.
- The distal wounds require skin closure only.
- Apply an impermeable dressing.

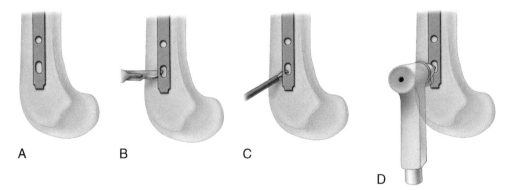

Figure 7-12 A, Distal femur showing the distal holes of the intramedullary nail. **B,** Lateral view of the distal femur with the scalpel blade overlying the center of the most distal hole. **C,** Lateral view of the distal femur with the drill tip lined up on the superior aspect of the hole. **D,** Lateral view of the distal femur with the drill tip directly in line with the superior aspect of the hole before drilling, to ensure the drill enters the hole perfectly without skiving.

BRIEF SUMMARY OF SURGICAL STEPS

- Room set-up (fracture table)
- Patient positioning (affected leg to longitudinal traction)
- Fracture reduction with fracture table via ligamentotaxis
- Prep and drape
- Refine reduction percutaneously or with open approach
- Achieve greater trochanteric starting point
- Femoral preparation with reaming
- Nail insertion
- Proximal targeting to achieve center-center position and optimal TAD
- Lag screw insertion
- Distal locking when indicated
- Closure

TECHNICAL PEARLS

- Preoperative planning is a must; usage of an intramedullary hip screw is ideally suited for the unstable intertrochanteric femur fracture, although it is acceptable for stable patterns as well
- Obtaining a traction view allows the surgical team to understand the intertrochanteric fracture pattern and have the appropriate implants and reduction tools available
- When positioning the patient for surgery on a fracture table, SAFETY FIRST; use multiple assistants on transfer to the ward bed, and secure the patient to the table before any fracture manipulation
- During draping, ensure that the sterile field extends well beyond the greater trochanter because the ultimate trajectory for the starting point and proximal incision can be significantly more cephalad especially in the larger patient
- Adducting the affected leg helps in the achievement of a greater trochanteric starting point, but be careful that the peroneal post does not cause fracture malreduction (varus, shaft lateralization)
- Achieve and maintain fracture reduction before and during the reaming process
- Be sure the guidewire is center-center in the distal femur to avoid anterior cortical penetration when using a long intramedullary hip screw
- Be sure there is not a mismatch between the radius of curvature of the nail chosen and the patient's native anterior bow of the femur to avoid anterior cortical penetration when using a long nail
- When inserting the nail, the anterior bow of the nail can be used to negotiate the proximal femur
- Final seating of the nail can cause a "wedge effect" and lead to varus and lateralization of the femoral shaft; to avoid this, ensure that the reamer carves out a path for the nail proximally; a ball-spike pusher on the shaft and usage of a reamer medializing tool helps avoid this pitfall (during percutaneous nailing)
- Use cannulated technique for precise lag screw placement into the head/neck segment; confirm with biplanar fluoroscopy center-center position with ideal tip to apex distance
- Distal locking is not indicated in all cases, except for patterns with subtrochanteric extension
- Placement of a drain in the starting point wound is recommended because occult muscular bleeding from reamer passage can lead to hematoma formation serving as a nidus for infection
- A biocclusive dressing is recommended to avoid the potential for contamination

EQUIPMENT REQUIRED

Fracture table
C-arm
Lead apron and thyroid shield for operators and ancillary staff
Reduction tools (ball-spike pusher, Schanz pins, reduction clamps (i.e., collinear clamp)
Drill/wire driver
Reaming system
Intramedullary hip screw implant system (intramedullary hip screw nail, proximal lag screw, distal locking screws, targeting guide with associated cannulas and guidewires)

COMMON PITFALLS

(When to call for the attending physician)

- A geriatric hip fracture is an end-of-life–type injury. Family counseling is a must regarding the seriousness of this fracture. Predictable loss of functionality and possible independence must be discussed. Further, the family should be prepared for the possibility of perioperative mortality.
- In the operating room, most osteoporotic hip fractures should adequately reduce with muscle relaxation and ligamentotaxis afforded by traction on a fracture table; call the attending physician if a decision is to be made for open fracture reduction.
- In contrast, most high-energy intertrochanteric fractures in the younger patient require an open reduction and may require the assistance of senior staff.
- A geriatric patient cannot afford a lengthy operation; use the 5-minute rule for obtaining a starting point. If the junior member of the team is having difficulties with this task, then turn over this critical portion of case to a senior member of the team.
- If you lose your reduction during nail insertion, request assistance in rereduction and reaming.
- If a geriatric patient is showing signs of medical instability, alert staff to expeditiously complete the operation or to make a decision to delay (resuscitate) or abort the operation.

POSTOPERATIVE PROTOCOL INCLUDING BRIEF REHABILITATION MILESTONES

The goal of operation in the geriatric host is pain control and immediate weight-bearing to improve survivorship by avoiding complications of prolonged recumbency. Patients are followed with serial x-rays until healing (approximately 4 months). Perioperative antibiotics are given to all patients. Prophylaxis for deep vein thrombosis is administered in the postoperative period. Younger patients with better cognitive and physical reserve may do well with restrictive weight-bearing if deemed appropriate based on fracture stability.

POSTOPERATIVE CLINIC VISIT PROTOCOL

After discharge from the hospital, patients are seen back in the office 2 weeks after surgery to ensure that they are actively involved in therapy and to ensure the wound has healed and fracture alignment has been maintained. Patients are again seen at 6-week intervals until successful rehabilitation and fracture healing is evident clinically and radiographically.

SUGGESTED READINGS

1. Anglen JO, Weinstein JN. Nail or plate fixation of intertrochanteric hip fractures: changing pattern of practice. A review of the American Board of Orthopaedic Surgery Database. *J Bone Joint Surg Am.* 2008;90(4):700-707. doi:10.2106/JBJS.G.00517.

2. Bridle SH, Patel AD, Bircher M, Calvert PT. Fixation of intertrochanteric fractures of the femur. A randomised prospective comparison of the gamma nail and the dynamic hip screw. *J Bone Joint Surgery Br.* 1991;73(2):330-334.

3. Azer E, Sands S, Siska P, et al. The "wedge effect" after intramedullary hip screw fixation for osteoporotic intertrochanteric fractures. Presented at the Annual Meeting of the Orthopaedic Trauma Association, 2010. Baltimore, MD.

4. Utrilla AL, Reig JS, Munoz FM, Tufanisco CB. Trochanteric gamma nail and compression hip screw for trochanteric fractures: a randomized, prospective, comparative study in 210 elderly patients with a new design of the gamma nail. *J Orthop Trauma.* 2005;19(4):229-233.

INTERTROCHANTERIC FEMUR FRACTURES
SLIDING HIP SCREW

Stephanie J. Swensen | Kenneth A. Egol

Intertrochanteric femur fractures account for approximately 250,000 fractures per year and represent a growing public health concern with the aging population in the United States. Most of these fractures occur in patients older than 65 years, and the fractures are more common in women (3 of every 4 fractures). Intertrochanteric fractures are most frequently the result of low-energy falls in the elderly. The cause of the fall must be investigated, and the patient should undergo a thorough medical evaluation on presentation. When an intertrochanteric fracture occurs in a younger individual, it is usually the result of a high-energy injury, such as a fall from height or motor vehicle collision.

Patients typically present after a fall with hip pain and inability to ambulate. Examination reveals shortening and external rotation of the affected extremity. A secondary examination is imperative to delineate any other injuries. Careful attention must be paid to the soft tissues to identify any degloving or pressure ulcers of the sacrum or heels. Radiographic assessment includes anteroposterior (AP) view of the pelvis, AP and cross table lateral views of the affected hip, and traction and internal rotation views to better delineate the fracture pattern. Magnetic resonance imaging (MRI) or computed tomographic (CT) scan is indicated in nondisplaced or occult fractures.

Operative fixation of intertrochanteric hip fractures has been found to significantly decrease mortality in elderly patients. Fracture implant selection for intertrochanteric femur fractures is determined by fracture stability. The Evans classification describes fracture patterns as stable or unstable, based on the integrity of the posteromedial bony cortex. The sliding hip screw is the most widely used device for both stable and unstable fracture patterns. The components of the device include a lag screw, a 130-degree to 150-degree side plate, and cortical screws to secure the plate to the bone. This construct allows controlled dynamic sliding of the proximal fragment along the lag screw, impacting into the distal fragment and stimulating fracture healing in response to dynamic loading of the bone. Therefore, early postoperative weight-bearing is essential for the success of this construct. Sliding hip screws are indicated for stable fracture patterns with an intact posteromedial cortex. Contraindications include lateral wall comminution and reverse obliquity fractures.

SURGICAL TECHNIQUE

Room Set-Up

- A fracture table is used.
- The C-arm fluoroscope is positioned from the contralateral side of the fracture table.

Patient Positioning

- The patient is positioned supine on a fracture table.
- A well-padded perineal countertraction post is placed in position.
- The patient's torso is brought down inferiorly on the table so that the perineum closely abuts the post.
- Ensure that there is no impingement of the labia or scrotum (Fig. 8-1).
- The contralateral lower extremity is either placed in flexion and external rotation in a well leg holder or placed in a scissor position with the nonfractured leg extended in a boot.
- The injured leg is wrapped with cotton undercast padding and placed in a foot-traction boot.
- Assess the positioning of the C-arm fluoroscope.
- Evaluate the AP and lateral images of the affected hip to ensure adequate visualization of the fracture, proximal shaft, femoral neck, and circumferential views of femoral head (Fig. 8-2).

Prepping and Draping

- The lateral aspect of the hip and thigh of the affected extremity is thoroughly prepped with chlorhexidine.
- Allow the preparation to dry before draping.
- The patient is draped with half sheets or a shower curtain (Fig. 8-3).
- Electrocautery device and suction tubing are placed in sterile pockets, and excess cords are passed over the shower curtain, away from the surgical field.

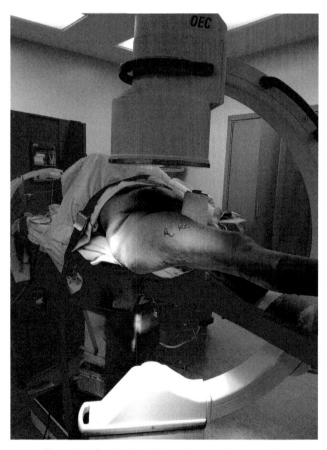

Figure 8-1 Positioning of the patient on a fracture table.

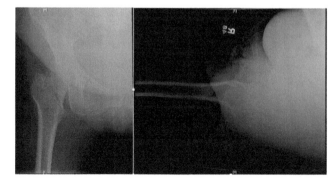

Figure 8-2 Anteroposterior and cross table lateral view of the affected hip.

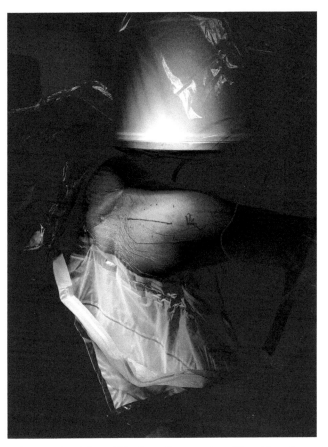

Figure 8-3 The patient is prepped and draped. The C-arm fluorscope is positioned from the contralateral side of the fracture table. Ensure adequate visualization of the fracture site on anteroposterior and lateral views of the affected hip.

Fracture Reduction

- Adequate reduction must be obtained and easily assessed with biplanar fluoroscopic views before prepping and draping the patient.
- Undisplaced fractures may only require slight internal rotation to place the femoral neck parallel to the floor.
- Gentle axial traction is initially placed to restore length and partially correct varus malalignment.
- Following reduction of the fracture the limb is internally rotated to bring the femoral neck en fosse.
- External rotation may be necessary for reduction of some fractures in which the proximal fragment is externally rotated from persistent attachment of external rotators.
  - Varus correction is obtained with additional traction or with abduction of the lower extremity.
  - Posterior sag is addressed with an adjustable pad that is added to the fracture table to apply anteriorly directed force.
  - Manual reduction of posterior sag can also be obtained with an external crutch or during surgery with a bone hook or periosteal elevator levering the shaft anterior.
- Adequate reduction is confirmed on both AP and lateral views to ensure no residual varus angulation, posterior sag, or malrotation.

Approach

- Straight lateral incision over the femur is used, beginning proximally at the palpable vastus lateralis ridge on the greater trochanter and extending distally (Fig. 8-4).

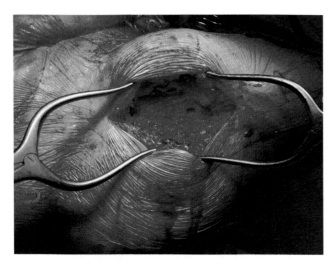

Figure 8-4 Straight lateral incision over the femur.

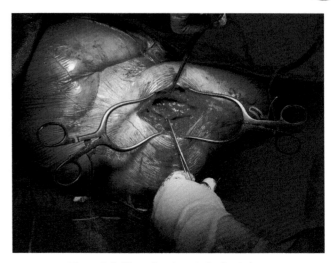

Figure 8-5 Dissection through the fascia lata.

- The dissection is carried through the fascia lata, avoiding the tensor muscle proximally and anteriorly (Fig. 8-5).
- Identify and ligate the first femoral perforator found approximately 4 to 6 cm distal to the trochanter.
- Incise the vastus lateralis fascia and muscle and bluntly dissect to the femoral shaft with a Cobb elevator.
- Identify and control any perforating vessels to the vastus lateralis and retract the vastus lateralis anteriorly to expose the femoral shaft (Fig. 8-6).
- Avoid extending the dissection medially to maintain adequate vascular supply to region of the fracture.

Guide Pin Positioning

- The entrance point for the guide pin is selected based on the angle of the plate.
- The entrance for a 130-degree or 135-degree plate is approximately 2 cm below the vastus lateralis ridge.
  - This level is identified by two landmarks: It is directly opposite the lesser trochanter and is at the same level as the insertion of most proximal fibers of the gluteus maximus tendon on the femoral shaft.
  - The entrance point is adjusted 1 cm proximal for lower angled devices or distal for higher angled devices from the 135-degree starting point for every 5-degree adjustment in measured neck-shaft angle.
- The correctly angled guide is placed at the guide pin insertion site midway between the anterior and posterior cortices of the femoral shaft (Fig. 8-7).
  - Alternatively, the guide pin may be drilled freehand.
- Fluoroscopic confirmation should be obtained to ensure that the guide lies flush on the lateral cortex of the femoral shaft before drilling (Fig. 8-8).
- Advance the guide pin with fluoroscopic guidance in both AP and lateral planes.
  - The pin should be center-center on both views and within 5 mm of subchondral bone.
- The position of the guide pin must be adjusted until central and deep placement is confirmed to allow screw purchase in the best bone.
  - Ensure that the tip-apex distance is less than 25 mm.
    - The tip-apex distance is the sum of the distance from the tip of the lag screw to the apex of the femoral head on an AP view and on a lateral view (Figs. 8-9 and 8-10).
- The interossesous length of the guide pin is measured with the ruler provided in the instrument set.
  - A 95-mm screw is typically used with a 135-degree plate.

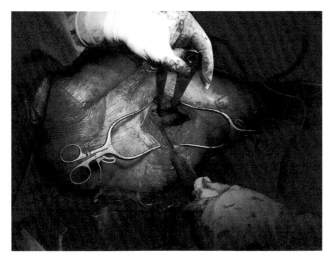

Figure 8-6 Incise the vastus lateralis fascia and muscle and bluntly dissect to the femoral shaft with a Cobb elevator.

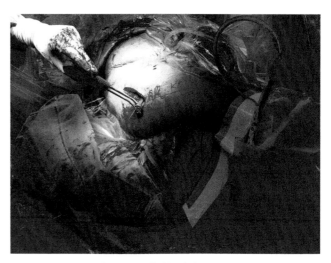

Figure 8-7 Guide pin insertion.

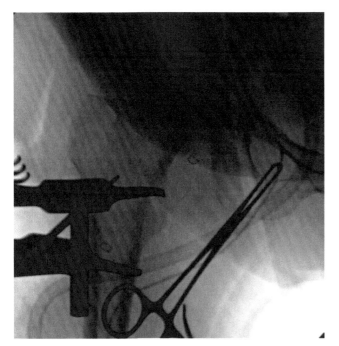

Figure 8-8 Guide pin advanced under direct fluoroscopic guidance.

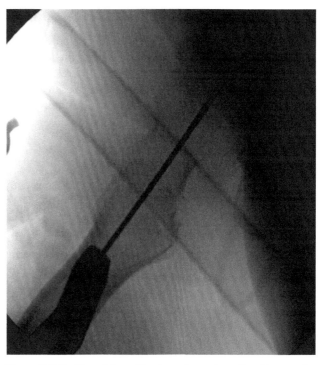

Figure 8-9 Position of the guide pin center-center with a tip-apex distance of less than 25 mm.

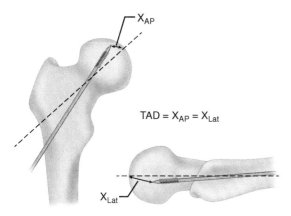

$$TAD = X_{AP} = X_{Lat}$$

Figure 8-10 The tip-apex distance *(TAD)* is estimated by measuring the distance from the tip of the guide pin to the apex of the femoral head on both anteroposterior *(X_{AP})* and lateral fluroscopic *(X_{Lat})* images.

- Ream the femoral neck and head over the guide pin with fluoroscopy with a triple diameter reamer.
  - The reamer is set to 5 mm less than the measured lag screw length so that the femoral head articular surface is not inadvertently violated during reaming.
- Tap the entire screw path to prevent femoral head foration with screw placement.
- A second guide pin can be advanced proximal to the original guide pin to act as a derotational pin, preventing rotation of proximal neck and head fragment with reaming and screw insertion (Fig. 8-11).

Implant Insertion

- A two-hole or four-hole side plate is typically chosen for fixation to the shaft.
- The cannulated lag screw is inserted over the guide pin with a centering sleeve.
- As lag screws are advanced in left-sided intertrochanteric fractures, the clockwise rotation may displace the fracture; however, with right-sided fractures, the screw may help reduce the fracture.
- Once proper positioning of the lag screw is confirmed fluoroscopically, the side plate is slid over the lag screw and seated over the lateral cortex (Fig. 8-12).
- Clamp the plate to the femoral shaft with reduction forceps and remove the guide-wire and derotational wire, if present.
- Release the traction and allow slight impaction of the fracture in the axial plane.
- Insert cortical screws to secure the plate to the femoral shaft.
- A compression screw inserted into the barrel of the lag screw and tightened to compress the fracture in the plane of the lag screw is rarely needed.
- Check alignment and implant position after completion of compression with fluoroscopy (Fig. 8-13).

Wound Closure

- Adequately débride any devitalized tissue and thoroughly irrigate the surgical field.
- Close the muscular, fascial, subcutaneous, and skin layers separately.

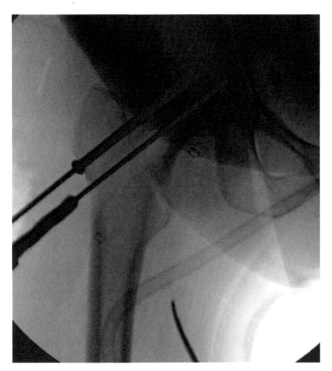

Figure 8-11 Placement of the derotational pin.

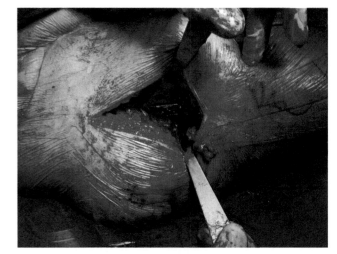

Figure 8-12 Implant insertion.

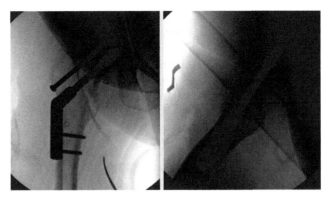

Figure 8-13 Final alignment and implant position.

BRIEF SUMMARY OF SURGICAL STEPS

- Position the patient on the fracture table with the large C-arm positioned from the contralateral side of the fracture table
- Reduce the fracture with gentle traction and internal rotation
- Confirm adequate reduction with anteroposterior and lateral views of the affected hip
- Straight lateral incision over the femur begins proximally at the vastus lateralis ridge; incise the vastus lateralis fascia and bluntly dissect to bone
- Insert the guide pin at the appropriate level for the correctly angled plate (level of lesser trochanter for 135-degree plate); the guide pin should be placed center-center and within 5 mm of subchondral bone
- Measure the the interosseous length of the guide pin and ream the femoral neck and head over the pin with fluoroscopy
- Insert cannulated lag screw over the guidewire and secure two-holed or four-holed side plate
- Release traction and allow slight impaction of fracture; insert compression screw into barrel of lag screw; confirm alignment and implant position with fluorscopy

REQUIRED EQUIPMENT

Fracture table

Large C-arm

Power drill

COMMON PITFALLS

(When to call for the attending physician)

- Inadequate preoperative fracture assessment: Fracture pattern must be carefully evaluated on anteroposterior and lateral radiographs to determine appropriate implant selection
- Failure to obtain acceptable fracture reduction
- Lateral cortical wall fracture
- Intraarticular or intrapelvic penetration with guide pin insertion
- Failure to place lag screw in center-center position and within 5 mm of subchondral bone
- Loss of reduction during lag screw insertion
- Inadequate screw-barrel engagement, preventing sliding
- Disengagement of the lag screw from the barrel

TECHNICAL PEARLS

- Ensure that all prominences are padded on the fracture table and that there is no impingement of the scrotum or labia
- Evaluate adqequate fracture reduction before prepping and draping the patient
- Use the correctly angled guide for the plate used to insert the guide pin and insert at the appropriate level
- Position the guide pin center-center and within 5 mm of subchondral bone
- Tip-apex distance should be less than 25 mm
- Insert a second guide pin proximal to the original pin to act as a derotational pin, if necessary
- Ream the femoral neck and head with fluoroscopy to prevent penetration and tap the entire screw path to prevent rotation
- Release traction and impact fracture before inserting the cortical screw into the plate

POSTOPERATIVE PROTOCOL

After surgery, the patient should be medically stabilized and the pain well-controlled. The patient should be weight-bearing as tolerated, with ambulation beginning as soon as medically feasible, ideally by postoperative day 1. Mechanical and chemical anti-coagulation therapy should be starter after surgery to prevent thromboembolic complications.

POSTOPERATIVE CLINIC VISIT PROTOCOL

The patient should return to clinic at 2, 6, and 12 weeks for repeat radiographs and clinical evaluation. Common complications of sliding hip screw fixation for intertrochanteric hip fractures include infection, wound dehiscence, loss of fixation with cut-out of lag screw from femoral head, and nonunion.

SUGGESTED READINGS

1. Andruszkow H, Frink M, Fromke C, et al. Tip apex distance, hip screw placement, and neck shaft angle as potential risk factors for cut-out failure of hip screws after surgical treatment of intertrochanteric fractures. *Int Orthop*. 2012;36(11):2347-2354.
2. Baumgaertner MR, Curtin SL, Lindskog DM, Keggi JM. The value of the tip-apex distance in predicting failure of fixation of peritrochanteric fractures of the hip. *J Bone Joint Surg Am*. 1995;77(7):1058-1064.
3. De Brujin K, den Hartog D, Tuinebreijer W, Roukema G. Reliability of predictors for screw cutout in intertrochanteric hip fractures. *J Bone Joint Surg Am*. 2012;94(14):1266-1272.
4. Goffin JM, Pankaj P, Simpson AH. The importance of lag screw position for the stabilization of trochanteric fracture with sliding hip screw: a subject-specific finite element study. *J Orthop Res*. 2013;31:596-600.
5. Hsu CE, Shih CM, Wang CC, et al. Lateral femoral wall thickness. A reliable predictor of post-operative lateral wall fracture in intertrochanteric fractures. *Bone Joint J*. 2013;95-B(8):1134-1138.
6. Kaplan K, Miyamoto R, Levine BR, Egol KA, Zuckerman JD. Surgical management of hip fractures: an evidence-based review of the literature. II: intertrochanteric fractures. *J Am Acad Orthop Surg*. 2008;16(11):665-673.
7. McLoughlin S, Wheeler DL, Rider J, et al. Biomechanical evaluation of the dynamic hip screw with two- and four-holed side plates. *J Orthop Trauma*. 2000;14:318-323.
8. Mohan R, Karthikeyan R, Sonanis SV. Dynamic hip screw: does side make a difference? Effects of clockwise torque on right and left DHS. *Injury*. 2003;31:697-699.
9. Parker MJ, Das A. Extramedullary fixation implants and external fixators for extracapsular hip fractures in adults. *Cochrane Database Syst Rev*. 2013;(2):CD000339.
10. Zuckerman JD, Skovron ML, Koval KJ, et al. Postoperative complications and mortality associated with operative delay in older patients who have a fracture of the hip. *J Bone Joint Surg Am*. 1995;77A:1551-1556.

CARPAL TUNNEL RELEASE

Hilton Phillip Gottschalk | Randip Bindra

CASE MINIMUM REQUIREMENTS

- N = 10

COMMONLY USED CPT CODES

- CPT Code: 64721—Neuroplasty or transposition; median nerve at carpal tunnel
- CPT Code: 29848—Endoscopy, wrist, surgical, with release of transverse carpal ligament
- CPT Code: 20526—Injection, therapeutic; carpal tunnel

COMMONLY USED ICD9 CODES

- 354.0—Carpal tunnel syndrome
- 719.24—Synovitis, hand
- 354.5—Multiple neuritis syndrome

COMMONLY USED ICD10 CODES

- G56.00—Carpal tunnel syndrome, unspecified limb
- G56.01—Carpal tunnel syndrome, right upper limb
- G56.02—Carpal tunnel syndrome, left upper limb

Carpal tunnel syndrome (CTS) is a common disorder with an incidence rate in the United States of 1 to 3 cases per 1000 persons per year and a prevalence rate of approximately 50 cases per 1000 persons. Patients present with pain in the volar wrist area and distal forearm, nighttime pain, numbness, and tingling within the median nerve distribution, which can include the thumb, index, and middle fingers and the radial side of the ring finger. Patients report daytime paresthesias when the wrist is placed in prolonged flexion or extension. Most patients describe waking up with stiffness in the fingers and the need to shake or wring their hands to alleviate the symptoms. In some cases, patients decribe weakness to the hand and dropping of objects; however, this may be indicative of more advanced disease process or combined ulnar neuropathy.

Several clinical tests have been described to help make the diagnosis of CTS. Durkan's median nerve compression test involves the examiner applying manual pressure over the median nerve at the carpal tunnel for more than 30 seconds. A positive result is numbness/tingling in the median nerve distribution. Other clinical tests include Tinel's sign, with percussion over the median nerve at the wrist and palm, and Phalen's test, with the wrist flexed by gravity for 60 seconds. Both tests are positive when the patient reports numbness or tingling within the median nerve distribution. Sensory testing that involves static or moving two-point discrimination is useful, as is Semmes-Weinstein monofilaments or vibrometry.

Electrodiagnostic testing involves nerve conduction measurements with or without electromyography and is helpful in confirming a diagnosis of carpal tunnel syndrome or eliminating other potential pathologies.

Nonsurgical treatment is commonly implemented first. This treatment involves immobilization of the wrist in a neutral position during the night and sometimes during the day. Oral medications and corticosteroid injections can be used as well. Additional modalities have been described including ultrasound therapy, ergonomic modifications, and nerve and tendon gliding exercises.

Surgical intervention involves release of the transverse carpal ligament. This procedure can be done in the more classic method of an open release, a "mini" open release, or an endoscopic release. The authors focus on the most common method of carpal tunnel release, which is the open method (Video 9-1).

SURGICAL TECHNIQUE

Room Set-Up

- The room is set up with a standard patient bed and a hand table.
- General anesthetic, regional anesthetic, or local anesthetic can be used.

Patient Positioning

- The patient is positioned supine with the affected extremity outstretched.
- Nonsterile tourniquet is recommended.
- Sequential compression devices are routinely placed on the lower extremities.

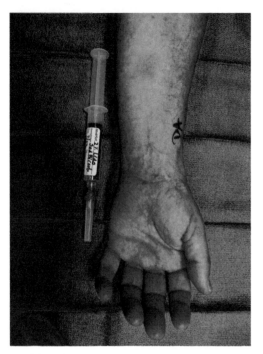

Figure 9-1 A 3-5-mL mixture of 2% lidocaine and sodium bicarbonate is used for local anesthetic.

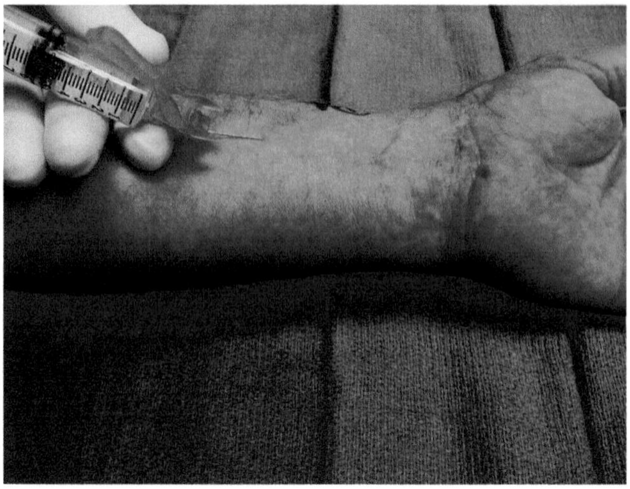

Figure 9-2 Care is taken to inject the local anesthetic just ulnar to the flexor carpi radialis tendon, in the distal forearm, but not into the median nerve.

Prepping and Draping

- A nonsterile tourniquet is applied.
- A plastic drape is placed around the tourniquet to prevent the preparation agent from getting underneath the tourniquet.
- A hand drape then is used.
- The skin is cleaned with appropriate preparation; the authors use an agent that contains chlorhexidine.
- If the procedure is performed with local anesthetic, 3 to 5 mL of 2% lidocaine with sodium bicarbonate is injected into the carpal tunnel in the distal forearm, with care taken not to inject into the median nerve (Figs. 9-1 and 9-2).
- Then, 3 to 5 mL of 2% lidocaine with sodium bicarbonate is injected around the incision (Fig. 9-3).
- Preoperative antibiotics can be given, as per the American Academy of Orthopaedic Surgeons (AAOS) Clinical Practice Guideline Summary (CPGS) recommendation "C."

General Principles

- The goal of surgery is to decompress the median nerve in the carpal tunnel.
- Complete division of the transverse carpal ligament and flexor retinaculum is crucial.

Incision

- The tourniquet is insufflated.
- A volar approach is used.
  - The approach is in line with the radial border of the ring finger.
  - The most distal extent is the Kaplan cardinal line, a line drawn obliquely across the palm from the ulnar border of the abducted thumb (Fig. 9-4).
  - The most proximal extent is to the level of the wrist crease.
- Incision length varies but is usually 2 to 3 cm (Fig. 9-5).
- In some patients, the incision can be made in a naturally occurring skin crease.

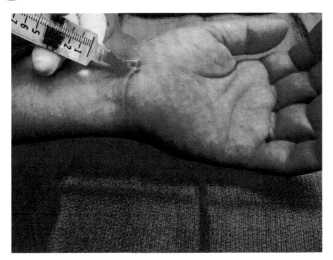

Figure 9-3 Three to five mL of 2% lidocaine with sodium bicarbonate then is injected around the incision.

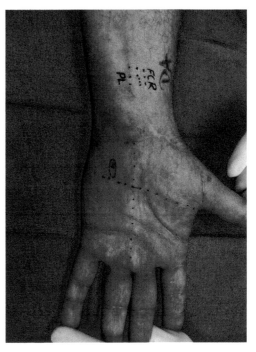

Figure 9-4 Appropriate landmarks are drawn from the radial border of the ring finger. The Kaplan cardinal line is drawn from the ulnar border of the abducted thumb.

Exposure

- A scalpel is used through skin and fat to the level of the palmar fascia.
- A self retractor (cricket) is placed to allow exposure of the palmar fascia.
- The fascia is incised longitudinally (in line with its fibers).
- Some patients may have muscle fibers below this layer, representing the palmaris brevis.
  - If muscle fibers are found, they should be divided layer by layer down to the transverse carpal tunnel, with special care taken not to injure the motor branch of the median nerve.
- The remaining muscle can be swept off with the scalpel to fully expose the transverse carpal ligament (TCL; Fig. 9-6).
- Before incising the TCL, the authors recommend using scissors to spread superficially above the TCL at the proximal extent of the incision where the wrist meets the forearm. This allows for ease later on when dividing the antebrachial fascia in the distal forearm.
- The self retractor can be advanced each step to better expose the TCL.

Incising the Transverse Carpal Ligament

- Palpate for the hook of the hamate, which is a good reference point for the ulnar border of the carpal tunnel.
- The authors recommend opening a small section of the TCL by using a #15 blade to push down on the transverse ligament just radial to the hamate.
  - This allows for better control, and one can feel the thickened ligament as one goes through it.
- In addition, take care to stay on the ulnar aspect of the TCL because this protects the median nerve from iatrogenic injury.
- Once the segment of TCL has been opened, some advocate placing a clamp or blunt instrument just under the TCL to allow for a surface to cut on and protection of deep structures (Fig. 9-7).
- If the steps are followed as stated previously, tenosynovium is encountered.

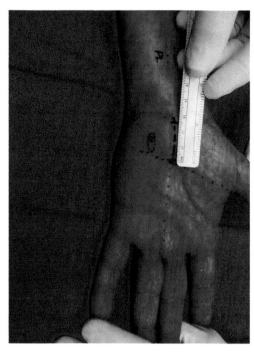

Figure 9-5 Incision length varies but is usually 2 to 3 cm.

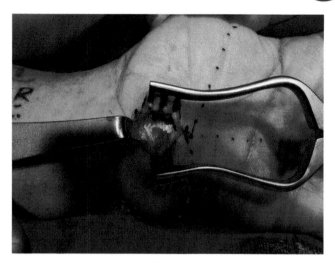

Figure 9-6 Muscle is swept off with the scalpel to fully expose the transverse carpal ligament.

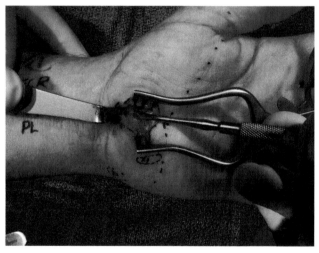

Figure 9-7 Once the segment of transverse carpal ligament has been opened, some advocate placing a clamp or blunt instrument just under the transverse carpal ligament to allow for a surface to cut on and for protection of deep structures.

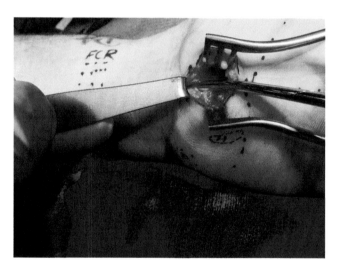

Figure 9-8 The authors recommend use of blunt scissors to incise the antebrachial fascia with direct visualization.

- A blunt retractor is used to better expose the TCL, which is further divided with direct visualization distally.
- Next, the remaining TCL is incised proximally with either scalpel or scissors.
  - The authors recommend use of blunt scissors to incise the antebrachial fascia with direct visualization (Fig. 9-8).
- Once fully decompressed, the median nerve should be visualized (Fig. 9-9).
- In patients with extensive tenosynovium, a portion of the synovium can be excised.
- The authors do *not* recommend internal neurolysis of the median nerve.
- The wound is copiously irrigated with normal saline solution.
- The tourniquet can be deflated, and points of bleeding identified and coagulated.
- The skin is closed with 4-0 nylon sutures.
- The wound is covered with Xeroform Petrolatum Wound Dressing (DeRoyal, Powell, TN), and a bulky dressing is applied.

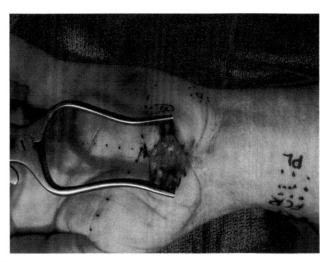

Figure 9-9 Once fully decompressed, the median nerve should be visualized.

BRIEF SUMMARY OF SURGICAL STEPS

- Volar approach in line with the radial border of the ring finger
- Incision 2 to 3 cm
- Incise palmar fascia in line with incision
- Spread superficially over transverse carpal ligament proximally at the junction of wrist and forearm
- Open a small segment of transverse carpal ligament ulnarly (just radial to hamate)
- Optional to place blunt instrument deep to transverse carpal ligament
- Completely incise transverse carpal ligament distal and proximal extents
- Release distal forearm antebrachial fascia with direct visualization

TECHNICAL PEARLS

- Drawing the landmarks (radial border ring finger and Kaplan cardinal line) is helpful
- Appropriate use of retractors aids in retracting fat and increasing visualization
- Before incising the transverse carpal ligament, spread above the transverse carpal ligament in the distal forearm to better identify the distal forearm antebrachial fascia
- Open a small section of the transverse carpal ligament on its ulnar border to prevent iatrogenic injury to the median nerve
- The transverse carpal ligament has a "gritty" feel to it and can be quite thick
- Use of a blunt instrument can help free any adhesions from the deep surface of the transverse carpal ligament
- The entire length of the transverse carpal ligament should be incised so that the flaps can be raised both radially and ulnarly
- Use of loupe magnification throughout is recommended

REQUIRED EQUIPMENT

Pneumatic tourniquet
Scalpel
Self retractor
Kleinert-Ragnell or other small blunt retractor
Metzenbaum scissors
4-0 Nylon sutures
Loupe magnification recommended

COMMON PITFALLS

(When to call for the attending physician)

- The incision seems too radial or ulnar
- The incision needs to cross the wrist crease
- Concern for motor branch of the median nerve crossing over the transverse carpal ligament
- Multiple incisions in the transverse carpal ligament
- Difficulty exposing the transverse carpal ligament distally or proximally
- Excessive tenosynovium, before excision
- Excessive bleeding; may be an arch injury

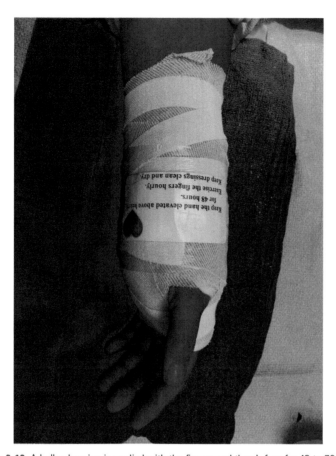

Figure 9-10 A bulky dressing is applied with the fingers and thumb free for 48 to 72 hours.

POSTOPERATIVE PROTOCOL

The palmar skin is thick and needs to be reapproximated well to leave a nice scar. A bulky dressing is applied with the fingers and thumb free for 48 to 72 hours (Fig. 9-10). The wrist is in a neutral position. The authors educate their patients on keeping the hand elevated for 24 to 48 hours after surgery. At the first follow-up visit (2 to 3 days after surgery), the dressing is removed and adhesive bandages are placed. The patient is instructed to keep the hand clean and dry for 7 to 10 days; after that, the incision can get wet.

The authors recommend early movement of the fingers to facilitate nerve gliding across the operative site. Limited weight-bearing on the affected extremity is advised; heavy lifting and forceful gripping are not recommended for 1 month. Return to work is discussed with the patient before surgery, and the decision is made conjointly with the physician and patient.

POSTOPERATIVE CLINIC VISIT PROTOCOL

The patient is seen 2 to 3 days after surgery to change the dressing. The next visit is around the 2-week mark to remove the sutures. In some patients, hand therapy is prescribed to aid with motion and scar management. The next follow-up visit is scheduled at 6 weeks after the operation, and extensive scar management can be implemented if needed.

SUGGESTED READINGS

1. Bury TF, Akelman E, Weiss AP. Prospective, randomized trial of splinting after carpal tunnel release. *Ann Plast Surg.* 1995;35:19-22.
2. Cook AC, Szabo RM, Birkholz SW, King EF. Early mobilization following carpal tunnel release: a prospective randomized study. *J Hand Surg [Br].* 1995;20:228-230.
3. Gelberman RH, Pfeffer GB, Galbraith RT, Szabo RM, Rydevik B, Dimick M. Results of treatment of severe carpal tunnel syndrome without internal neurolysis of the median nerve. *J Bone Joint Surg Am.* 1987;69:896-903.
4. Keith MW, Masear V, Amadio PC, et al. Treatment of carpal tunnel syndrome. *J Am Acad Orthop Surg.* 2009;17:397-405.
5. Verdugo RJ, Salinas RS, Castillo J, Cea JG. Surgical versus non-surgical treatment for carpal tunnel syndrome. *Cochrane Database Syst Rev.* 2003;(3):CD001552.

CHAPTER 10

SPINE DECOMPRESSION AND POSTERIOR SPINE FUSION

Nicholas M. Brown | Howard S. An

Many disease processes may lead to the need for spinal decompression and fusion. The spinal cord and nerve roots are most commonly compressed by a herniated disk, surrounding soft tissues, or osteophytes. Fusion may be necessary for spondylolisthesis, instability after decompression, pseudarthrosis, or progressive deformity from degenerative, idiopathic, neurologic, or iatrogenic causes. In general, spinal decompression is performed when a neurologic structure is being compressed, and fusion is necessary for instability that results from either the underlying disease process or the extent of the decompression. The most classic indication for posterior spinal fusion with decompression is degenerative spondylolisthesis associated with spinal stenosis, which most commonly occurs at the L4-L5 level.

Degenerative spondylolisthesis arises from instability as a result of intervertebral disk and facet joint degeneration. In many individuals, these changes are asymptomatic. However, nerve root compression may result in radicular pain, numbness, or weakness. Symptoms of neurogenic claudication such as lower extremity cramping and weakness may be present and are typically relieved with spinal flexion. Further, the degeneration and resultant motion between the spinal elements may cause mechanical back pain. Patients with less severe symptoms, isolated herniated disk, or stable spondylolisthesis may only need decompression, but patients with unstable listhesis and those who need a more extensive decompression may require fusion to stabilize the spine. The Spine Patient Outcomes Research Trial (SPORT) is a recent randomized prospective study that showed the efficacy of decompressive surgery in the setting of degenerative lumbar spinal stenosis.

SURGICAL TECHNIQUE

Room Set-Up

- A Jackson table is placed in the center of the room.
- A portable x-ray device should be available.
- Depending on the surgeon preference and complexity of the case, neuromonitoring should be considered.

Patient Positioning

- Anesthesia is induced and the patient is intubated before placement in the prone position.
- The patient is positioned prone on the Jackson table with the abdomen hanging free to decrease venous pressure (Fig. 10-1). Ensure that all bony prominences are appropriately padded, including pelvis, knees, ankles, and elbows.
- Arms should have less than 90 degrees of flexion to prevent neurapraxia.

COMMONLY USED CPT CODES

- CPT Code: 22612—Arthrodesis, posterior or posterolateral technique, single level; lumbar (with lateral transverse technique, when performed)
- CPT Code: 22800—Arthrodesis, posterior, for spinal deformity, with or without cast; up to six vertebral segments
- CPT Code: 63005—Laminectomy with exploration or decompression of spinal cord or cauda equina, without facetectomy, foraminotomy, or discectomy (e.g., spinal stenosis), one or two vertebral segments; lumbar, except for spondylolisthesis
- CPT Code: 63012—Laminectomy with removal of abnormal facets or pars interarticularis with decompression of cauda equina and nerve roots for spondylolisthesis, lumbar (Gill-type procedure)
- CPT Code: 63017—Laminectomy with exploration or decompression of spinal cord or cauda equina, without facetectomy, foraminotomy, or discectomy (e.g., spinal stenosis), more than two vertebral segments; lumbar
- CPT Code: 63030—Laminotomy (hemilaminectomy), with decompression of nerve root(s), including partial facetectomy, foraminotomy, or excision of herniated intervertebral disc; one interspace, lumbar

Continued

- CPT Code: 63042—Laminotomy (hemilaminectomy), with decompression of nerve root(s), including partial facetectomy, foraminotomy, or excision of herniated intervertebral disc, reexploration, single interspace; lumbar
- CPT Code: 63047—Laminectomy, facetectomy, and foraminotomy (unilateral or bilateral with decompression of spinal cord, cauda equina, or nerve root[s]; e.g., spinal or lateral recess stenosis), single vertebral segment; lumbar

COMMONLY USED ICD9 CODES

- 724.2—Pain lower back, low back pain
- 722.52—Disc degeneration, other intervertebral disk degeneration, lumbar region
- 722.1—Disc herniation, other intervertebral disk displacement, lumbar region
- 724.3—Sciatica, sciatica, unspecified site
- 724.02—Spinal stenosis, spinal stenosis, lumbar region
- 738.4—Spondylolisthesis, spondylolisthesis, site unspecified

COMMONLY USED ICD10 CODES

- M54.5—Low back pain
- M51.36—Other intervertebral disk degeneration, lumbar region
- M51.26—Other intervertebral disk displacement, lumbar region
- M54.30—Sciatica, unspecified site
- M48.06—Spinal stenosis, lumbar region
- M43.1—Spondylolisthesis, site unspecified

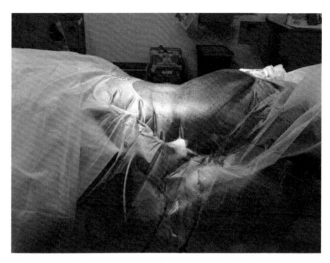

Figure 10-1 The patient is positioned prone on a Jackson table, with careful padding of any bony prominences. Adhesive nonsterile drapes are placed, and the surgical site is prepped.

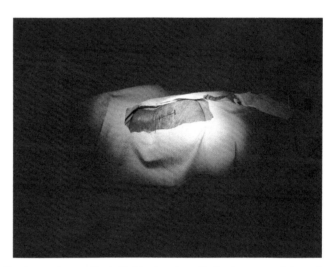

Figure 10-2 Draping continues with sterile blue towels and iodine-impregnated clear adhesive dressing, and final drapes are placed.

Prepping and Draping

- The surgical site is shaved if necessary, and the patient is prepped and draped (Fig. 10-2).
- First, place nonsterile adhesive drapes widely demarcating the surgical field. The authors' method is to clean the skin with alcohol and then with a chlorhexidine prep stick. Sterile blue towels then are stapled to the skin on the perimeter of the surgical field. Iodine-impregnated adhesive drapes are placed directly on the sterile field. The final drape then is placed around the sterile field. An adhesive lining typically is on the underside of this drape to help it attach to the outer aspect of the sterile field.

Approach

- Consider passing a needle lateral to the spinous process to confirm the appropriate level.
- A midline skin incision is made over the involved area, and dissection proceeds down through subcutaneous fat to the level of the fascia with either a scalpel or electrocautery. Maintenance of tension on the tissues helps with dissection. Self-retaining retractors are positioned to allow visualization.

- The fascia is split with either a scalpel or electrocautery and retracted with the self-retaining retractor. The lumbar muscles are elevated to expose the vertebrae with a Cobb elevator in one hand to retract and peel back the tissues and with electrocautery in the other hand.
- Once the spine is exposed, x-ray is again used to verify that decompression and fusion will occur at the correct level.

Decompression

- The interspinous ligament and spinous processes typically are removed with a rongeur for visualization. In addition, consider headlamp, loupes, or magnification at this point (Video 10-1).
- A laminotomy is then performed with a Kerrison rongeur. Consider first thinning the lamina with a high-speed burr. The ligamentum flavum is left undisturbed at this point to protect the underlying neurologic structures. This is performed by placing the Kerrison rongeur teeth only around the osseous lamina and leaving the underlying ligamentum flavum intact.
- A medial facetectomy is performed, followed by removal of the ligamentum flavum. A Kerrison rongeur is used for these steps.
- A full decompression then is performed, with any compressive pathology addressed. This may include a herniated disk, osteophytes, facet capsular tissue, synovial cysts, or posterior longitudinal ligament hypertrophy (Fig. 10-3). This tissue is typically removed with a Kerrison rongeur.

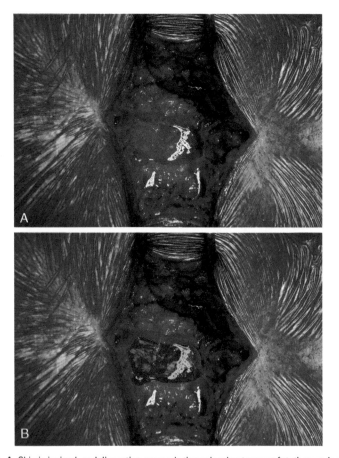

Figure 10-3 A, Skin is incised, and dissection proceeds through subcutaneous fat, then underlying fascia. The lumbar muscles are elevated. Decompression then proceeds according to the individual compressive pathology that is causing the patient's symptoms. In this case, a wide decompression was performed at L4-L5; the lamina and underlying ligamentum flavum have been removed. **B,** The area of decompression has been outlined in this image.

Hardware Placement

- Ensure that the dorsal bony anatomy is fully exposed. The starting point for each pedicle screw varies slightly at each spinal level and is based on each patient's individual anatomy. A general reference point in the lumbar spine is at the intersection of a horizontal line from the transverse process and 2 mm lateral to the pars.
- Decorticate the posterior entry point with a 4-0 burr.
- A "gearshift" pedicle probe is used to cannulate the pedicle by applying light pressure and avoiding breach of a cortical wall.
- A flexible ball-tip probe is used to identify all four walls and the base of the tract to ensure integrity of the canal. A hemostat is placed on the probe to measure the depth of the canal.
- The tract is then tapped, typically 1 mm smaller than the anticipated screw diameter. However, in the presence of poor bone quality, this step may be skipped.
- Sound the tract again with the flexible ball-tip probe to again ensure no cortical disruption.
- After all pedicle screw tracts have been created, the screws are placed (Fig. 10-4), followed by the interconnecting rods (Fig. 10-5).

Fusion

- The transverse processes, lateral facet joint, and pars are decorticated with a 4-0 burr. The area is irrigated during decortication to avoid thermal injury and preserve the quality of bone generated, which may be used as local graft.
- Bone graft is placed to aid in fusion. This can be iliac crest autograft, local autograft (from bone removed from burring, laminectomy, and spinous process removal), bone morphogenic protein (BMP), demineralized bone matrix (DBM), or allograft. Iliac crest, although recognized as the gold standard, is currently used less often because of morbidity associated with its harvest. The most commonly used approach, and that used by the authors, is to primarily use local autograft with additional allograft or DBM to provide more volume and osteoinductivity (from DBM). The use of BMP is somewhat controversial.

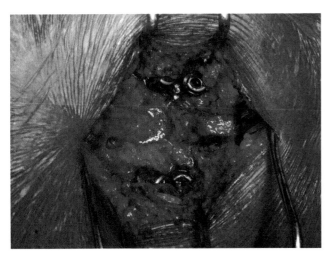

Figure 10-4 Hardware placement, if needed for stability, proceeds with burr decortication of the pedicle screw entry site, with a gearshift probe to cannulate the pedicle, verify wall integrity with a ball-tip probe, measure depth, tap, and place the screw. In this case, the screws were placed in the pedicles of L4 and L5.

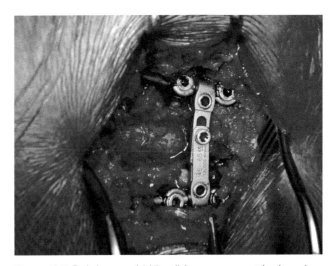

Figure 10-5 Rods between L4-L5 pedicle screws are put in place along with cross connectors. Further decorticate with a burr as needed for fusion, with subsequent placement of bone graft (iliac crest autograft, local autograft, allograft, demineralized bone matrix, or bone morphogenic protein are options). Obtain hemostasis; irrigate; place a drain if necessary; subsequently close fascia, subcutaneous tissue, and skin; and place a sterile dressing.

Closure

- Hemostasis is obtained, the wound is irrigated, and a subfascial drain may be placed if necessary.
- The fascia is closed with absorbable braided suture, the subcutaneous tissue is closed with interrupted absorbable braided suture, and the skin is approximated with a running subdermal stitch. The skin incision is sealed with 2-octyl cyanoacrylate, and a sterile dressing is placed.

BRIEF SUMMARY OF SURGICAL STEPS

- Room set-up
- Patient positioning
- Prep and drape
- Approach
- Decompression
- Hardware placement
- Fusion
- Closure

REQUIRED EQUIPMENT

Fluoroscopy
Basic spine tray
Pedicle screws, rods
Bone graft or bone graft substitute
High-speed burr

TECHNICAL PEARLS

- The key to performing laminectomy for multilevel spinal stenosis is adequate decompression of all the affected nerve roots with central laminectomy and undercutting the facet joints to preserve stability of the motion segments.
- The pars should be preserved at all levels. The pars in the upper lumbar spine is relatively more medial; therefore, laminectomy should be narrower in the upper lumbar spine as compared with the low lumbar spine.
- Spinal stenosis is mainly at the level of facet joints and lateral recess; therefore, laminectomy should be slightly wider at the facet joints and narrower at the pars.
- Overall, the pathoanatomy of nerve root compression varies from patient to patient, and it is important to determine the exact nature of nerve root compression and strategies to safely decompress the affected nerve roots while preserving stability of the motion segments.

COMMON PITFALLS

(When to call for the attending physician)

- Inadequate decompression
- Neurologic injury
- Wrong level surgery
- Durotomy
- Postoperative cauda equina syndrome

POSTOPERATIVE PROTOCOL

The patient is mobilized early to maintain function, increase strength and flexibility, decrease the risk of deep venous thrombosis, minimize atelectasis, and promote bowel function. If a drain was placed, it is removed once output is less than 30 to 50 mL per 8-hour shift. Diet is advanced slowly as bowel function returns. The patients should be monitored closely for urinary retention. This is commonly the result of the effects of anesthesia, pain medications, recent surgery, and relative immobility, but cauda equina syndrome must always be ruled out. Postoperative bracing is at the surgeon's discretion, although is less commonly used.

POSTOPERATIVE CLINIC VISIT PROTOCOL

The patient's initial follow-up visit is within the first 2 weeks for a wound check. Anteroposterior and lateral standing radiographs are obtained at this time. The patient then is followed at 6 weeks, 12 weeks, and 6 months after surgery, with x-rays obtained at each visit. Physical therapy is initiated at 2 weeks after surgery if necessary. The patient should limit bending, lifting, and twisting (BLT) for the first 12 weeks after surgery.

SUGGESTED READINGS

1. Cauchoix J, Benoist M, Chassaing V. Degenerative spondylolisthesis. *Clin Orthop Relat Res*. 1976; 115(115):122-129.
2. Majid K, Fischgrund JS. Degenerative lumbar spondylolisthesis: trends in management. *J Am Acad Orthop Surg*. 2008;16(4):208-215.
3. Weinstein JN, Lurie JD, Tosteson TD, et al. Surgical versus nonsurgical treatment for lumbar degenerative spondylolisthesis. *N Engl J Med*. 2007;356(22):2257-2270.

OPEN REDUCTION INTERNAL FIXATION BIMALLEOLAR ANKLE FRACTURE

David Walton | Marc A. Zussman

Fractures of the ankle are the most common intraarticular fractures of a weight-bearing joint. Their ubiquitous nature requires all orthopaedic surgeons to be facile in both nonoperative and surgical treatment. However, because of the pervasiveness of these fractures, the significance of the injury and treatment strategy are often undervalued. Every patient with an ankle fracture should be approached with care; a detailed history and physical examination provide significant information in planning a treatment strategy.

The complexity in the treatment of ankle fractures arises in the variability of presentation. The fractures range from simple standing-height twisting injuries to high-energy injuries, as in an automobile collision. In addition, the ankle is a highly congruent modified hinge joint that does not tolerate malalignment well. Displacement of the tibiotalar joint by just 1 mm increases the overall contact stresses by 40% and leads to significant risk of posttraumatic arthritis. With this in mind, each ankle fracture must be carefully assessed for the specific characteristics of the fracture and host, with care devoted to bone quality, comminution, presence of additional fractures, and soft tissues about the injured ankle.

Most ankle fractures can be defined with the Lauge-Hansen classification, which describes several patterns of injury that predict transmission of energy causing the fracture. In each subcategory, the bones or ligaments fail in a specific pattern that can require specific treatment strategies. This chapter focuses on supination external rotation bimalleolar ankle fractures, an injury pattern that accounts for up to 75% of ankle fractures. Classically, the lateral followed by the medial malleolus is anatomically reduced and stabilized to restore articular congruity. This is followed by syndesmotic fixation to stabilize the distal tibiofibular articulation when unstable.

CASE MINIMUM REQUIREMENTS

- N = 15 Ankle fracture fixation

COMMONLY USED CPT CODES

- CPT Code: 27766—Open reduction internal fixation medial malleolus
- CPT Code: 27792—Open reduction internal fixation lateral malleolus
- CPT Code: 27814—Open reduction internal fixation bimalleolar ankle fracture
- CPT Code: 27822—Open reduction internal fixation trimalleolar fracture; medial and lateral malleolus only
- CPT Code: 27823—Open reduction internal fixation trimalleolar fracture, medial, lateral, and posterior lip fixation
- CPT Code: 27829—Open treatment of distal tibiofibular joint (syndesmosis) disruption

SURGICAL TECHNIQUE

Room Set-Up

- The operating table with a radiolucent distal end is in standard position with the patient's head toward the anesthesia station.
- The instrument table and scrub technician are on the ipsilateral side of the surgical extremity or at the foot of the bed, depending on the surgical theater orientation.
- Fluoroscopy should be positioned to enter the surgical field from the contralateral side.

Patient Positioning

- The patient is placed supine on a radiolucent table.
- The surgical extremity is placed on a radiolucent ramp or stack of blankets for fluoroscopic ease.
- A bump is placed under the ipsilateral hip to obtain static neutral position of the surgical extremity.

Prepping and Draping

- A thigh tourniquet is applied to the surgical extremity.
- An impervious U-drape is used to secure the tourniquet and isolate the surgical field before the extremity is prepared.
- If no open wounds or abrasions exist, the leg is prepped initially in a nonsterile manner with alcohol, followed by sterile chlorhexidene-based prep solution. When abrasions or open wounds are present, a povidone-iodine–based wet prep solution should be used.
- Draping proceeds with a sterile down sheet, followed by an upward U-drape, and then a downward U-drape.
- A cohesive self-adherent bandage is applied around the forefoot and the toes to isloate the toes from the surgical field.
- An aperture drape then is used as the final drape for the surgical field.
- The distal leg is placed on sterile towels or sheets to suspend the heel off the bed to avoid anterior translation of the talus in the mortise (Fig. 11-1).

Preoperative Considerations

- In cases in which reduction reads will be difficult or the syndesmosis is suspected to be compromised, contralateral radiographs are useful to obtain, including anterioposterior, lateral, and mortise views before surgery. These views allow the surgeon to have confidence in appropriate length, rotation, and appearance of the ankle mortise and syndesmosis if the intraoperative reduction is uncertain.
- Radiographs should be carefully assessed for posterior malleolar fractures, Chaput fragments, and osteochondral lesions (OCD), which could require operative treatment. In cases in which the size or orientation of a posterior malleolar fracture or Chaput fragment is uncertain, a computed tomographic (CT) scan can provide further information regarding the portion of articular surface and the character of the fracture. If treatment of this fracture is indicated, the surgical approach may need to be modified accordingly.
- Before intervention with anesthesia, the skin overlying the planned surgical incisions should be inspected in the preoperative holding area for fracture blisters, excessive swelling, and other skin abberations that would increase the risk of postsurgical infection or preclude safe surgical intervention. Surgery should be delayed

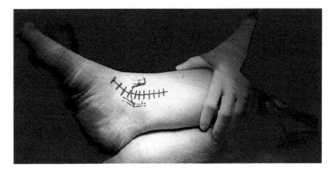

Figure 11-1 The bump is placed proximal to the heel to prevent anterior translation of the talus in the mortise.

until evidence of satisfactory healing of the soft tissues, including resolution of fracture blisters, epithelialzation of abrasions, or presence of the wrinkle sign at the operative site.

- Host factors should be considered during preoperative planning. Patients with significant medical comorbidities, history of wound healing problems, or preinjury compromised soft tissue should be considered at high risk for hardware implantation. Fixation strategies can be amended to minimize the risk of hardware problems, such as low-profile implants, external fixation, or intramedullary fixation.
- The anesthesia staff administers appropriate preoperative prophylactic antibiotics.

Lateral Malleolus

- The fibula is exposed with a straight lateral approach. Before surgial incision, the entire distal one third of the fibula is palpated and marked with a surgical marker. When appropriate, the leg should be exsanguinated and the tourniquet set at 250 mm Hg or 100 mm Hg greater than the systolic blood pressure. After this, the surgical incision is placed in the midline, centered over the fracture as proximal and distal as necessary for direct plating (Fig. 11-2, *A*). If the fracture cannot be palpated, fluoroscopy can be used to localize the fracture site. With a scalpel, the skin is sharply incised and carried down into the subcutaneous tissues. Electrocautery is used judicioulsy for superficial bleeders. After this, blunt dissection with Metzenbaum scissors is performed in the distal aspect of the wound over the distal fibula. A safe extraperiosteal plane is created and carried proximally, with careful evaluation of the soft tissues for the presence of the superficial peroneal nerve

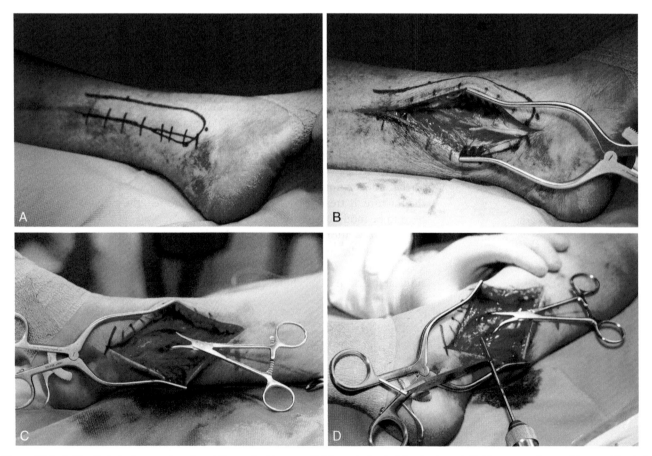

Figure 11-2 A, The fibula is drawn out, and a midline, or in this case, slightly posterior, incision is planned. **B,** The peroneal musculature and fascia is retracted to protect the superficial peroneal nerve during the procedure. **C,** A reduction forceps is used to hold the fracture or manipulate the fragments into position. **D,** An anterior-to-posterior or a posterior-to-anterior (as seen in this image) lag screw is placed as perpendicular to the fracture line as possible (please note Figures A-B are of the right ankle and Figures C-D are of the left ankle).

Continued

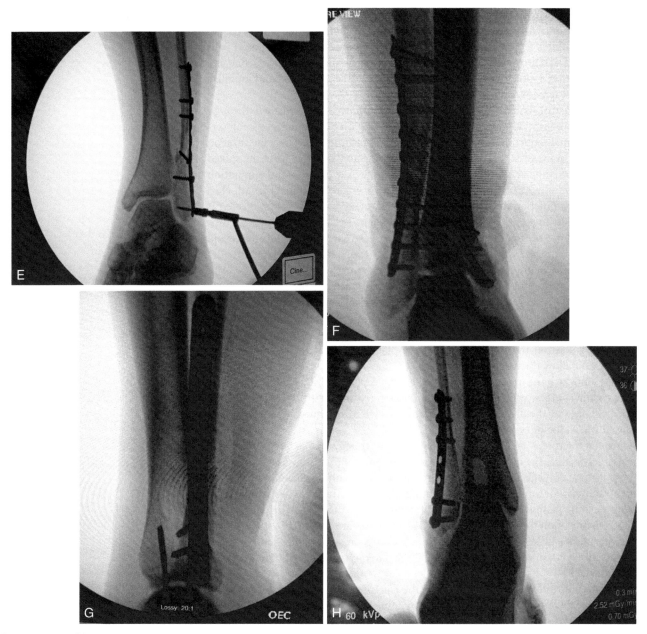

Figure 11-2, cont'd **E,** Care is taken to avoid penetration past the second cortex during placement of the distal cancellous screws. **F** and **G,** The optimal position of the medial malleolar screws is shown, parallel and into each colliculus without impingement onto the posterior tibial tendon. **H,** External rotation view shows medial widening and insufficiency of the syndesmosis.

(SPN). The SPN should be coursing from posterior to anterior over the fibula, approximately 5 cm proximal to the ankle joint or 7 cm proximal to the tip of the fibula. Then, the peroneal fascia, if intact from the injury, should be sharply divided and the peroneal tendons and musculature retracted posteriorly (Fig. 11-2, *B*). When encountered, the SPN carefully should be freed from soft tissue attachments to allow it to be mobilized as needed without tension anteriorly out of the direct surgical field. The SPN should be known and protected throughout the duration of the case.

- The facture site then is isolated. With a combination of a dental pick, Freer elevator, small rongeur, curette, and bulb irrigation, the fracture site is gently cleared of hematoma and soft tissue as needed. Care is taken to avoid damage to the cortical ends because they are crucial in reduction. With a #15 blade scalpel, the cortical edges of the fracture are then cleared of 1 to 2 mm of periosteum for a cortical read of the reduction. The posterior and medial spikes frequently can be caught in soft tissues and inhibit reduction. Anteriorly, the fracture site should be exposed with care to avoid extensive detachment of the distal syndesmotic ligaments that are often encountered near the fracture site. Care must be taken to dissect and mobilize the fracture fragments only as needed.

- Once the fracture is mobilized, the reduction maneuver is performed through several techniques. With oblique fractures, depending on bone quality, a small serrated or pointed reduction forceps can be used. This technique requires the surgeon to lightly grasp the proximal and distal fragments at equal distance from the spiked ends and in a singular motion, with a combination of pronation and supination and radial and ulnar deviation, to reverse the displacement and regain length (Fig. 11-2, C). Manipulation of the foot through traction and external rotation often is helpful to assist the translation of the distal fragment. This maneuver can be cumbersome and put the fragile reduction points at risk, so care must be taken to avoid comminution of the fracture. When the fracture is transverse, two serrated reduction forceps can be used to manually reduce the fracture.

- A push-pull technique can be used if extensive shortening of the fracture cannot be overcome with simple manual traction. This involves applying the desired plate in the distal fragment and securing it with two points of fixation, followed by placement of a unicortical screw proximal to the site of plating. After this, a lamina spreader is used at the proximal end of the plate to distract the fracture, regain length, and allow fracture reduction.

- In cases in which the fracture is unable to be reduced, inspection of the fluoroscopic images for sources, which could block reduction, is important. Occasionally, the medial gutter or the distal tibia-fibula space needs to be débrided because of interposed soft tissue or bone.

- Once the fracture is reduced, the internal fixation strategy is dependent on several variables, such as the quality of bone, comminution, soft tissue envelope, and other host factors. In general, oblique fractures are treated with lag screw fixation and neutralization or antiglide posterior plating. Transverse fractures are treated with compression plating, and comminuted fractures are treated with bridge plating. These Association for Osteosynthesis (AO) techniques are beyond the scope of this chapter; however, during their application, the surgeon should allow empty screw holes for syndesmotic fixation through the lateral construct if later deemed necessary.

- In supination external rotation injuries, the fracture is oblique and amenable to either lateral plating or posterior antiglide plating. When lateral plating is chosen, the lag screw is initially placed independent of the plate, usually in anterior to posterior fashion, perpendicular to the fracture (Fig. 11-2, D). When antiglide plating is chosen, the lag screw preferably is placed through the plate in a posterior to anterior fashion, again perpendicular to the fracture. This is done through AO technique with a 3.5-mm lag screw in which the near cortex is overdrilled with a 3.5-mm drill bit, followed by placement of the 2.5-mm soft tissue guide into the drill hole. The far cortex is drilled with a 2.5-mm drill. The appropriate 3.5-mm cortical screw is then placed across the screw track after countersinking as necessary. In small fragments, a 2.7-mm lag screw, with the proper drills, can be used. In addition, if the initial lag screw does not have adequate purchase, a partially threaded 4.0-mm cancellous screw can be used as a "bail out."

- When a lateral plate is used, the distal screws must be unicortical to avoid penetrating the distal tibiofibular joint. These screws are usually fully threaded 4.0-mm cancellous screws. Other screws into the plate are typically 3.5-mm (Fig. 11-2, E).

Medial Malleolus

- The medial malleolus is approached through a longitudinal incision along the midline of the medial tibia. It is carried 1 to 2 cm distal to the end of the bone to allow access to the tip of the anterior colliculus. The skin is incised sharply, but care is taken to keep the sharp dissection superficial as the saphenous neurovascular bundle courses along the incision.

- With blunt dissection, the neurovascular bundle is identified, mobilized, and retracted anteriorly if encountered. The fracture site then is identified with sharp dissection. The fracture site then can be booked open with a dental pick to assess the articular surface of the talar dome.
- These fracture fragments are often small, and the reduction may be difficult to assess. Fluoroscopic imaging is crucial for adequate reduction and should be gauged with the articular surface of the tibia and lateral radiographs.
- The fracture site must be adequately débrided of soft tissue and hematoma for proper reduction. Often periosteum is caught in the fracture site, which impedes precise reduction. The débridement is done as with the lateral malleolus. Care must be taken to protect the structures posterior to the medial malleolus, most intimately, the posterior tibial tendon and the neurovascular bundle.
- One to 2 mm of periosteum then are sharply débrided off both ends of the fracture as needed to provide a cortical read for reduction, which is obtained with a dental pick or pointed reduction forceps.
- The reduction is maintained with the use of a 0.062-inch K-wire or with pointed reduction forceps. With use of the reduction forceps, a small pilot hole should be created proximal to the fracture site on the medial aspect of the exposed tibia to provide one point of fixation for the forceps. The other tine of the forceps is placed on the tip of the colliculus. Once fluoroscopic imaging has confirmed the reduction, internal fixation is performed.
- The construct in which the medial malleolus is treated depends on the features of the fracture and the host. A popular technique is with preferably two screws applied in retrograde fashion into the tibial metaphysis. The location of these screws should be parallel to one another on the lateral radiograph and oblique along the tibia on the anteroposterior radiograph as perpendicular as possible to the fracture (Fig. 11-2, *F*). Care should be taken to avoid the articular surface. The anterior screw should be at the anterior colliculus, and the second should be no further posterior than the center of the intercollicular groove to avoid damage to the posterior tibial tendon (Fig. 11-2, *G*). The screws generally are partially threaded 4.0-mm cancellous screws, 40 to 50 mm in length; however, modifications are made to adapt to host differences. The authors do not prefer the routine use of washers with screw fixation because they can be prominent and get caught in the soft tissues, impeding appropriate fracture compression.
- In patients with poor bone quality and in fractures in which only one screw can be used, consideration for an antirotational K-wire or a bicortical fixation can be given. A 3.5-mm cortical screw can be placed across the fracture to engage the posterolateral tibial cortex. In vertical medial malleolar fractures, AO technique advocates for buttress plating. This can be achieved with a 3.5-mm plate or a minifragment plate. In fragments that are too small to be adequately controlled with screw fixation tension, a band technique or locked minifragment plating can be used.

Syndesmoses

- Syndesmotic disruption occurs in 10% of all ankle fractures. During surgery, the syndesmosis is assessed after ankle fixation is achieved. This is done most commonly with a Cotton test or an external rotation test. The Cotton test, or the modified Cotton test, is done with an attempt to cause distal tibia-fibula diastasis by directly pulling on the fibula laterally with a bone hook. If a widening of more than 1 to 2 mm is found with fluoroscopic imaging, the syndesmosis is believed to be disrupted. The external rotation test stresses the distal tibia-fibula articulation with applying an external rotational force about the foot while stabilizing the distal leg and assessing the same space for widening (Fig. 11-2, *H*).
- When the syndesmosis is disrupted, fixation is approached laterally to medially either with suture button fixation or screw fixation. When a lateral fibula plate has been used for ankle fixation, it is used for fixation of the syndesmosis as well. A

large pointed reduction clamp is placed across the distal tibiofibular joint, with one end on the distal tibia and one end on the distal fibula. With the clamp, the distal tibiofibular joint is reduced. Syndesmotic reduction can be accurately assessed with comparisons with the contralateral extremity obtained before surgery. If no images were obtained, on a true lateral, the distal tip of the fibula should be anterior to the posterior border of the diaphyseal tibia. The heel must not rest on the bed during reduction and fixation because this anteriorly displaces the talus and may malreduce the syndesmosis (Fig. 11-3, *A*). Although the technique is controversial, overtightening of the syndesmosis can be avoided with the fixation performed with the ankle in dorsiflexion.

- Choice of syndesmotic fixation ranges significantly without clear superiority. The authors prefer endobutton fixation or one 3.5-mm positional screw placed across four cortices; however, others propose two screws from 3.5 to 4.5 mm in diameter

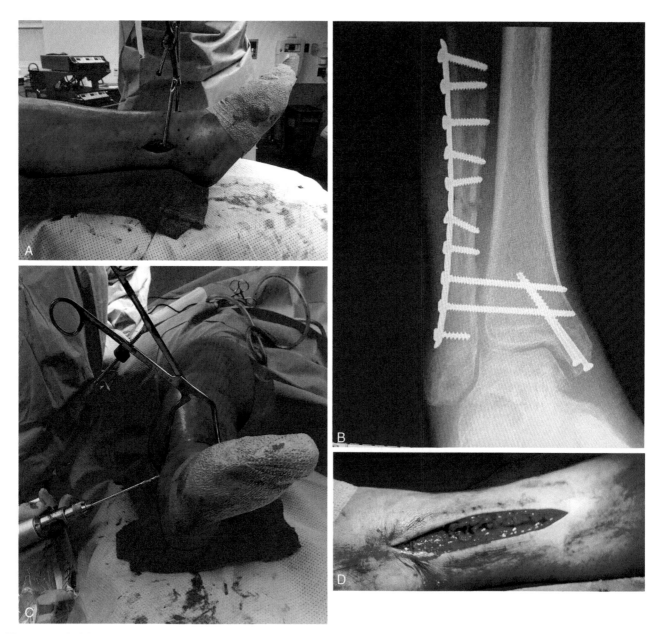

Figure 11-3 A, A large periarticular reduction clamp is placed onto the plate laterally and through a stab incision medially parallel to the joint line for syndesmotic reduction. **B,** X-rays show the optimal distance of syndesmotic screws from the joint line. **C,** The leg should be placed close to the edge of the table to allow the surgeon to drop the hand to the floor and to allow for the proper anterior trajectory of the syndesmotic fixation. **D,** Care is taken to close the fascia over the hardware to reduce hardware prominence.

and three or four cortices. The screws should preferably be placed about 2 cm proximal and parallel to the tibiotalar joint (Fig. 11-3, *B*). If a lateral fibula plate is used, the screws or endobuttons should be placed through the plate; however, lateral malleolar lag screws may preclude optimal placmement. The screw or endobuttons should be aimed approximately 25 to 40 degrees anteriorly to engage centrally in the tibia (Fig. 11-3, *C*). With use of endobuttons, the knots should be cut with 1-cm to 2-cm length to enable them to be laid flat as they can become symptomatic if left proud.

- A standard layered closure follows for both the medial and the lateral side after copious irrigation. Care is taken to cover the hardware, especially on the lateral side with the peroneal fascia or musculature (Fig. 11-3, *D*). This is followed by subcutaneous and skin closure.

BRIEF SUMMARY OF SURGICAL STEPS

- Lateral dissection with mobilization of superficial peroneal nerve
- Lateral malleolar fracture débridement and reduction
- Lag screw fixation
- Neutralization or antiglide plate application
- Medial dissection with mobilization of saphenous nerve and vein
- Medial malleolar fracture débridement and reduction
- 4.0-mm cannulated screw fixation
- Cotton or external rotation test for syndesmotic stability
- Placement of syndesmotic fixation
- Placement in short leg and sugar tong splint in neutral dorsiflexion
- Layered closure
- Final fluoroscopic images are obtained and saved

TECHNICAL PEARLS

- Carefully identify superficial peroneal nerve on lateral approach
- Carefully débride soft tissues around the fracture as needed; if reduction is difficult, more exposure and débridement may be needed
- Avoid comminuting fibula during reduction
- If unable to reduce the lateral fracture, assess for the need to débride the tibia-fibula space or medial and lateral gutters
- Avoid posterior placement of medial malleolar screws to avoid damage to the posterior tibial tendon and neurovascular bundle
- When placing syndesmotic screws, elevate the distal leg on towels or blankets to allow hand to drop to desired angle and prevent malreduction

REQUIRED EQUIPMENT

| Small fragment plate and screw set |
| Cannulated 4.0-mm screw set |
| K-wire set |
| Fluoroscopy with radiolucent table |
| Large pointed reduction clamps |
| Small pointed and serrated reduction forceps |

COMMON PITFALLS

(When to call for the attending physician)

- Unable to reduce fibular fracture
- Fibula comminutes with reduction
- Fibular lag screw does not achieve purchase
- Unable to reduce the medial malleolus
- Medial malleolar fragment comminutes
- Syndesmosis does not reduce with application of clamp

POSTOPERATIVE CLINIC VISIT PROTOCOL

After surgery, all ankles are placed in a three-sided splint with neutral dorsiflexion and are encouraged to be elevated. The patients are kept non–weight-bearing. At 10 to 14 days after surgery, the patients are seen in clinic and radiographs are obtained out of the splint. The wounds are examined, sutures or staples are removed, and sterile adhesive strips are applied if appropriate. The patients then are transitioned into either a controlled ankle motion (CAM) boot or short leg cast depending on bone quality, ankle stability, and patient compliance.

The patient returns at 6 weeks for repeat radiographs and clinical examination. At this time, if not already in one, the patient is transitioned to a CAM boot that allows removal for active and passive range of motion. The radiographs are assessed for

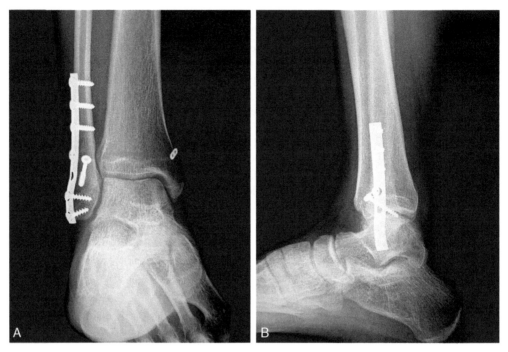

Figure 11-4 A and **B,** Mortise and lateral views postoperatively demonstrate maintenance of reduction of the syndesmosis.

appropriate healing, and the patient is advanced to gradual full weight-bearing over the next 2 to 4 weeks, depending on bone quality fracture fixation and type of syndesmotic fixation if present. Physical therapy is initiated often at this time for progressive strengthening, range of motion, and proprioception on a case-by-case basis.

The patient typically is seen again at 12 weeks after surgery for routine radiographs and assessment of healing, gait, and the need for further therapy and evaluation of syndesmotic and symptomatic hardware possibly requiring future removal. If hardware is removed, the patient should be followed with radiographs for at least 6 weeks of weight-bearing to ensure no rediastasis (Fig. 11-4). At this point, the patient is released to participate in contact activities if full strength of the dynamic ankle stabilizers is seen. The final follow-up visit is usually 6 months after surgery.

SUGGESTED READINGS

1. Clare MP. A rational approach to ankle fractures. *Foot Ankle Clin.* 2008;13(4):593-610.
2. Duscher D, Wenny R, Entenfellner J, Weninger P, Hirtler L. Cutaneous innervation of the ankle: an anatomical study showing danger zones for ankle surgery. *Clin Anat.* 2013;27(4):653-658.
3. Jensen SL, Andresen BK, Mencke S, Nielsen PT. Epidemiology of ankle fractures. A prospective population-based study of 212 cases in Aalborg, Denmark. *Acta Orthop Scand.* 1998;69(1):48-50.
4. Lloyd J, Elsayed S, Hariharan K, Tanaka H. Revisiting the concept of talar shift in ankle fractures. *Foot Ankle Int.* 2006;27(10):793-796.
5. Pakarinen H, Flinkkilä T, Ohtonen P, et al. Intraoperative assessment of the stability of the distal tibiofibular joint in supination-external rotation injuries of the ankle: sensitivity, specificity, and reliability of two clinical tests. *J Bone Joint Surg.* 2011;93(22):2057-2061.
6. Ricci WM, Tornetta P, Borrelli J. Lag screw fixation of medial malleolar fractures: a biomechanical, radiographic, and clinical comparison of unicortical partially threaded lag screws and bicortical fully threaded lag screws. *J Orthop Trauma.* 2012;26(10):602-606.
7. de Souza LJ, Gustilo RB, Meyer TJ. Results of operative treatment of displaced external rotation-abduction fractures of the ankle. *J Bone Joint Surg Am.* 1986;68(4):633-634.
8. Shibuya N, Davis ML, Jupiter DC. Epidemiology of foot and ankle fractures in the United States: an analysis of the National Trauma Data Bank (2007 to 2011). *J Foot Ankle Surg.* 2014;53(5):606-608.
9. Summers HD, Sinclair MK, Stover MD. A reliable method for intraoperative evaluation of syndesmotic reduction. *J Orthop Trauma.* 2013;27(4):196-200.
10. Wukich DK, Kline AJ. The management of ankle fractures in patients with diabetes. *J Bone Joint Surg.* 2008;90(7):1570-1578.

ANKLE ARTHRODESIS

James Albert Nunley | David Walton

The ankle joint is rarely affected by primary osteoarthritis. Most tibiotalar arthritis seen results from trauma, neuropathic disease, or other inflammatory conditions. Although in the last several decades increased interest in total ankle arthroplasty has been seen as a result of improvements in design and surgical technique, the current gold standard for the treatment of ankle arthritis continues to be tibiotalar fusion, especially in young, high-demand patients, such as patients involved in heavy labor occupations or impact recreational activities.

Historically, ankle arthrodesis had been disparaged because of the high rate of pseudarthrosis that leads to recurrent deformity. Initially, external fixation was used, which was ideal for patients who had poor wound healing potential; further, external fixation afforded the ability to adjust the fusion after surgery. However, the transition to modern internal fixation techniques has resulted in improved rates of fusion and superior outcomes because of improved biomechanics. The addition of anterior plating to transarticular screws has been shown to increase the biomechanical rigidity of the construct, causing many surgeons to supplement traditional two or three crossed-screw techniques with an anterior plate. This chapter discusses the authors' preferred technique for ankle fusion, with double anterior compression plating with both anterolateral and anteromedial locking plates.

SURGICAL TECHNIQUE

Room Set-Up

- The operating table is in standard position with the patient's head toward the anesthesia station.
- The instrument table and the scrub technician are on the contralateral side of the surgical extremity or at the foot of the bed, depending on the surgical theater orientation.
- Fluoroscopy should be positioned to enter the surgical field from the ipsilateral side.

Patient Positioning

- The patient is placed supine on a radiolucent table.
- The surgical extremity is placed on a radiolucent ramp or stack of blankets for fluoroscopic ease.
- A bump is placed under the ipsilateral hip to obtain static mortise position of the ankle.

Prepping and Draping

- Thigh tourniquet is applied to the surgical extremity.
- An impervious U-drape is used to secure the tourniquet and isolate the surgical field before prepping the extremity.

- The leg is then prepped with chlorhexidine-based preparation solution.
- Draping proceeds with a sterile down sheet, followed by an upward U-drape and then downward U-drape.
- A coadhesive bandage is applied around the forefoot and the toes to isolate the toes from the surgical field; alternatively, a sterile surgical glove or other means of isolating the toes from the operative field can be used.
- An aperture drape then is used as the final drape for the surgical field.

Preoperative Considerations

- A thorough history and physical examination should be obtained before surgical planning to aid in surgical incision placement. Particular attention should be paid to any previous incisions. The soft tissues should be examined for a safe surgical corridor. The ankle may be approached anteriorly, medially with an osteotomy, laterally with an osteotomy, or posteriorly.
- Any and all deformities should be noted; if present, they may necessitate supplemental procedures or planning to provide a plantigrade foot when the tibiotalar joint becomes fused.
- Patients with conditions that could affect wound healing should be counseled to improve any patient-specific factors to bolster the success rate of fusion.
- Patients who have diabetes mellitus should be counseled about tight glucose control. Patients who smoke should be counseled regarding the risks to their health and the negative effects smoking would have on the success of the procedure.
- Preoperative radiographs should be obtained, including weight-bearing anterior-posterior (AP), mortise, lateral, and standing mechanical axis views for preoperative planning (Fig. 12-1).

Anterior Approach

- A utilitarian anterior approach is used to access the tibiotalar joint. The incision is placed approximately 1 cm lateral to the tibial crest, beginning 10 cm proximal to the tibiotalar joint line and carried distally to the talonavicular joint.
- Full-thickness skin flaps are created, and care should be taken because the superficial peroneal nerve is found subcutaneous often at, or just proximal to, the tibiotalar joint. This should be identified and retracted laterally.

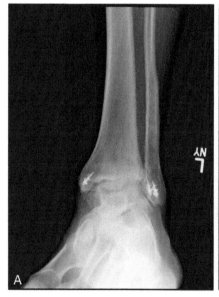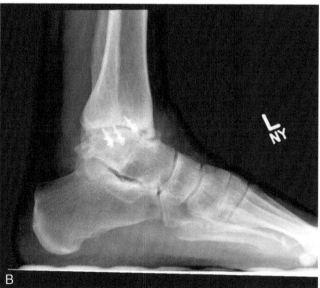

Figure 12-1 Tibiotalar joint space loss on both the anteroposterior **(A)** and the lateral **(B)** views with evidence of previous instability procedures performed.

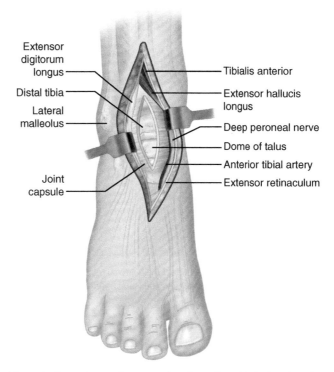

Extensor digitorum longus

Distal tibia

Lateral malleolus

Joint capsule

Tibialis anterior

Extensor hallucis longus

Deep peroneal nerve

Dome of talus

Anterior tibial artery

Extensor retinaculum

Figure 12-2 Schematic shows the anterior approach to the ankle, with the location of several important tendinous and neurovascular structures.

- The extensor retinaculum then is exposed. This is sharply incised over the extensor hallucis longus (EHL) tendon, which is immediately lateral to the tibialis anterior (TA) tendon.
- Care is taken to avoid disrupting the TA sheath.
- The interval between the EHL and the TA is identified, and the EHL is retracted laterally and the TA medially (Fig. 12-2).
- The neurovascular bundle then is identified and carefully retracted laterally.
- Sharply, a capsulotomy is made, which extends proximally and distally along the anterior tibia and talus, elevating the periosteum. This is carried medially and laterally with a small elevator to expose the entire tibiotalar joint, including the medial and lateral gutters.
- A deep Gelpi retractor is used for visualization, but retractors that place pressure on the wound edges are never used (Fig. 12-3, *A*).
- Next, a ¼-in straight osteotome is used to resect the anterior osteophytes from the distal tibia. This allows for greater exposure to the articular surfaces and assists with obtaining the proper tibiotalar position.

Fixation

Joint Preparation
- With a small laminar spreader or pin distractor, the joint then is widened to provide room to prepare the arthrodesis surfaces.
- With a sharp chisel and various curettes, any remaining cartilage is resected.
- During this process, the subchondral bone is preserved for structural support.
- The medial and lateral gutters are also prepared.
- With a 2.5-mm drill, the subchondral bone then is perforated to promote fusion.
  - K-wires are not used because they cause more necrosis than a drill bit.
- The bony architecture is preserved to reduce shortening and deformity.

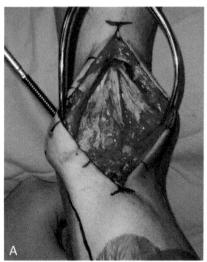
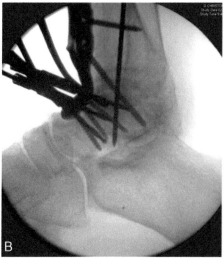
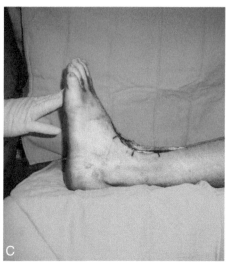

Figure 12-3 A, Deep Gelpi retractors used to protect the neurovascular bundle laterally and tibialis anterior tendon medially. Note the skin edges are free from pressure ischemia. **B,** Radiographic and **C,** clinical demonstration of neutral tibiotalar alignment.

- In cases of significant bone loss or deformity, bone graft is used to assist in correction and fusion.

Joint Reduction

- In general, the optimal position for the tibiotalar joint is in neutral dorsiflexion, 5 to 7 degrees of valgus and 5 to 10 degrees of external rotation, or comparable with the contralateral extremity that should be examined before entering the operating room.
- This position should be confirmed clinically and with fluoroscopy (Fig. 12-3, *B* and *C*).
- The body of the talus should be in line with the central axis of the tibia on the lateral radiograph.
  - There is a tendency for the talus to subluxate anteriorly; this should be avoided to preserve optimal biomechanics of the foot.
- Because of the wear patterns in posttraumatic arthritis, additional resection of the posterior tibial articular surface often is necessary to maintain the proper position of the tibiotalar joint in the sagittal plane.
- Once the proper alignment is obtained, the position is held temporarily with 2.5-mm K-wires from the central portion of the anterior tibial into the posterior talus (Fig. 12-4, *A* and *B*).

Internal Fixation

- Multiple techniques are available for fixation of the tibiotalar arthrodesis.
- In simple cases without significant deformity or bone loss, some authors suggest isolated crossed screw fixation in which two or three cannulated, partially threaded screws are placed across the tibiotalar joint.
- More contemporary strategies use anterior compression plating to provide greater rigidity at the fusion site, which allows for use in cases with significant deformity and extensive bone grafting (Tarkin and colleagues, 2007).
- Depending on the fusion system used, transarticular fixation can be used as part of the plate construct or independent to it.
- The authors' preferred technique uses double anterior compression plating with both anterolateral and anteromedial locking plates for improved biomechanical stability (Kestner, 2013).
- Specific steps between systems vary; however, concepts are similar.
- When bone grafting is to be used, it should be placed into the joint space before application of the plates.

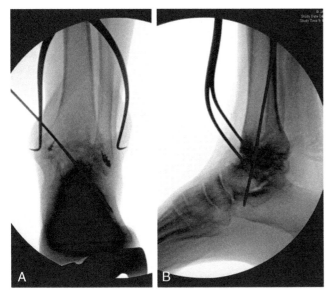

Figure 12-4 **A,** Anteroposterior and **B,** lateral radiographs show K-wire maintenence of reduction placed proximal medially to distal laterally.

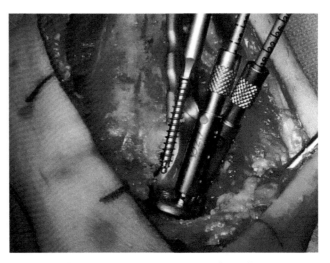

Figure 12-5 The plate is first reduced to the talus while being held in netural reduction, aligning the proximal portion of the plate flush onto the tibia.

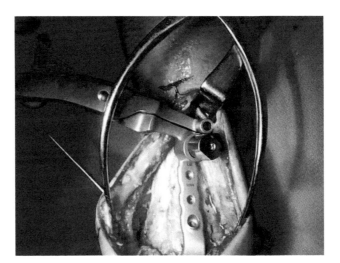

Figure 12-6 After placement of a unicortical screw onto the tibia proximal to the plate, a compression forceps can be used to compress the previously secured talus to the distal tibia.

- Initially the anterolateral plate is fixated to the talus (Fig. 12-5).
- A unicortical screw then is placed proximal to the desired plate location.
  - This allows compression forceps to gain purchase when applied to the plate and this screw (Fig. 12-6).
- At this time, the temporary fixation K-wires should be removed to allow compression along the desired plane.
- Proximal locking screws achieve fixation into the tibia.
- The joint fixation then is augmented with a nonlocking transarticular screw through the plate from the tibia into the talus, gaining stability of the grafted sites.
- During the process of compression, care should be taken to maintain the desired alignment.
- After this, the anteromedial plate is applied statically as the construct has been previously compressed (Fig. 12-7, *A*).
- The construct can be augmented by further transarticular screw fixation as indicated (Fig. 12-7, *B*).

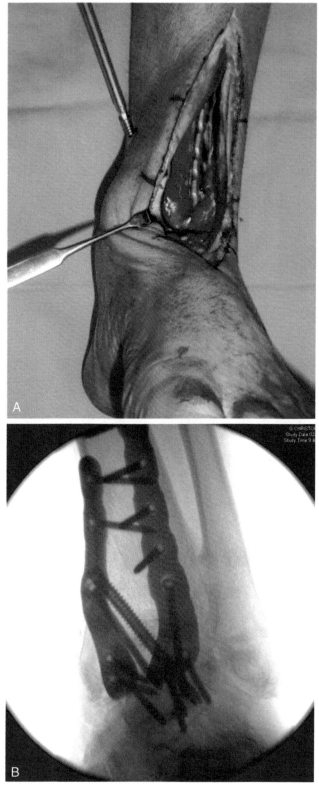

Figure 12-7 **A,** If there is room, anterorlateral and anterormedial plates can be used; the anterolateral plate is placed first in compression, followed by the anteromedial statically. **B,** Note the transarticular screws on the mortise intraoperative radiograph.

Closure

- Closure is performed in a layered manner, with independent closing of the capsule, extensor retinaculum, subcutaneous layer, and skin.
- Covering the hardware with the capsule can be challenging; however, this does decrease adhesions, especially if tendon sheaths have been violated.
- Sterile dressings then are applied, and a well-padded three-sided short leg splint is applied in neutral dorsiflexion.

BRIEF SUMMARY OF SURGICAL STEPS

- Prep and drape with bump under ipsilateral hip
- Anterior exposure of tibiotalar capsule
- Capsulotomy and exposure of tibiotalar joint
- Joint preparation
- Appropriate reduction of tibiotalar joint
- Application of anterior plates
  - Lateral first with placement of screws into talus
  - Compression across plate fusion interface
  - Lock proximal into tibia
  - Transarticular screw fixation
- Closure
- Three-sided splint application in neutral

REQUIRED EQUIPMENT

| Fluoroscopy |
| Radiolucent operating table |
| Small fragment plates and screws |
| Small osteotomes |
| Large cannulated screws |
| Anterior tibial precontoured plates |
| Suture for closure |
| Splint material |

COMMON PITFALLS

(When to call for the attending physician)

- Unexpected bone loss in tibial plafond or talus
- Tibiotalar joint does not reduce appropriately
- After resection, unable to dorsiflexion ankle to neutral
- Difficulty obtaining symmetric compression of tibiotalar joint
- Tibiotalar joint does not compress
- Inadequate bone stock for screw purchase
- Soft tissue does not cover plate

TECHNICAL PEARLS

- Avoid disruption of tendon sheaths during approach to reduce postoperative adhesions
- During joint preparation, avoid disruption of subchondral architecture to mainatain anatomic reduction
- Thoroughly clear cartilage posteriorly and into gutters to maximize fusion surface area
- Avoid overcompression, which will produce gapping at the posterior aspect of the tibiotalar joint
- Bone graft should be placed before hardware for access to contoured locations
- Careful dissection of capsule and closure allows plate coverage to avoid adhesions
- Meticulous repair of extensor retinaculum prevents bow stringing of anterior tendons
- Splinting in neutral dorsiflexion assists in preventing postoperative equinas contracture

POSTOPERATIVE PROTOCOL

The patient remains in the postoperative splint for the first 2 to 3 weeks. The goals are to control pain and swelling with icing and elevation and learn activities of daily living (ADLs) while immobilized. Education is focused on proper crutch use and active hip and knee range of motion. At 2 to 3 weeks, the patient is seen in clinic for the initial postoperative visit. Sutures are removed if the wound is fully healed. The patient is placed into a non–weight-bearing cast or controlled ankle motion (CAM) boot and is kept non–weight-bearing with instructions to maintain hip and knee active range of motion and perform ADLs.

At 6 weeks, the patient is seen in clinic and the cast is removed. Radiographs are obtained to assess for fusion. At this time, depending on the radiographic signs, the

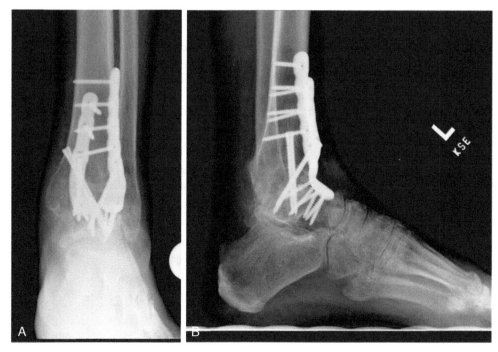

Figure 12-8 A, Anteroposterior and **B,** lateral postoperative weight-bearing radiographs obtained in the clinic show fusion consolidation and neutral tibiotalar joint.

patient is transitioned to a fracture boot and allowed to start progressive weight-bearing (Fig. 12-8). During the next 4 to 6 weeks, the patient is instructed to progress to full weight-bearing in the fixed angle boot only. Patients are instructed to begin stationary cycling with the boot and core exercises. Goals are to continue to protect the fusion mass while improving strength of the surgical extremity.

At 12 to 14 weeks, the patient is instructed to start weaning the fracture boot and begin gait training. Patients are encouraged to begin swimming if the wound is healed. The patient is also to begin low-level balance and proprioception exercises with a physical therapist. The goals are to recover core, hip, and knee strength and to reduce apparent limp.

At 16 weeks, radiographs are obtained and assessed for fusion. If fusion appears appropriate, the patient may return to previous low-level activities. The patient's gait should be observed and assessed for the need for rocker sole shoe.

SUGGESTED READINGS

1. Buck P, Morrey BF, Chao EY. The optimum position of arthrodesis of the ankle. A gait study of the knee and ankle. *J Bone Joint Surg Am.* 1987;69(7):1052-1062.
2. Kestner CJ, Glisson RR, Nunley JA. A biomechanical analysis of two anterior ankle arthrodesis systems. *Foot Ankle Int.* 2013;34(7):1006-1011.
3. King HA, Watkins TB, Samuelson KM. Analysis of foot position in ankle arthrodesis and its influence on gait. *Foot Ankle Int.* 1980;1(1):44-49.
4. Mann RA, Rongstad KM. Arthrodesis of the ankle: a critical analysis. *Foot Ankle Int.* 1998;19(1):3-9.
5. Maurer RC, Cimino WR, Cox CV, Satow GK. Transarticular cross-screw fixation. A technique of ankle arthrodesis. *Clin Orthop Relat Res.* 1991;268:56-64.
6. Moeckel BH, Patterson BM, Inglis AE, Sculco TP. Ankle arthrodesis. A comparison of internal and external fixation. *Clin Orthop Relat Res.* 1991;268:78-83.
7. Monroe MT, Beals TC, Manoli A. Clinical outcome of arthrodesis of the ankle using rigid internal fixation with cancellous screws. *Foot Ankle Int.* 1999;20(4):227-231.
8. Plaass C, Knupp M, Barg A, Hintermann B. Anterior double plating for rigid fixation of isolated tibiotalar arthrodesis. *Foot Ankle Int.* 2009;30(07):631-639.
9. Tarkin IS, Mormino MA, Clare MP, Haider H, Walling AK, Sanders RW. Anterior plate supplementation increases ankle arthrodesis construct rigidity. *Foot Ankle Int.* 2007;28(2):219-223.
10. Thomas RH, Daniels TR. Ankle arthritis. *J Bone Joint Surg Am.* 2003;85-A(5):923-936.

HINDFOOT AND MIDFOOT FUSION

Christopher E. Gross | Steven L. Haddad

The hindfoot consists of the subtalar (talocalcaneal), talonavicular, and calcaneocuboid joints. Functionally, the hindfoot allows for inversion and eversion and pronation and supination, which helps the lower extremity walk over uneven surfaces. During early stance phase, the subtalar joint is responsible for converting tibial internal rotation into foot pronation and calcaneal eversion. The primary indication for a subtalar fusion is for pain from instability, deformity, or arthritis of the joint. Subtalar arthritis in isolation is often posttraumatic in nature and can be from talus or calcaneal fractures. A subtalar fusion may also be a part of correcting a fixed valgus deformity in a patient with stage III posterior tibialis tendon dysfunction. Other indications include failed talocalcaneal coalition resection, failed medial calcaneal osteotomy, or failed spring ligament reconstructions.

The Lisfranc joint complex (midfoot) supports the transverse arch of the foot. Its strength and stability are inherent to its bony and ligamentous anatomy. The middle cuneiform is recessed in relation to the medial and lateral cuneiforms. This recess allows for the second metatarsal to articulate with five osseous structures (which include the three cuneiforms and the first and third metatarsals). Coronally, the bases of the second, third, and fourth metatarsals are trapezoidal and make up a "Roman arch" configuration, which further enhances stability. During gait, the midfoot and the Chopart joint (also known as the midtarsal joint, consisting of the calcaneocuboid and talonavicular articulations) allow for load transmission from the hind to the forefoot. The Chopart joint is flexible during heel strike (increases efficiency of gastroc-soleus complex) and rigid during toe-off, which then transfers the forward movement through to the tarsometatarsal (TMT) joints.

Midfoot arthritis is a debilitating condition characterized by midfoot instability, severe functional impairment, and pain. The most common cause of midfoot arthritis is posttraumatic arthritis, followed by primary osteoarthritis and other inflammatory processes. A midfoot fusion is an option for those with failed nonoperative treatment for arthritis or those who have a primary Lisfranc ligamentous injury. This arthrodesis requires fixation of the first, second, and sometimes third TMT joints along with their intercuneiform joints.

SURGICAL TECHNIQUE

Room Set-Up

- A C-arm or mini C-arm fluoroscope is needed.
- If a full-sized C-arm is needed, it should be placed on the same side of the operative table so that anteroposterior (AP) ankle, lateral foot, and axial (hindfoot alignment view) calcaneal radiographs are easily taken.
- If the mini C-arm is used, it can be placed on the operative side as well.
- If a mini C-arm is used, the surgeon must take extra care to ensure appropriate hindfoot alignment because of the limited field of view.
- The scrub technician should set up the equipment near the foot of the bed or on the opposite side of the operative table from the involved extremity.

Patient Positioning

- For a subtalar or hindfoot fusion, place the patient supine with a significant bump underneath the ipsilateral buttocks to slightly internally rotate the foot.
  - In addition, the operation is facilitated by having the involved extremity placed on multiple flat blankets to provide a solid operating surface while keeping the leg elevated above the opposite extremity to faciliate lateral radiographs.
  - Some surgeons may also use a "sloppy" lateral decubitus (semilateral) position to accomplish the same internal rotation (Fig. 13-1).
    - One must ensure that if this position is used, the greater trochanter, axilla, and fibular neck are well padded.
- For a midfoot fusion, place the patient supine with enough padding under the thigh to ensure the foot is at neutral.
  - Again, the operation is facilitated by having the involved extremity placed on multiple flat blankets to provide a solid operating surface while keeping the leg elevated above the opposite extremity to facilitate lateral radiographs.

Prepping and Draping

- A thigh pneumatic tourniquet should be placed in the setting of a hindfoot fusion.
  - Note that a patient must be under general or spinal anesthesia or have a femoral and sciatic block for the tourniquet to be tolerable that proximal on the leg.
- A calf pneumatic tourniquet or esmarch tourniquet may be used for a midfoot arthrodesis.
- The operative leg then is provisionally cleaned with a scrub brush with soap and water.
- This is patted dry.
- The leg then is held in the air by a surgical assistant or with a mechanical leg holder.
- A chlorhexidine gluconate and isopropyl skin preparation is applied.
- A drop sheet is then placed below the extemity.
- A sterile impervious U-drape is placed as far proximally as the leg was prepped.
- An impervious stockinette then is rolled over the operative limb.
- An impervious split drape is unfolded over the patient.
- The leg is the placed through a drape with a limb fenestration.
- The drape is unfolded toward the feet.

Anesthesia Options

- Most importantly, the femoral and sciatic divisions must be blocked.
- A number of permutations achieve this goal.
- Hindfoot fusion:
  - General (or spinal) + popliteal block
  - General (or spinal) + popliteal + muscle relaxation
  - Femoral + sciatic block; popliteal + saphenous
  - Femoral + popliteal
- Midfoot fusion:
  - Popliteal + saphenous + conscious sedation

Midfoot Fusion

- Before the tourniquet is inflated, palpate and mark the dorsalis pedis. This helps to identify the direction and location of the neurovascular bundle (Fig. 13-2).
- A 5-cm longitudinal incision is made directly over the second metatarsal (MT) and Lisfranc joint. Proximally, the superficial peroneal nerve may be encountered. Protect the nerve and retract it. Use of a C-arm (or mini C-arm) is appropriate to confirm the appropriate location of the proposed incision as it is often further lateral in the foot than anticipated.

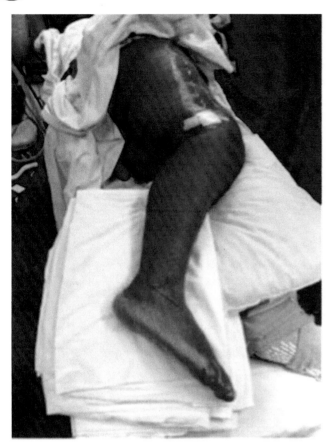

Figure 13-1 Patient positioned in the sloppy lateral position.

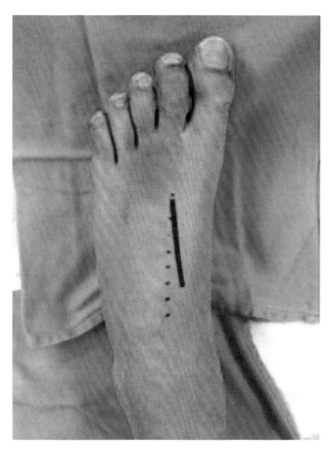

Figure 13-2 Marking of the dorsalis pedis pulse and incision site before surgery.

- Distally, one finds the neurovascular bundle (deep peroneal nerve and dorsalis pedis; Fig. 13-3). At this point, the dorsalis pedis sends a large branch (first proximal perforating artery) through the first web space.
- Locate the first and second tarsometatarsal (TMT) joints. Débride the cartilage and a small amount of the subchondral bone with a small rongeur, osteotome, microsaw, or curettes.
- Next, make a second incision over the medial border of the fourth MT to expose the third through fifth TMT joints (Fig. 13-4).
- Ensure that one can completely reduce all the joints after all cartilage and subchondral bone is removed. Reduction of deformity is critical to achieve an optimal result.
- Next, reduce the first TMT joint before anything else as the forefoot is usually displaced laterally and the first MT may interfere with reduction of the second MT.
- The original location of the first TMT joint is sometimes difficult to appreciate as the medial cuneiform is eroded dorsolaterally.
- Provisionally reduce the TMT joint with a 0.062-in K-wire and compare it with the position of the first TMT joint on the contralateral foot (either from a preoperative image or intraoperative fluoroscopy; Fig. 13-5).
- Reposition the first ray in relation to medial cuneiform posteromedially and then confirm on AP and lateral images.
  - Simulated weight-bearing with a flat box is helpful to check the alignment in the sagittal plane.
  - The goal is to reduce the talo-first metatarsal angle to 0 degrees.
  - There is a tendency is to make the ray lateral and valgus; therefore, in some cases with more severe deformity, it may be best to fuse the first TMT in slight varus.

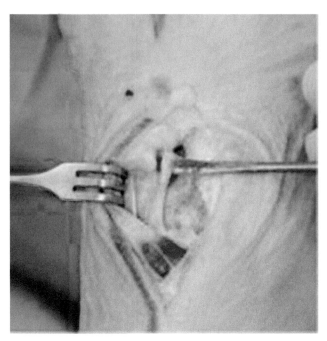

Figure 13-3 Intraoperative identification of the neurovascular bundle (deep peroneal nerve and dorsal pedis).

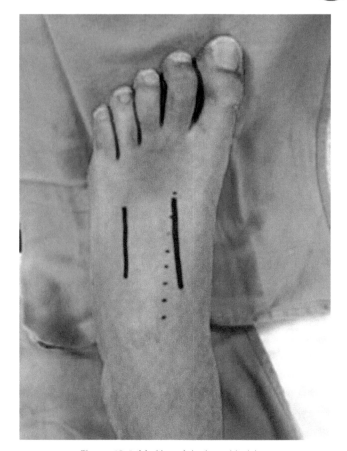

Figure 13-4 Marking of the lateral incision.

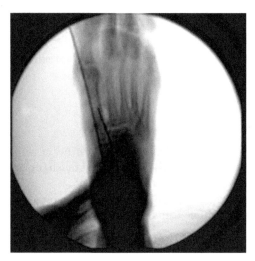

Figure 13-5 Provisional reduction of the first tarsometatarsal joint with 0.062-in K-wires.

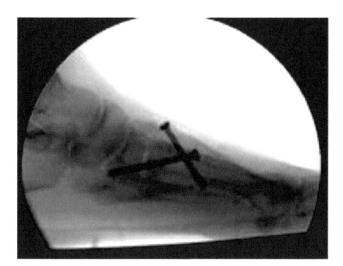

Figure 13-6 Definitive fixation of the first tarsometatarsal joint with 2 × 3.5–mm cortical screws.

- The correct plantar flexion and adduction alignment is important to achieve.
- The TMT fusion may need to be supplemented with a small medial tension plate (2.7-mm direct compression plate [DCP]; Fig. 13-6).
- Next, place a small lateral distractor (a 2-mm Schanz pin) into the calcaneus and the second pin into the proximal fourth and fifth MT.
- Lengthen the lateral side and débride the third through fifth TMT joints along the way.

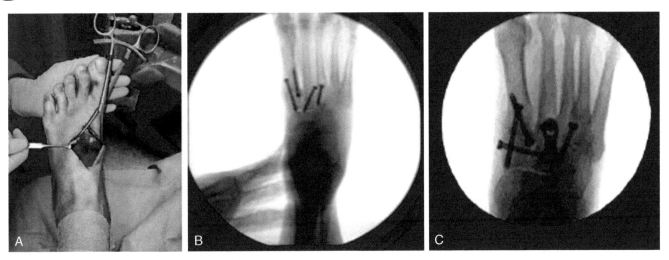

Figure 13-7 While the lisfranc complex is reduced **(A)**, the 2.7-mm or 2.5-mm threaded lag screws are inserted from the base of the second metatarsal into the middle cuneiform **(B)**, the medial cuneiform to the base of the second metatarsal, and the base of the first metatarsal to the medial cuneiform **(C)**.

- Reduce the forefoot such that the second MT rests in the mortise.
- Provisionally fix the second TMT with 0.054-in K-wires.
- Next place 2.7-mm or 2.5-mm threaded lag screws from the base of the second MT into middle cuneiform, medial cuneiform to the base of second MT, and the base of first MT to medial cuneiform (Fig. 13-7).
- Reduce the third TMT and then fixate it with a 3.5-mm cortical screw from the base of the third MT to the lateral cuneiform.
- Supplement all fusion sites with plate fixation as necessary to achieve stability and promote fusion.
- Ensure the plates conform well to the bone surface to avoid distortion of the fusion sites as the plates are applied to the bone.
- Reduce and hold the fourth/fifth TMT with K-wires.
  - If these joints are not salvageable, then perform an interpositional arthroplasty and stabilize with K-wires.
- If the intertarsal articulations are to be fused as well, then place a screw from the medial side of the medial cuneiform across the intercuneiform joints. If a broad joint fusion is required through both the naviculocuneiform and the tarsometatarsal joints, plate fixation often spans the entire construct.
- The subcutaneous and skin then are closed with simple braided sutures and nylon sutures, respectively, in a vertical mattress pattern.

Subtalar Fusion

- With the lateral approach, make a 6-cm longitudinal incision centered over the sinus tarsi from the tip of the fibula to the fourth MT. This helps to avoid the intermediate branch of the superficial peroneal nerve (Fig. 13-8).
- Incise the skin and isolate the visible vessels; then, coagulate them.
- Retract the nerve superiorly if seen.
- Identify the peroneal tendon sheath and fat in the sinus tarsi.
- The fascia of the extensor digitorum brevis (EDB) is incised along the lines of the skin incision.
- Sharply incise the sinus tarsi fat pad to expose the tarsal canal.
- Identify the posterior facet of the subtalar (ST) joint lateral to tarsal canal (Fig. 13-9). The anterior tubercle is located anteriorly. From here, the bifurcate ligament has two limbs that extend to the navicular and cuboid.

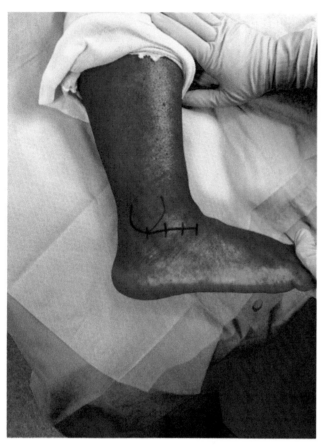

Figure 13-8 Planned incision for the subtalar arthrodesis.

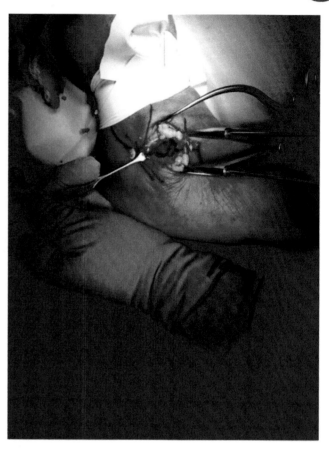

Figure 13-9 Dissect the extensor digitorum brevis as a distally based flap off the calcaneus.

- Using a Key elevator, subperiosteally dissect along the posterior facet. As best as possible, try to preserve the blood supply to the talus within the sinus tarsi.
- Protect the peroneal tendons by retracting them posteriorly with a small Hohmann retractor.
- With a laminar spreader without teeth, distract and débride the posterior facet, which runs inferiorly to superiorly, as the surgeon progresses posteriorly.
- Placement of the lamina spreader directly in the posterior lateral corner of the posterior facet is helpful to gain better visualization of middle and anterior facets. This may also assist with reduction in a valgus deformity hindfoot.
- After adequate débridement of the posterior facet, débride the dorsal anterior surface of the calcaneus and inferior lateral talar neck. Again, respect the blood supply to the talus.
- Use a 3.5-mm drill bit to fenestrate the subchondral bone. Pack the subtalar joint with either autograft or cancellous allograft and then bring the calcaneus into neutral/slight valgus with respect to the tibia.
- A combined aiming device may be used to direct a guidewire through a small incision at the apex of the heel through the posterior facet of the subtalar joint.
- A cannulated drill is then passed over the guidewire across the ST joint.
- Compression fixation may be achieved with a partially threaded 7.3-mm cancellous cannulated screw.
  - Thus, the calcaneus is aligned with respect to the talus at 5 degrees of valgus.
  - Confirm this with an axial view of the calcaneus with the C-arm.
  - Be sure to include the tibia in this view so that appropriate aligment is achieved.

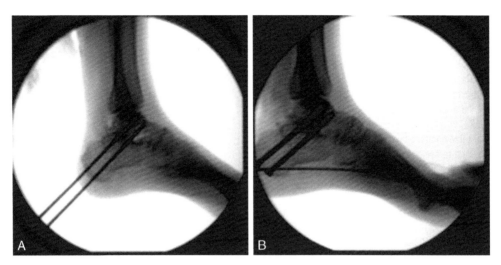

Figure 13-10 **A,** A combined aiming device may be used to direct a guidewire through a small incision at the apex of the heel through the posterior facet of the subtalar joint. Final screw construct of the subtalar arthrodesis **(B).**

- If extra stability or compression is needed, a second screw can be placed through the same heel incision in a similar fashion (Fig. 13-10). This also controls rotation across the subtalar joint.
- If concerns still exist about the fusion construct, a third dorsal to plantar screw can be placed.
- The arthrodesis site may be supplemented with additional autogenous bone (distal tibia, iliac crest, or anterior process of the calcaneus) or allograft.
- At this point, the hindfoot is evaluated. If the hindfoot is in excessive varus or valgus alignment, a separate calcaneal osteotomy may be necessary. This requires the osteotomy to be performed before screw fixation across the subtalar joint and should be planned at the time of provisional fixation with the guidewires for the cannulated drill bit.
- The extensor digitorum brevis and fat of the sinus tarsi are now reapproximated over the fusion site.
- The subcutaneous and skin are then closed with simple braided suture and vertical mattress nylon, respectively.

BRIEF SUMMARY OF SURGICAL STEPS

Midfoot Arthrodesis

- First incision: Over second metatarsal and tarsometatarsal joint
- After locating the neurovascular bundle, débride the first and second tarsometatarsal joints
- Second incision: Over medial border of the fourth metatarsal and tarsometatarsal joint
- Remove additional tarsometatarsal cartilage
- Reduce and fix the first tarsometatarsal joint
- Place a small distractor on the lateral foot and distract
- Débride the cartilage of the third through fifth tarsometatarsal joints
- Place 2.7-mm or 2.5-mm fully threaded lag screws from base of second metatarsal into middle cuneiform, medial cuneiform to base of second metatarsal, and base of first metatarsal to medial cuneiform
- Supplement with plate fixation as appropriate to achieve stability
- Pin the fourth and fifth tarsometatarsal joints

Subtalar Arthrodesis

- Make an incision centered over the sinus tarsi from tip of fibula to fourth metatarsal
- Identify the peroneal tendon sheath and fat in the sinus tarsi
- Locate fascia of the extensor digitorum brevis and incise along lines of skin incision
- Dissect off the extensor digitorum brevis as a distally based flap off the calcaneus and sharply
- Incise the sinus tarsi fat pad to expose the tarsal canal, taking care to preserve talus blood supply.
- Identify the posterior facet of the subtalar joint lateral to tarsal canal and débride the cartilage
- The calcaneus then is brought into neutral with respect to the tibia
- A combined aiming device may be used to direct a guidewire through a small incision at the apex of the heel through the posterior facet of the subtalar joint
- A cannulated drill is then passed over the guidewire across the subtalar joint
- Compression fixation is then achieved with one to two partially threaded 7.3-mm cancellous screws

TECHNICAL PEARLS

Midfoot Arthrodesis

- Before surgery, radiograph the contralateral foot to see the patient's native anatomy
- Before the tourniquet is inflated, palpate and mark the dorsalis pedis
- Reduce the first tarsometatarsal joint first, as the forefoot is displaced laterally and the first ray may interere with reduction of the second tarsometatarsal joint
- Fuse the first tarsometatarsal joint in slight varus and try to maintain correct plantar flexion and adduction alignment
- Evaluate for plate fixation; often screw fixation is insufficient into the softer bone of the cuneiforms

Subtalar Arthrodesis

- Only the posterior facet needs to be débrided; however, it must have all cartilage denuded and the subchondral bone feathered with an osteotome
- Dissect the extensor digitorum brevis as a distally based flap as this facilitates soft-tissue coverage over the arthrodesis site
- Fuse the joint in 5 degrees of valgus
- Try to avoid solely arthrodese dorsal to plantar as some sugeons have reported talar avascular necrosis

REQUIRED EQUIPMENT

Midfoot Arthrodesis

Foot and hand trays
McGlamry instrument tray
Small fragment set and mini fragment set

Subtalar Fusion

5-mm Pineapple burr
Large fragment set with 3.2-mm drill bit (long)
Two 6.5-in lamina spreaders
Hand tray for small Hohmann retractors, Littlers, Senn retractors, small Key elevator, osteotomes, Freer

COMMON PITFALLS

(When to call for the attending physician)

- If any neurovascular bundle is disrupted
- When positioning the arthrodesis sites for the midfoot fusion
- When positioning the subtalar joint for final fixation
- To check the final position of the hindfoot after a subtalar arthrodesis because an additional calcaneal osteotomy may be necessary; check for this before placing definitive screw fixation across the subtalar joint

POSTOPERATIVE PROTOCOL

After closure, the patient is placed in a either a bulky postmold splint (midfoot arthrodesis) or a bulky postmold and sugar tong splint (subtalar fusion). Alternatively, controlled ankle motion (CAM) boot application is acceptable with rigid fixation, which facilitates compression wrapping to minimize incision complications. In this event, the patient is still restricted to non–weight-bearing precautions. Both surgeries can be done on an outpatient basis as long as the patient is healthy and has adequate pain control. If not, the patient is usually admitted overnight for pain control with a patient-controlled analgesia pump. If the patient is admitted, perioperative prophylactic antibiotics should be administered. The patient is discharged when the pain is controlled and the patient can reasonably ambulate with crutches (usually after a gait training physical therapy session), with weight-bearing on the affected extremity avoided.

POSTOPERATIVE CLINIC VISIT PROTOCOL

Week 1: Wound check at no later than 4 days after surgery.

Week 2: Continuance of compression wraps for 2 weeks if that path is chosen. Immobilization with casting from 2 weeks until 6 weeks after surgery. The sutures may come out if the incision is healing well at 2 weeks, before cast application. Midfoot fusions tend to have more edema and a higher wound complication rate because of the location of the incision (emphasizing the compression wrap protocol in extensive cases). The patient is to remain non–weight-bearing until at least postoperative week 6.

Week 6: Remove the K-wires from the midfoot arthrodesis. X-rays are performed to ensure the hardware is in good position and there is radiographic evidence of healing. A computed tomographic (CT) scan is usually performed at this time to assess percentage of fusion. Partial weight-bearing is allowed for 6 additional weeks in a CAM boot, followed by a transition out of the durable medical equipment into a hard-soled shoe. Patients should be full weight-bearing by 12 weeks, or sooner if the CT scan indicates successful fusion developing.

3 Months: X-rays are performed to analyze the fusion construct. Cycling and swimming are encouraged. Physical therapy may be instituted if contractures are present (toes in the midfoot fusion, ankle in the subtalar fusion). Again, a CT scan may be used to confirm sufficient fusion.

6 Months: X-rays are performed and should show a sufficient arthrodesis construct. At this point, the patient should be able to resume impact activities.

SUGGESTED READINGS

1. de Palma L, Santucci A, Sabetta SP, Rapali S. Anatomy of the Lisfranc joint complex. *Foot Ankle Int.* 1997;18:356-364.
2. Gellman H, Lenihan M, Halikis N, Botte MJ, Giordani M, Perry J. Selective tarsal arthrodesis: an in vitro analysis of the effect on foot motion. *Foot Ankle.* 1987;8:127-133.
3. Ly TV, Coetzee JC. Treatment of primarily ligamentous Lisfranc joint injuries: primary arthrodesis compared with open reduction and internal fixation. A prospective, randomized study. *J Bone Joint Surg Am.* 2006;88:514-520.
4. Mann RA, Beaman DN, Horton GA. Isolated subtalar arthrodesis. *Foot Ankle Int.* 1998;19:511-519.
5. Patel A, Rao S, Nawoczenski D, Flemister AS, DiGiovanni B, Baumhauer JF. Midfoot arthritis. *J Am Acad Orthop Surg.* 2010;18:417-425.
6. Saltzman CL, Fehrle MJ, Cooper RR, Spencer EC, Ponseti IV. Triple arthrodesis: twenty-five and forty-four-year average follow-up of the same patients. *J Bone Joint Surg Am.* 1999;81:1391-1402.
7. Sangeorzan BJ, Veith RG, Hansen ST Jr. Salvage of Lisfranc's tarsometatarsal joint by arthrodesis. *Foot Ankle.* 1990;10:193-200.
8. Sarrafian SK. Biomechanics of the subtalar joint complex. *Clin Orthop Relat Res.* 1993;17-26.
9. Watson TS, Shurnas PS, Denker J. Treatment of Lisfranc joint injury: current concepts. *J Am Acad Orthop Surg.* 2010;18:718-728.

CHAPTER 14

CLOSED REDUCTION FOREARM AND WRIST (ADULT)

Sophia A. Strike | Dawn M. LaPorte

Adult forearm and wrist fractures include distal radius fractures, both bone metaphyseal and shaft fractures, and associated injuries. When displaced greater than acceptable standards of alignment, these fractures require initial closed reduction regardless of potential definitive surgical management. Nondisplaced or minimally displaced fractures require immobilization and close radiographic and clinical follow-up for continued nonoperative management. Displaced fractures fall into one of two categories: 1, those that may be reduced to a stable pattern within acceptable standards of alignment for continued nonoperative management; and 2, those that are inherently unstable fracture patterns and, in the setting of specific patient factors (age, hand dominance, functional level, medical comorbidities), need operative fixation regardless of the ability to obtain an adequate reduction.

A thorough skin check and neurovascular examination must be performed before manipulation of any fracture. Open fractures necessitate urgent surgical débridement. Swelling, paresthesias, pulse changes, and disproportionate pain are all concerning for compartment syndrome and should be noted. These signs necessitate contacting an attending physician immediately for decompression. Fractures of the forearm and wrist can be accompanied by ipsilateral hand and elbow fractures; thus, the entire extremity should be examined clinically and the adjacent joints imaged radiographically.

Distal radius fractures are one of the most common upper extremity fractures and present most often in young males with high-energy injuries and in older females with a low-energy mechanism. Historically, distal radius fractures were almost exclusively treated nonoperatively, and despite the advent of surgical technology that allows for near-anatomic reduction, an understanding of closed reduction and nonoperative management is important for any orthopaedic surgeon.

The critical facet of nonoperative management of distal radius fractures relies on restoring normal anatomy, which is determined with three key radiographic parameters: volar tilt (average, 11 degrees), radial height (average, 11 mm), and radial inclination (average, 23 degrees). Restoration of anatomy has been shown in multiple studies to correlate with improved functional outcomes. Colles' fractures are distal radius fractures with dorsal displacement, dorsal comminution, radial shortening, and usually an associated ulnar styloid fracture. Smith's fractures have volar displacement, and Barton's (volar or dorsal) fractures involve an intraarticular fracture of the lip of the distal radius with proximal (volar or dorsal) displacement of the fragment and the carpus. These eponyms are useful when describing distal radius fractures to a colleague or attending physician, although a detailed description of the fracture pattern, including angulation and displacement, is usually adequate.

Ulnar shaft fractures are commonly a result of direct trauma, as in the termed "nightstick" injury, which involves a distal two-third shaft fracture of the ulna. These injuries can also be seen in cases of physical abuse and should provoke at least consideration of abuse as the inciting cause. Nondisplaced ulnar shaft fractures or those

CASE MINIMUM REQUIREMENTS

- N = 20 Closed reduction of wrist and forearm fractures

COMMONLY USED CPT CODES

- CPT Code: 25565—Closed treatment of radial and ulnar shaft fractures; with manipulation
- CPT Code: 25605—Closed treatment of distal radial fracture (e.g., Colles' or Smith's type) or epiphyseal separation, includes closed treatment of fracture of ulnar styloid, when performed; with manipulation
- CPT Code: 25520—Closed treatment of radial shaft fracture and closed treatment of dislocation of distal radioulnar joint (Galeazzi's fracture/dislocation)
- CPT Code: 25505—Closed treatment of radial shaft fracture; with manipulation
- CPT Code: 25535—Closed treatment of ulnar shaft fracture; with manipulation
- CPT Code: 25624—Closed treatment of carpal scaphoid; with manipulation
- CPT Code: 25690—Closed treatment of lunate dislocation; with manipulation
- CPT Code: 25680—Closed treatment of transscaphoperilunar type of fracture dislocation; with manipulation
- CPT Code: 25675—Closed treatment of distal radioulnar dislocation with manipulation

with less than 10 degrees of angulation and less than 50% displacement can be treated nonoperatively with functional bracing. Both bone forearm fractures in adults are almost exclusively treated with operative fixation. Initial closed reduction and immobilization remains necessary for displaced fractures for patient comfort and for soft tissue management. The Galeazzi's fracture variant should be specifically mentioned because these fractures involve a distal radius fracture with concomitant distal radioulnar joint (DRUJ) injury and require reduction. Elbow injuries associated with forearm fractures include Monteggia's (proximal ulna fracture and associated radial head dislocation) and Essex-Lopresti (radial head fracture and associated interosseous membrane injury) variants. These variants are not explicitly discussed in this chapter but should be considered in evaluation of any patient with a forearm fracture.

SURGICAL TECHNIQUE

Room Set-Up

- Finger traps or a gauze bandage roll, intravenous (IV) pole or elevated hook for hanging fingers, 5-lb to 10-lb weights for traction, and splint and cast supplies should be available.
- Local analgesia, a 25-gauge to 30-gauge needle, and a 5-mL or 10-mL syringe for administration should be accessible.
- A mini C-arm and a fluoroscopy or radiology technician should also be available.

Patient Positioning

- The patient should be positioned supine on the bed.
- The ipsilateral shoulder should be flush with the side of the bed, and the injured arm should be entirely off the bed (Fig. 14-1).

Prepping and Draping

- No sterile draping is necessary.
- The thumb and radial fingers should be placed in a finger trap or hung with Kerlix from the IV pole or hook (Fig. 14-2).
- The shoulder should remain at the same height as the supine patient with the elbow flexed at approximately 90 degrees and the hand pointing directly toward the ceiling (see Fig. 14-1).

Hematoma Block

- Identify the fracture location with gentle palpation of the forearm and wrist.
  - Alternatively, the mini C-arm can be used to localize the fracture site if palpation proves difficult because of body habitus or degree of swelling.
- Aspirate 5 to 10 mL of lidocaine (1% without epinephrine), dosed appropriately based on the patient's weight, into a 10-mL syringe with a large-bore needle and replace with a 25-gauge or 30-gauge needle for administration.
- Insert the needle at the fracture site on the *dorsal* side of the wrist.
- Aspirate before injection of lidocaine and look for a slow return of blood, which is suggestive of insertion at the fracture hematoma as opposed to a blood vessel.
- Insert the needle into the fracture hematoma and periosteum to provide local analgesia, injecting a weight-appropriate amount of lidocaine (maximum 4.5 mg/kg/dose).
- Allow 3 to 5 minutes for the analgesic effects of the lidocaine to occur.

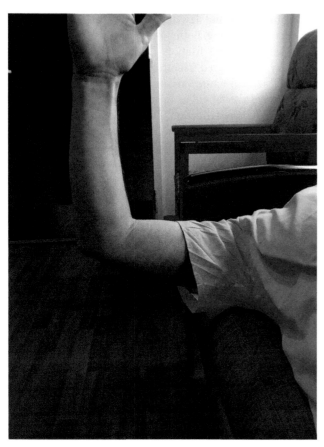

Figure 14-1 Shoulder and elbow position at 90 degrees of flexion with the patient in the supine position.

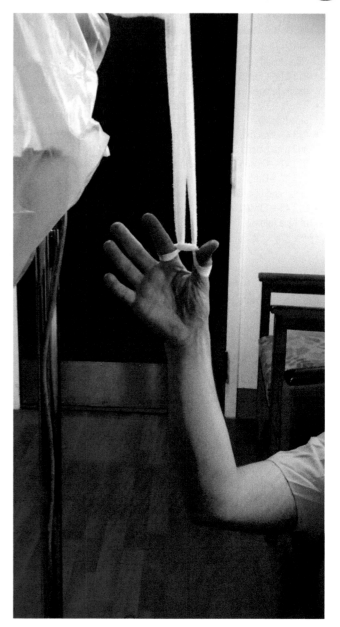

Figure 14-2 Placement of the thumb and radial finger in a gauze bandage (in the absence of a finger trap) for appropriate ulnar deviation of the hand during reduction.

Fracture Reduction

- Before beginning patient positioning and hematoma block, the radiographs should be closely reviewed to determine specific fracture pattern, the direction of displacement (volar or dorsal), shortening, radial and ulnar deviation, and comminution.
- After the local analgesia has taken effect, hang weights from the antecubital fossa to provide traction along the forearm; use 5-lb to 10-lb weights based on patient size.
- For substantially shortened fractures, hanging traction for 10 to 15 minutes allows for muscular fatigue that facilitates reduction (Video 14-1).
  - Traction also makes use of ligamentotaxis to assist with reduction.
- Begin reduction by re-creating the direction of displacement and accentuating the presenting deformity.
- An adequate hematoma block allows for substantial force to be used during reduction.

Fractures	Acceptable Tolerances
Distal Radius	Less than 5 mm of radial shortening
	Radial inclination angle greater than 10 degrees
	Dorsal tilt less than 10 degrees
Ulnar Shaft	Less than 50% displacement
	10-15 degrees of angulation
Radial Shaft	None
Both bone forearm	None

Figure 14-3 Acceptable tolerances for alignment of common forearm fractures.

- Ideally one attempt at reduction is adequate.
  - Reassuring the patient that one attempt with maximal force leads to fewer attempts at reduction is helpful.
- Manipulation of the fracture opposite the initial deformity then is performed to achieve anatomic reduction.
- After the initial reduction, radiographs in traction are recommended.
  - These views allow both closer evaluation of the fracture pattern with the forearm in maximal traction and evaluation of the initial reduction.
- At this point, if fracture reduction is adequate (Figure 14-3 shows acceptable tolerances for various forearm and wrist fractures), immobilization can be placed (see subsequent).
- If fracture reduction is inadequate, another attempt at reduction should be performed.
- No more than three attempts at reduction are recommended.
- If an acceptable reduction is not achieved after three attempts at reduction, surgical intervention is likely necessary.

Immobilization

- After an acceptable reduction has been achieved, some form of immobilization must be applied to maintain the reduction.
- The most commonly used forms of immobilization for distal radius fractures are bivalved short forearm cast and sugar-tong splint.
  - Both of these forms of immobilization accommodate for swelling of the affected forearm.
  - The sugar-tong splint is also used for forearm fractures and associated elbow pathology.
- An appropriate three-point mold must be applied to maintain a reduction.
  - One point must be focused on counteracting the direction of initial deformity and tendency for displacement (most commonly dorsal) with two points surrounding this primary mold for stability (Fig. 14-4).
- For forearm shaft fractures, a straight ulnar border (cast application only) and pronation of the forearm tightens the interosseous membrane and facilitates reduction of the fracture (Fig. 14-5).
  - An interosseous mold should also be applied with cast immobilization to tighten the interosseous membrane.
- Ulnar deviation of the hand and wrist and volar translation of the carpus (invoking ligamentotaxis) facilitates restoration of radial height and inclination and volar tilt in reduction of Colles' fractures.
  - Similar principles of counteracting the deforming force should be applied as appropriate to other variants of distal radius fractures.
- Taking the arm out of traction for mold application may allow for increased mobility of the forearm and improved technique for applying a mold at a specific location.
- Radiographs must always be obtained after splint or cast application and molding to evaluate maintenance of reduction.

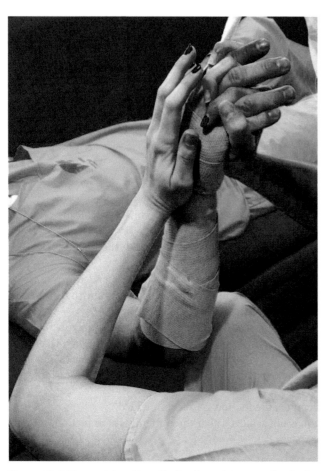

Figure 14-4 Three-point mold application for maintenance of reduction in splint or cast.

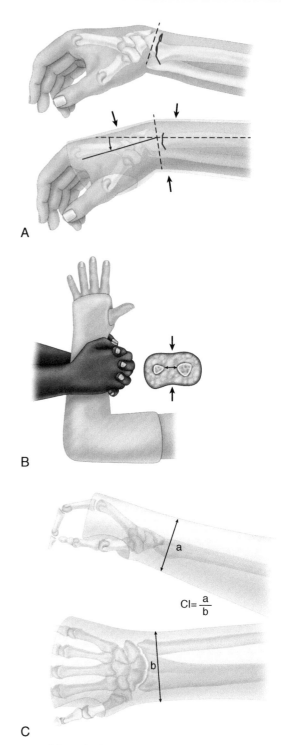

Figure 14-5 Schematic shows appropriate cast or splint molding techniques for **(A)** typical dorsally angulated distal radius fracture and **(B)** both bone forearm fracture interosseus mold. The cast index **(C)** is calculated by dividing the sagittal cast width *(a)* by the coronal cast width *(b)* at the fracture site.

BRIEF SUMMARY OF SURGICAL STEPS

- Position patient supine with shoulder at edge of bed
- Administer local analgesia
- Place fingers into finger trap
- Apply weights for traction
- Manual reduction
- Radiographs (in traction)
- Repeat manipulation if necessary
- Application of immobilization and radiographs

REQUIRED EQUIPMENT

Finger traps or gauze bandage roll, intravenous pole
Weights, 5 to 10 lbs
Lidocaine or short-acting local analgesia
Syringes and needles for injection of local analgesia
Cotton roll, plaster or fiberglass, elastic bandage

TECHNICAL PEARLS

- A good hematoma block that provides complete local analgesia allows for maximal force to be used in manipulation while patient comfort is maintained
- Allowing the forearm to hang in traction relaxes local musculature and facilitates fracture manipulation
- A three-point mold is necessary for maintaining reduction of any forearm or wrist fracture

COMMON PITFALLS

(When to call for the attending physician)

- Open fractures
- Clinical signs of compartment syndrome
- Inadequate reduction after three attempts
- Loss of reduction at follow-up visit
- New-onset numbness or tingling in the median nerve distribution/signs of acute carpal tunnel syndrome
- Multiple ipsilateral fracture or concomitant carpal fractures

POSTOPERATIVE PROTOCOL

The most important aspects of care after fracture reduction and immobilization include pain control and splint or cast maintenance. Patients should be instructed on appropriate splint or cast care and the importance of compliance. Elevation for control of swelling is highly recommended. Symptoms of tight splinting or casting and compartment syndrome should be discussed thoroughly to prevent complications of immobilization.

POSTOPERATIVE CLINIC VISIT PROTOCOL

Patients for whom an acceptable closed reduction is obtained and maintained after closed reduction and application of immobilization can be sent home from the emergency room or clinic. The initial follow-up visit in clinic should be at 7 days or less to allow repeat radiographic evaluation to ensure an acceptable reduction has been maintained. This allows early surgical intervention if necessary. In addition, the patient needs a skin check and placement into a cast if nonoperative treatment is used. Patients who are treated nonoperatively should be followed with weekly clinic visits for the first 2 weeks to follow the radiographic status of the fracture and ensure adequate control of swelling and skin maintenance. After the initial two visits, 6-week and 12-week clinic visits followed by a final 6-month visit are adequate. Patients should be switched to a removable splint at 6 weeks, at which time they can begin active and active-assisted range of motion at the wrist.

SUGGESTED READINGS

1. Bong MR, Egol KA, Leibman M, Koval KJ. A comparison of immediate postreduction splinting constructs for controlling initial displacement of fractures of the distal radius: a prospective randomized study of long-arm versus short-arm splinting. *J Hand Surg [Am]*. 2006;31(5):766-770.
2. Lafontaine M, Hardy D, Delince P. Stability assessment of distal radius fractures. *Injury*. 1989; 20(4):208-210.

3. Lichtman DM, Bindra RR, Boyer MI, et al. American Academy of Orthopaedic Surgeons clinical practice guideline on the treatment of distal radius fractures. *J Bone Joint Surg Am*. 2011;93(8):775-778.

4. Lichtman DM, Bindra RR, Boyer MI, et al. Treatment of distal radius fractures. *J Am Acad Orthop Surg*. 2010;18(3):180-189.

5. McQueen MM, Hajducka C, Court-Brown CM. Redisplaced unstable fractures of the distal radius: a prospective randomised comparison of four methods of treatment. *J Bone Joint Surg Br*. 1996;78(3): 404-409.

6. Young CF, Nanu AM, Checketts RG. Seven-year outcome following Colles' type distal radial fracture. A comparison of two treatment methods. *J Hand Surg [Br]*. 2003;28(5):422-426.

ADULT DISTAL HUMERUS FRACTURES
OPEN REDUCTION INTERNAL FIXATION

Miguel S. Daccarett | Todd Gaddie | Philipp N. Streubel

Distal humerus fractures most frequently occur as a consequence of high-energy trauma in young males or after simple falls in elderly females. In most instances, frank displacement is present and leads to deformity and functional limitation. Physical examination should include assessment of the soft tissue envelope to rule out open fractures and a careful neurovascular examination. All major upper extremity nerves, including the radial, ulnar, and median nerves, are at risk for injury.

Fractures are best classified according to the AO (Association for Osteosynthesis)/ OTA (Orthopaedic Trauma Association) system. Extraarticular fractures are classified as type A fractures. Fractures in which only a part of the articular surface has been disconnected from the proximal shaft are classified as type B (partial articular), and intraarticular fractures in which there is no continuity between the articular surface and the proximal shaft are classified as type C fractures (complete articular). Only stable nondisplaced fractures and those that occur in patients too sick to undergo surgery should be treated nonoperatively.

Operative treatment requires careful preoperative planning. From an anatomic perspective, the trochlea and capitellum are connected to the humeral shaft via medial and lateral columns, which are separated by the olecranon fossa posteriorly and the coronoid and radial fossae anteriorly. Operative fixation of the distal humerus requires detailed reconstruction of the normal anatomy with provision of a stable construct to allow for early range of motion as healing occurs. Dual plating is recommended in most instances in either parallel or 90-90 configurations. With parallel plating, plates are placed straight medially and straight laterally; in the 90-90 configuration, one plate is placed straight medially and the second plate is placed posteriorly onto the lateral column. In the setting of extraarticular fractures with satisfactory bone stock, single posterolateral plating can be performed.

SURGICAL TECHNIQUE

Room Set-Up

- The operating table is turned (typically 90 degrees) so that the operative extremity is aiming toward the center of the room.
- With the patient in the lateral decubitus position, the anesthesia team is located toward the back of the patient, at either the area of the patient's head or legs, on the opposite side of the surgeon.
- A standard C-arm is used to come in from the head of the bed. Alternatively, a mini C-arm can be used. Before prepping, it should be confirmed that posteroanterior (PA) and lateral images can be obtained.
- The right-handed surgeon stands on the left, the first assistant stands to the right of the extremity, and the scrub technician stands in the back (Fig. 15-1).

COMMONLY USED ICD10 CODES

- S42.41—Simple supracondylar fracture without intercondylar fracture of humerus
- S42.42—Comminuted supracondylar fracture without intercondylar fracture of humerus
- S42.45—Fracture of lateral condyle of humerus
- S42.46—Fracture of medial condyle of humerus

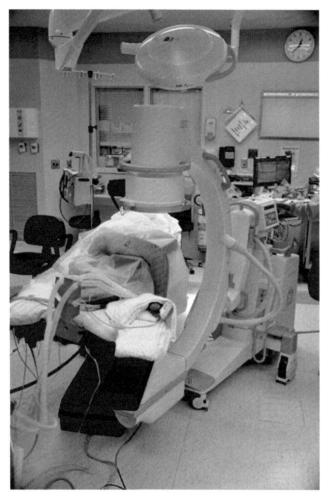

Figure 15-1 Intraoperative photograph shows room set-up, including C-arm. Anesthesia is to the back of the patient. Surgeon is to the left and assistant to the right of the elbow. Scrub technician is in the back of the surgeons.

Patient Positioning

- The authors' preference is to position the patient in the lateral decubitus position with the operative extremity facing up. Alternatively, the patient may either be placed prone, or supine with the arm across the chest. The following sections describe the authors' approach with the patient in the lateral decubitus position.
- A gel roll is placed under the contralateral axilla to protect the brachial plexus.
- The operative arm is placed over a radiolucent arm support.
- The contralateral arm is flexed at the shoulder to avoid interference with the operative extremity during imaging.
- A sterile tourniquet is placed on the proximal arm after prepping.
- For lengthy procedures, a urinary catheter is recommended.
- One should confirm that adequate images can be obtained once positioning has been completed.

Prepping and Draping

- Prepping solution is alcohol-based chlorhexidine solution if not contraindicated. Complete formal scrub is performed in the setting of open wounds or dirty skin. A chlorhexidine-based soap is preferred in this setting.
- Sterile U-drapes are placed at the level of the axilla, leaving the upper extremity distal to the shoulder exposed, followed by an upper extremity drape.

- A sterile tourniquet is applied and connected with a sterile tube extension.
- An impervious stockinette is placed over the hand, and an elastic wrap is used to hold it in place. An opening is cut into the tip of the stockinette to avoid pooling of fluid on the inside.
- An iodine-impregnated adhesive incise drape may be placed on the skin. "Tiger stripes" are drawn across the surgical field before the drape is placed to aid in closure.

Operative Approaches

- Paratricipital (medial or lateral) approach: Recommended mainly for type A (Figs. 15-2 and 15-3), type B, and simple type C (Fig. 15-4) fractures.
  - Type B fractures that involve the anterior trochlea and capitellum cannot be reached through this approach.

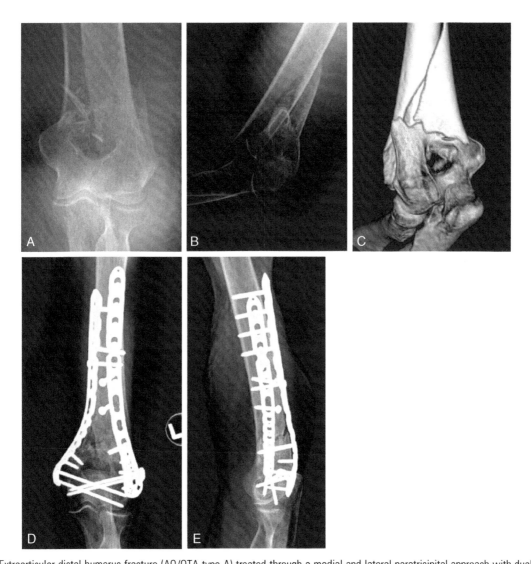

Figure 15-2 Extraarticular distal humerus fracture (AO/OTA type A) treated through a medial and lateral paratricipital approach with dual 90-90 plates. Note the presence of a large spiral butterfly fragment at the medial metadiaphysis (**A** and **B**, anteroposterior and lateral injury radiographs; **C**, posterolateral view of three-dimensional computed tomographic renderings; **D** and **E**, anteroposterior and lateral views at 3 months with healed fracture). An olecranon osteotomy was not required. The proximal plate ends are staggered longitudinally to avoid the creation of a potential stress riser. Dissection and identification of the radial and ulnar nerves was required. Plates are positioned in a 90-90 configuration, with one medial and the other posterior on the lateral column. This specific plate design has an anterior extension for the posterolateral plate to allow screws placed from laterally to medially. In this case, special length plates were used because of the comminution present at the metadiaphysis. Screw length and number were maximized distally, staying clear of the olecranon fossa. Independent lag screws were used outside of the plate for preliminary fixation of the butterfly fragment.

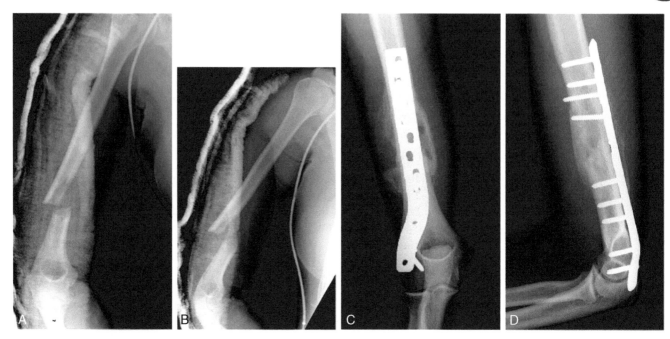

Figure 15-3 Distal humeral shaft fracture treated with a posterolateral plate construct with a lateral paratricipital approach (**A** and **B**, anteroposterior and oblique lateral injury radiographs; **C** and **D**, anteroposterior and lateral radiographs at 3 months with healed fracture). Given the sturdier geometry of this implant, fixation can be reliably obtained with a single plate. Dissection of the ulnar nerve is not required. However, the radial nerve has to be identified before fracture reduction and fixation. Distally, care should be taken to avoid screw tip penetration through the articular surface of the capitellum.

- Triceps splitting: Recommended for the same fracture patterns as the paratricipital approach.
- Olecranon osteotomy: Extensile approach to the distal humerus.
  - Appropriate for most fractures, including complex intraarticular fractures (Figs. 15-5 and 15-6).
- Fractures that involve the capitellum and anterior trochlea may require additional windows to the anterior aspect of the distal humerus.
  - This is best achieved through Kaplan's interval (extensor origin split) laterally or Hotchkiss' over-the-top approach (flexor pronator peel) medially.

Paratricipital

- An incision centered over the humerus is started 10 cm proximal to the olecranon tip and continued to 3 cm distal to the olecranon tip.
- Full-thickness skin flaps, including the triceps fascia, are raised medially and laterally off the underlying triceps to the level of the medial and lateral intermuscular septae, respectively.
- The ulnar nerve is identified medially between the triceps and the medial intermuscular septum distally to the level of the medial epicondyle. It can be protected with a Penrose drain for location during the remainder of the procedure. Of note, with use of a posterolateral plate construct, the medial component of the paratricipital approach is not required.
- Laterally, the radial nerve may be identified as it pierces the lateral intermuscular septum 10 cm proximal to the lateral epicondyle. The lateral brachial cutaneous nerve originates off of the radial nerve. It can be easily identified on the deep aspect of the lateral triceps fascia and followed proximally to localize the radial nerve. The triceps is lifted off the lateral and medial intermuscular septae and epicondyles. Distally the anconeus is lifted off the lateral epicondyle to gain access to the lateral column.

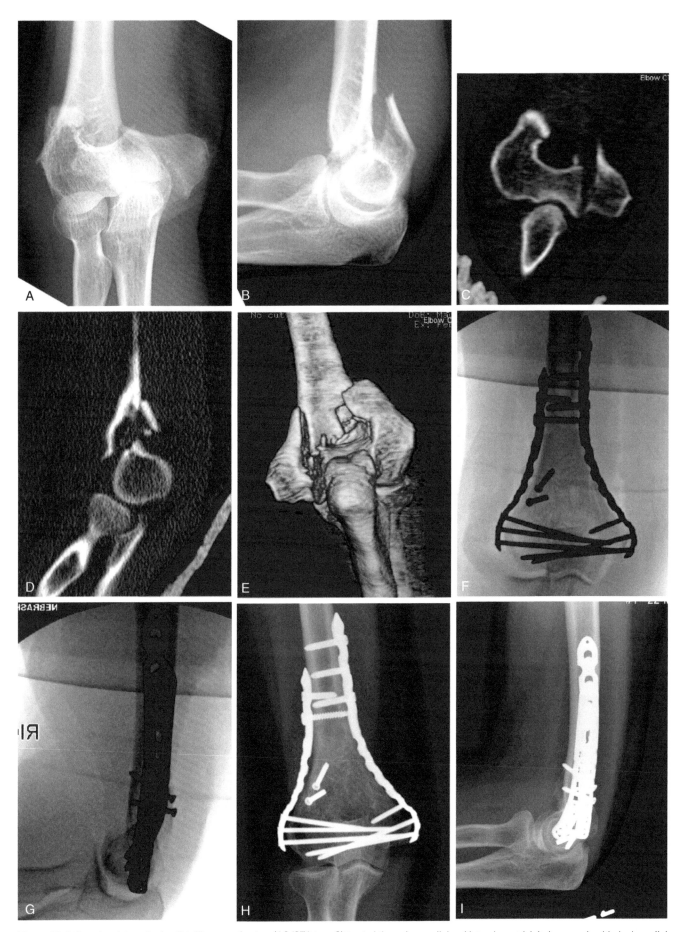

Figure 15-4 Complete intraarticular distal humerus fracture (AO/OTA type C) treated through a medial and lateral paratricipital approach with dual parallel plates. Note the simple split into the distal segment just medial to the trochlea (**A** and **B**, anteroposterior and lateral injury radiographs; **C** and **D**, coronal and sagittal computed tomographic reconstructions; **E**, posterior view of three-dimensional computed tomographic renderings; **F** and **G**, immediate postoperative anteroposterior and lateral fluoroscopy images; **H** and **I**, anteroposterior and lateral views at 3 months with healed fracture). An olecranon osteotomy was not performed. The proximal plate ends are staggered longitudinally to avoid the creation of a potential stress riser. Posterior to anterior lag screws were used outside of the plate for preliminary fixation of the lateral column. Distally, plates are placed to maximize screw number and length.

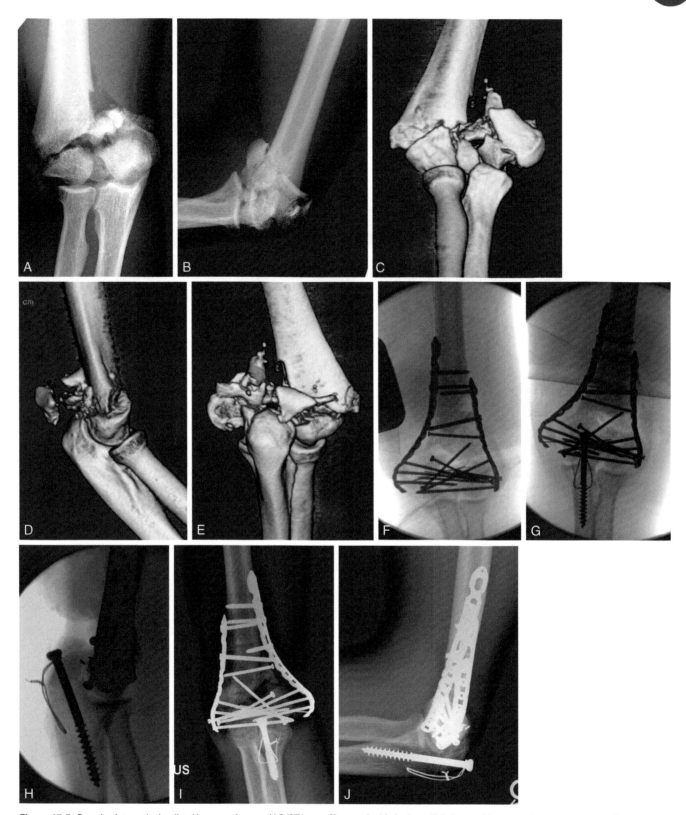

Figure 15-5 Complex intraarticular distal humerus fracture (AO/OTA type C) treated with dual parallel plates with a transolecranon approach. The olecranon osteotomy was fixed with a 6.5-mm screw and a tension band construct (**A** and **B**, anteroposterior and lateral injury radiographs; **C, D,** and **E**, anterior, lateral, and posterior views of three-dimensional computed tomographic renderings; **F**, intraoperative anteroposterior fluoroscopy image showing final humeral fixation before fixation of osteotomy; **G** and **H**, immediate postoperative anteroposterior and lateral fluoroscopy images showing humeral and ulnar fixation; **I** and **J**, anteroposterior and lateral views at 3 months with healed fracture and osteotomy). Note the use of free K-wires and multiple long small fragment screws to aid in fixation of intraarticular fracture fragments. Proximally, plates are staggered to avoid creation of a stress riser. Distally, screw number and length are maximized.

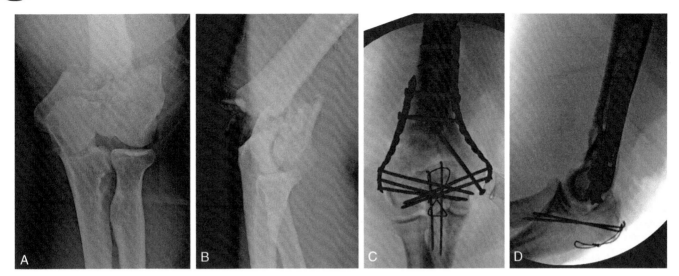

Figure 15-6 Complex intraarticular distal humerus fracture (AO/OTA type C) treated with dual parallel plates with a transolecranon approach. The olecranon osteotomy was fixed with a tension band construct with K-wires (**A** and **B**, anteroposterior and lateral injury radiographs; **C** and **D**, immediate postoperative anteroposterior and lateral fluoroscopy images showing humeral and ulnar fixation). Note that K-wires are placed parallel to each other and are directed clear of the proximal radioulnar joint.

- The medial collateral ligament of the elbow originates at the anteroinferior aspect of the medial epicondyle. The lateral collateral ligament originates at the lateral aspect of the lateral epicondyle and capitellum. These ligaments should not be disrupted during surgical exposure.
- The triceps is finally elevated off the posterior surface of the humerus.

Triceps Split
- Incision is similar to that in the paratricipital approach as described previously.
- Limited full-thickness flaps are raised off triceps fascia.
- The triceps split uses the interval between the long and lateral head of the triceps and incises the medial head along its fibers.
- The proximal border of the medial head is the spiral groove that holds the radial nerve. Dissection should therefore proceed carefully proximally.
- The split is completed distally to the level of the olecranon. Exposure may be maximized with subperiosteal elevation of the triceps tendon of the olecranon. Distal extensions of the extensor mechanism remain intact through the flexor carpi ulnaris medially and the anconeus laterally.

Olecranon Osteotomy
- Exposure is started as for the paratricipital approach as described previously.
- Once the triceps has been released off the intermuscular septae, medial and lateral capsulotomies are performed at the level of the greater sigmoid notch of the proximal ulna to identify the "bare area."
- An apex distal chevron osteotomy is made with an oscilating saw for 90% of the depth of the olecranon. The final 10% are cracked while levering with the use of an osteotome. This aids in obtaining interdigitation of the fragments and aids in osteotomy fixation.
- At this point, the extensor mechanism can be reflected proximally, fully exposing the distal humerus.
- Final fixation is preferentially achieved with a tension band construct. Alternatively, plate and screw fixation may be used. If a plate is to be used, the most proximal screw can be predrilled to help anatomically align the osteotomy at the conclusion of the case.

Fracture Fixation

- Fixation systems are variable and include both locking and nonlocking constructs. Precontoured plates are the mainstay of fixation currently. As an example, the Synthes (DePuy Synthes, Westchester, PA) system can be used, with 3.5-mm cortical screws in the shaft and 2.7-mm locking screws going into the articular segment. Locking screws are not necessary in this setting, especially with younger patients.
- Reduction and fixation starts with the distal articular segment. Provisional fixation is obtained with K-wires.
  - For reduction, large pointed reduction clamps can be used to get compression through an articular split but also medially and laterally across the supracondylar area, which is prone to nonunions.
    - A lobster claw helps to keep the plates opposed to bone. To prevent the plates sliding off posteriorly and thereby loosing "parallelicity," a 0.062-inch K-wire can be placed through the plate to lock it into position in the sagittal plane when applying the clamp (keeping it from sliding).
    - When performing the reduction, manipulation of the forearm in both flexion-extension and pronation-supination can aid in neutralizing deforming forces and facilitating reduction.
    - Placement of a bump on the anterior aspect of the distal arm can aid in correcting angulation in the sagittal plane.
    - Starting reduction at the articular segment and then progressing to the shaft segment can be helpful.
- The distal articular segment is provisionally fixed to the shaft with one medial and one lateral K-wire.
  - Small pieces of articular comminution can be stabilized to a larger piece with 0.045-in or 1.1-mm pins that are cut flush to the cortical surface.
    - Placement of these pins should be as peripheral (as close to subchondral bone) as possible to avoid interference with later screw placement.
    - Pins may be either threaded or smooth; the authors prefer the latter.
  - Placement of a locking guide (Fig. 15-7) sitting on the left (lateral) aspect of the bone can be useful in confirming radiographically that screw trajectory is going to be appropriate.
    - With use of nonlocking screws, this can be done by checking with a drill bit on the surface of the bone with fluoroscopic visualization.
    - Lag screws (in lag mode) are not typically necessary. If screws are placed after a reduction clamp has been tightly applied to compress the fracture fragments, primary healing is typically achieved.
- Plates are provisionally fixed onto the shaft, and reduction and adequate implant positioning are confirmed radiographically.
- As many screw holes as possible should be lined up along the bone distally to maximize screw fixation through the plate. Adequate alignment in the sagittal plane is necessary to allow for central screw placement and maximize screw length.
- The articular segment should be lined up in the sagittal plane so that the anterior humeral cortical line bisects the capitellum.
- Plates are fixed to the articular segment maximizing screw length and number. This is done while compression is obtained with a clamp between the fragments and plate.
- Final proximal plate fixation is obtained proximally, while compression is provided between the articular and shaft segment.
- Olecranon osteotomy fixation is performed with tension band wiring or plate and screw fixation.
- Closure is completed.

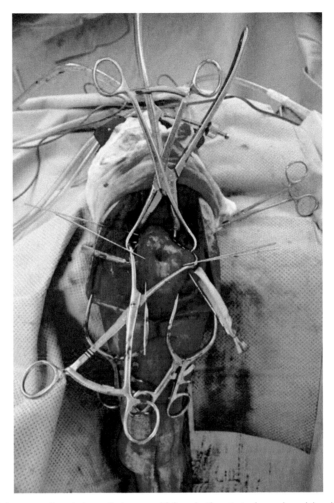

Figure 15-7 Intraoperative photograph shows multiple reduction strategies and provisional fracture fixation, including the use of large pointed reduction clamps to get compression through articular split and also medially and laterally across supracondylar area; lobster claw to help keep plates opposed to bone; and the use of 0.062-inch K-wires placed through the plate to lock it into position in the sagittal plane to avoid plate slippage. Note placement of a locking drill guide on the left (lateral) aspect of the bone, which can be useful in confirming radiographically that screw trajectory is going to be appropriate. Finally, note the Penrose drain medially around the ulnar nerve.

BRIEF SUMMARY OF SURGICAL STEPS

- Room set-up
- Patient positioning
- Confirm that adequate imaging can be obtained
- Prep and drape
- Arm exsanguination and tourniquet insufflation
- Posterior approach
- Ulnar nerve identification
- Fracture débridement and reduction
- Provisional K-wire fixation
- Final fixation with dual column plates (90-90 versus parallel plating); consider posterolateral plate for simple extraarticular fractures
- Radiographic confirmation of reduction and adequate hardware placement
- Fixation of olecranon osteotomy if performed
- Consider ulnar nerve transposition
- Closure

REQUIRED EQUIPMENT

Bipolar cautery
Loupe magnification during nerve exposure
Retractors including Senn, army-navy, Hohmann, mini Hohmann, Weitlaner, and Gelpi
Vascular loop or Penrose drain
Tenotomy scissors
Sagittal saw, if osteotomy planned
Large and small pointed fracture reduction forceps
Assortment of K-wires (0.035-inch, 0.047-inch, 0.062-inch, and 0.079-inch)
2.7-mm and 3.5-mm implant and instrument set
Screws with lengths of at least 55 mm for the articular segment
Elbow plating system of choice (medial, lateral, posterolateral, and olecranon plates); alternatively, plates can be contoured with 3.5-mm implants
18-gauge wire and 0.062-inch K-wires for osteotomy fixation; consider large screw or plate

TECHNICAL PEARLS

- Use of a sterile tourniquet helps in maximizing proximal exposure and allows for easy removal if needed
- Ensure that proper fluoroscopic views can be obtained before prepping and draping
- Ulnar and radial nerves should be located depending on the surgical approach used
- Small articular fragments may be fixed with small K-wires cut flush within the construct
- Elbow flexion and extension may aid in aligning fracture fragments during reduction
- Reduction of anterior articular fragments may be achieved by hinging major articular fragments around collateral ligaments
- Compression should be achieved between articular fragments and at the supracondylar level
- Maximize screw length and number distally
- Avoid blocking motion with screws placed through the olecranon or radial and coronoid fossae
- If fixing an olecranon osteotony with plates, preliminary implant positioning may be done before performing the osteotomy to make reduction and fixation easier

COMMON PITFALLS

(When to call for the attending physician)

- Inability to locate radial or ulnar nerves
- Inability to reduce the fracture anatomically
- Suboptimal plate placement

POSTOPERATIVE PROTOCOL

A posterior splint or bulky Jones dressing is placed during surgery and is maintained for the immediate postoperative period. Patients are kept in-house for 24 hours for perioperative antibiotics and pain control. The extremity is kept elevated on a pillow with the elbow extended. This aids in minimizing skin/flap complications. Radiation therapy (for heterotopic ossification prophylaxis) is not recommended in the acute setting.

At discharge, the patient is encouraged to maintain active range of motion of the shoulder, wrist, and hand. Local ice and extremity elevation is continued for the first 4 days.

At 4 days, the dressing is removed and a compressive stockinette is applied by the occupational therapist. A custom-made posterior long arm splint is fabricated by an occupational therapist with the elbow at 90 degrees of flexion and the forearm and wrist in neutral.

In noncomplicated cases, early motion is started. Active and active-assisted elbow extension and forearm pronation and supination are begun with the patient upright with the arm adducted by the side at all times out of the brace. Elbow flexion is performed gravity-assisted in the supine position with the shoulder forward-flexed 90 degrees. Passive range of motion is started at 6 weeks.

In complex cases, patients are maintained in the posterior splint for 3 weeks full-time, with no motion. Active range of motion is started thereafter after the previously stated protocol.

At 6 weeks, the splint is weaned, and passive motion and static progressive extension splinting is added as needed.

At 10 weeks, gentle progressive strengthening of the elbow and forearm is added.

Work conditioning may be required for laborers.

Gradual return to full activity and sports is allowed at 14 weeks.

POSTOPERATIVE CLINIC VISIT PROTOCOL

First clinic visit: 10 to 14 days. First visit goals are to assess the wound and confirm normal neurovascular examination results. Stitches are removed if the incision appears to be healing appropriately, and rehabilitation is started as described previously. No radiographs are obtained at this visit.

Second clinic visit: 6 weeks. This visit allows for a repeat inspection of the wound and evaluation of active and passive range of motion. The first postoperative radiographs are obtained at this visit. If the patient has an unacceptable range of motion, initiation of static flexion/extension splints may begin at this time. If radiographic evidence of fracture healing is noted at this time, dynamic splinting may be initiated. No pushing, pulling, or lifting is allowed.

Third clinic visit: 3 months. Range of motion (active and passive) is assessed. Repeat radiographs are also performed. If radiographic and clinical union is obtained, the patient may progress to full use of the arm without limitations.

If radiographic and clinical union has not been achieved, the patient should continue weight restrictions and follow up until radiographic evidence of union is noted on a monthly basis.

If functional range of motion (at least 100-degree arc from 30 degrees short of full extension to 130 degrees of flexion) has not been obtained at 6 months after surgery despite a carefully executed rehabilitation plan, consideration of surgical capsular release may be considered.

SUGGESTED READINGS

1. Coles CP, Barei DP, Nork SE, Taitsman LA, Hanel DP, Bradford Henley M. The olecranon osteotomy: a six-year experience in the treatment of intraarticular fractures of the distal humerus. *J Orthop Trauma.* 2006;20(3):164-171.

2. Doornberg J, Lindenhovius A, Kloen P, van Dijk CN, Zurakowski D, Ring D. Two and three-dimensional computed tomography for the classification and management of distal humeral fractures. Evaluation of reliability and diagnostic accuracy. *J Bone Joint Surg Am.* 2006;88(8):1795-1801.

3. Doornberg JN, van Duijn PJ, Linzel D, et al. Surgical treatment of intra-articular fractures of the distal part of the humerus. Functional outcome after twelve to thirty years. *J Bone Joint Surg Am.* 2007;89(7):1524-1532.

4. Dubberley JH, Faber KJ, Macdermid JC, Patterson SD, King GJ. Outcome after open reduction and internal fixation of capitellar and trochlear fractures. *J Bone Joint Surg Am.* 2006;88(1):46-54.

5. Erpelding JM, Mailander A, High R, Mormino MA, Fehringer EV. Outcomes following distal humeral fracture fixation with an extensor mechanism-on approach. *J Bone Joint Surg Am.* 2012;94(6):548-553.

6. Guitton TG, Doornberg JN, Raaymakers EL, Ring D, Kloen P. Fractures of the capitellum and trochlea. *J Bone Joint Surg Am.* 2009;91(2):390-397.

7. Hamid N, Ashraf N, Bosse MJ, et al. Radiation therapy for heterotopic ossification prophylaxis acutely after elbow trauma: a prospective randomized study. *J Bone Joint Surg Am.* 2010;92(11):2032-2038.

8. Nauth A, McKee MD, Ristevski B, Hall J, Schemitsch EH. Distal humeral fractures in adults. *J Bone Joint Surg Am.* 2011;93(7):686-700.

9. Ruan HJ, Liu JJ, Fan CY, Jiang J, Zeng BF. Incidence, management, and prognosis of early ulnar nerve dysfunction in type C fractures of distal humerus. *J Trauma.* 2009;67(6):1397-1401.

10. Sanchez-Sotelo J, Torchia ME, O'Driscoll SW. Complex distal humeral fractures: internal fixation with a principle-based parallel-plate technique. *J Bone Joint Surg Am.* 2007;89(5):961-969.

INTRAMEDULLARY NAILING OF FEMORAL SHAFT FRACTURES

Lisa K. Cannada | Jesse Seamon

Fractures of the femoral shaft are high-energy injuries often associated with significant traumatic events, such as motor vehicle or motorcycle accidents, falls from heights, and motor vehicles striking pedestrians. Not surprisingly, these injuries can be associated with significant other orthopaedic, head, and visceral injuries that can affect the treatment of these patients. Ipsilateral limb injuries can include femoral neck fractures and knee ligament injuries, along with lower extremity fractures. Less common mechanisms of femoral shaft fractures include bisphosphonate-related stress fractures, pathologic fractures, and low-energy torsional injuries in elderly patients.

The gold standard for treatment is placement of a rigid, statically locked intramedullary nail, which results in union greater than 95% of the time. Although great debate exists about the optimal starting point, proper technique and adherence to basic principles can maximize chances of a good outcome. In the adult patient, open or percutaneous plating is reserved for rare scenarios in which the intramedullary canal is unable to accept a nail because of size, previous trauma, or the presence of implants (total hip, stemmed total knee) that cannot be removed.

Current clinical challenges include accurate intraoperative determination of femoral shaft rotation and length, minimization of fluoroscopy usage during freehand techniques for placement of interlocking screws, and timing of fixation in the patient with multiple injuries.

SURGICAL TECHNIQUE

Room Set-Up

- The room should be large enough to allow for adequate space for a C-arm, instrument tables, and an operative table without excessive crowding.
- Place the C-arm in the room on the opposite side from the fractured limb.
- Position the table off-center in the room, closer to the side of the C-arm, to allow for extra space between the operative table and the instrument table.
- Place the base component of the C-arm at the end of the table to ensure easy viewing of x-rays while performing the case.

Patient Positioning

- The supine position is the most commonly used and allows for the easiest fluoroscopy and determination of overall alignment (Fig. 16-1).
- The lateral position can be helpful for more proximal fractures in which excessive proximal fragment flexion can be exacerbated in the supine position (Fig. 16-2).
- The lateral position can be helpful for obese patients in whom an antegrade nail is placed, as excessive hip fat falls to the side and increased hip adduction can be achieved to improve accessibility to the starting point (Fig. 16-3).

CASE MINIMUM REQUIREMENTS

- N = 25 Operative treatment of femoral and tibial shaft fractures

COMMONLY USED CPT CODES

- CPT Code: 27506—Open treatment of femoral shaft fracture, with or without external fixation, with insertion of intramedullary implant, with or without cerclage or locking screws
- CPT Code: 27507—Open treatment of femoral shaft fracture with plate/screws, with or without cerclage

COMMONLY USED ICD9 CODES

- 821.0—Fracture of shaft or unspecified part of femur closed
- 821.1—Fracture of shaft or unspecified part of femur open
- 821.2—Fracture of lower end of femur closed
- 821.3—Fracture of lower end of femur open

COMMONLY USED ICD10 CODES

- S72.1—Pertrochanteric fracture
- S72.2—Subtrochanteric fracture of femur
- S72.3—Fracture of shaft of femur
- S72.4—Fracture of lower end of femur
- S72.8—Other fracture of femur
- S72.9—Unspecified fracture of femur

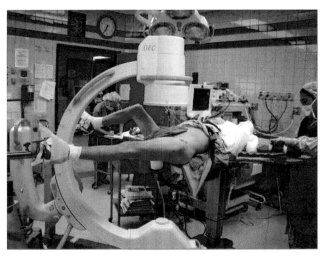

Figure 16-1 A patient is positioned supine on a fracture table with the contralateral extremity in a well leg holder and fractured extremity taped into a traction boot. Note that the C-arm is opposite to the injured leg to allow for unobstructed access to the injured limb during fluoroscopy.

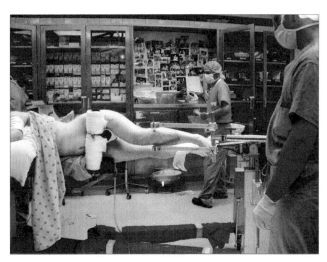

Figure 16-2 A patient is positioned laterally on a fracture table with a distal tibial traction pin in use to apply traction to the leg. No traction boot is necessary in this scenario.

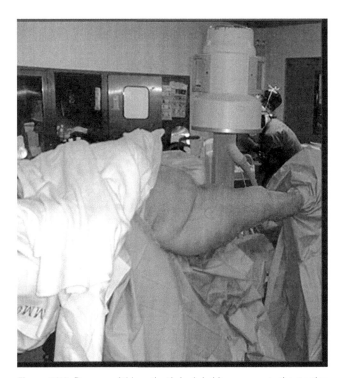

Figure 16-3 Because of this patient's body habitus, access to the starting point is quite difficult in the supine position. Options include switching to the lateral position or considering a retrograde nail if the fracture pattern is amenable.

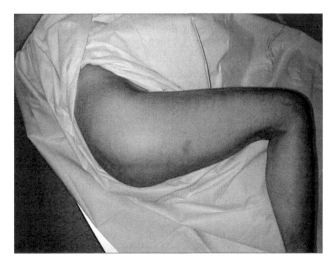

Figure 16-4 The fractured extremity is prepped leg "free" in the lateral position. The surgical assistant can freely move the leg in space, making reduction maneuvers easier but maintenance of the reduced position more difficult.

- Table options include a fracture table or a Jackson table; both have many variations with respect to attachments and traction options. (See the subsequent Fracture Table and Jackson Table sections.)
- Of note, the leg may be prepped "free" or "fixed."
  - If prepped free, the foot is not constrained in a boot and the leg may be moved by an assistant into any position.
  - If prepped fixed, the foot is in a traction boot; therefore, movement of the limb is more limited with the advantage of the ability to maintain a fixed position of the extremity (compare Fig. 16-1 with Fig. 16-4).

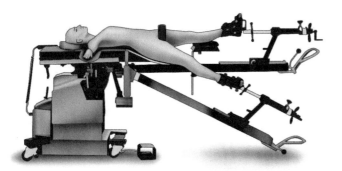

Figure 16-5 Picture of a fracture table. Note the metal beams projecting from the midportion of the table with a traction boot attachment for holding the fracture extremity and providing static traction and rotational adjustments.

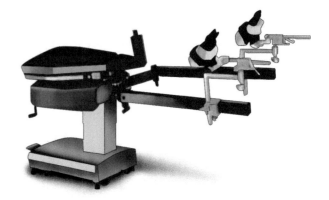

Figure 16-6 Close-up view of the fracture boot attachment on the fracture table. Care should be taken to pad the foot and ensure that it is well fixed in the boot to prevent loss of traction during the operative procedure.

Prepping and Draping

- On a fracture table, prep and drape from the bottom of the rib cage proximally to the fibular head distally to allow for adequate working space.
- On a Jackson (flat top) table, prep from the anterior superior iliac spine (ASIS) proximally and prep the entire leg.
  - With a Jackson table, consider prepping both legs in to better judge rotation and length.

Fracture Table Set-Up (Figs. 16-5 and 16-6)

- A table with two large beams that support a boot and traction set-up with a perineal post should be used.
- Tables range from very basic to more complex tables, such as the Hana (Mizuho OSI, Union City, CA) table and others that are used for anterior total hip arthroplasty.
- The fractured extremity can be placed in a traction boot to allow for traction and rotation of the fracture, and the fracture can be statically held in that position by the table.
  - Care should be taken to pad the foot and ankle with sufficient cotton undercast padding before placement in the traction boot.
  - Confirm that the reduction can be visualized *before* prepping by taking antero-posterior (AP) and lateral C-arm views.
  - If adequate length cannot be obtained, place the leg in skeletal traction and use a bow for set-up and pulling traction to assist reduction.
- The uninjured, or well, leg may be scissored into adduction and hip extension with a traction boot or flexed, abducted, and externally rotated into a well leg holder.
- The arm of the injured side should be crossed over the body and placed on an arm holder or on a pillow and blankets and then secured across the body with tape.
- Care should be taken to ensure adequate foot perfusion and lack of leg swelling in the well leg holder; this should be checked by the circulating nurse every 30 minutes during the case.
- A separate drape for the C-arm may be used.
- For proximal fractures, reduction aids may be necessary.
  - These aids include a ball-tip pusher, rigid reamer or equivalent, cannulated reduction finger, and use of a crutch with a sterile cover to reduce the posterior sag.

Jackson Table (Fig. 16-7)

- This radiolucent flat top table with various attachments available to allow for static traction on the limb may also be used without these attachments for "limb free" positioning.
- In general, the patient is positioned supine or "lazy" lateral with a bump underneath the hip on the side of the fracture.
- The patient should be positioned on the table so that the injured side is at the very lateral edge of the table if an antegrade nail is planned to allow for ease of access to the starting point.
- The arm of the injured side should be crossed over the body and placed on an arm holder or on a pillow and blankets and then secured across the body with tape.
- If a retrograde nail is planned, *radiolucent triangles* are necessary to allow for appropriate positioning of the limb for nail insertion.
- An assistant needs to hold traction and assist with fracture reduction.
- Alternatively, a traction pin may be used with a sterile rope and weight hung off the end of the table or through a table attachment such as a traction tower or pipe bender (Fig. 16-8).
- A lateral position may be used to assist with reduction of subtrochanteric femur fractures, as this can reduce deforming forces on the proximal fragment.

Surgical Incision: Antegrade Nail

- Greater trochanteric starting point: In a thin patient, one is able to palpate the greater trochanter and the ASIS.
- The incision is in line with the midpoint of the greater trochanter longitudinally, beginning 10 to 15 cm proximal to the tip of the greater trochanter; total incision length is about 3 to 5 cm.
  - The incision may be even more proximal in obese patients.
  - Incision closer to the greater trochanter (too distal) may result in a surgical approach not in line with the femoral bow and may result in eccentric reaming.
- Sharp dissection with a #10 blade scalpel is carried down through the skin, subcutaneous tissue, and fascia lata.

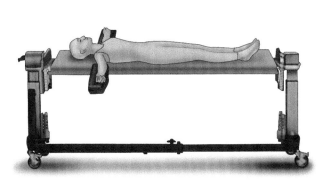

Figure 16-7 A classic Jackson table is shown. The carbon fiber top of the table is radiolucent. Various attachments are available for the end of the table to facilitate skeletal or boot traction of the injured extremity.

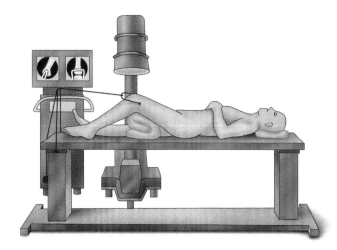

Figure 16-8 Patient is placed on a radiolucent table with the knee flexed approximately 30 degrees under a leg roll. Image intensifier is placed on side opposite the operative extremity, and a monitor just inferior to the image intensifier. Once the Steinmann pin is inserted and the traction bow is tightened, a rope with weight can be placed over a crossbar attached to the table to maintain reduction.

- The fascia lata need to be divided more distally than the skin incision (slightly underminded).
- A finger then may be bluntly advanced to feel the tip of the greater trochanter and surrounding gluteus medius tendon.

Surgical Incision: Retrograde Nail (Fig. 16-9)

- The incision is made either directly in line with the patellar tendon or just medial to it, per surgeon preference.
- Make a longitudinal incision from the distal pole of the patella to the tibial tubercle.
- Sharp dissection is taken down through the skin, subcutaneous tissue, and bursa.
- The paratenon is sharply incised over the patellar tendon, and medial and lateral flaps can be raised for closure at the end of the case.
- The paratenon is identified by its horizontal fibers, and the true patellar tendon is identified by its longitudinal fibers.
- The tendon may be split longitudinally through the center in line with its fibers, or a medial parapatellar incision may be made.
- The fat pad of the knee joint then is encountered; this may be excised or partially split to allow for access to the intercondylar notch.

Antegrade Femoral Nails: Key Points (Figs. 16-10, 16-11, and 16-12)

- This approach is applicable to all diaphyseal femoral fractures, including subtrochanteric and peritrochanteric variants.
- The starting point may be the greater trochanter or the piriformis fossa, depending on nail design.
- For trochanteric entry point nails, the starting point is generally the tip of the greater trochanter, 4 to 6 degrees of axis from the anatomic axis of the femur on the AP view and directly in line with the center of the femoral canal on the lateral view.

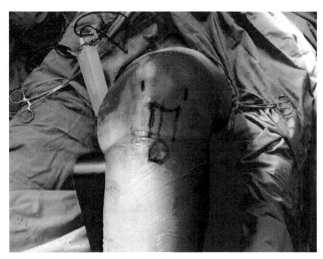

Figure 16-9 Planned incision for starting a retrograde nail. Note the flexed position of the knee over a radiolucent triangle. The incision is made in between the nose of the patella and the tibial tubercle; the patellar tendon may be split, or a medial parapatellar split may be chosen.

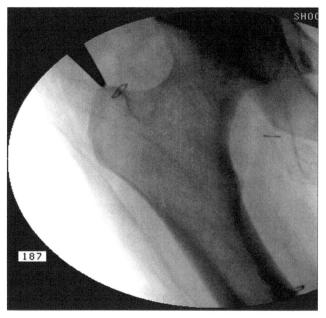

Figure 16-10 Anteroposterior fluoroscopic project shows the starting point for a trochanteric entry femoral nail at the tip of the greater trochanter, 4 to 10 degrees of axis from the femoral canal depending on the specifications of the specific nail used.

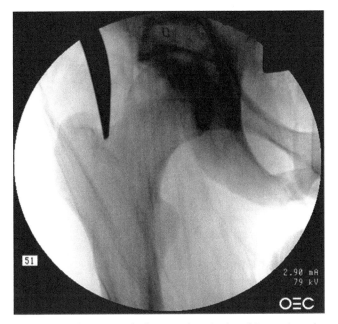

Figure 16-11 Anteroposterior fluoroscopic projection of the starting point for a piriformis entry nail with the awl positioned in the piriformis fossa.

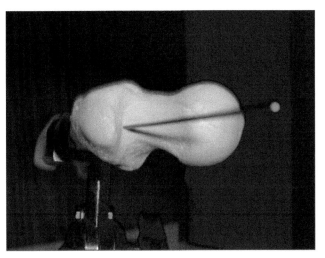

Figure 16-12 Axial view on a sawbone shows the starting point for a piriformis entry antegrade femoral nail.

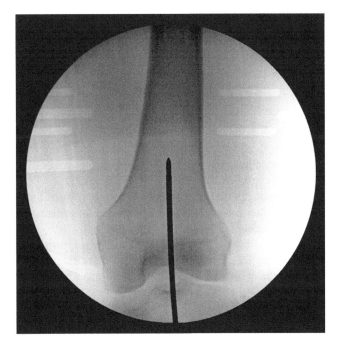

Figure 16-13 A guidewire has been placed through the starting point for a retrograde femoral nail on the anteroposterior projection; the starting point is just medial to the central apex of the intercondylar notch.

- For piriformis entry point nails, the starting point is the piriformis fossa, which is directly in line with the femoral canal on both views.
- Carefully read the technique guide for any nail with a trochanteric starting point, as entry points vary slightly depending on the proximal bend of the nail.

Retrograde Femoral Nails (Figs. 16-9, 16-13, 16-14, and 16-15)

- This approach is applicable to all diaphyseal femoral shaft fractures and distal femoral metaphyseal fractures where adequate bone stock remains to obtain purchase with distal interlocking screws.

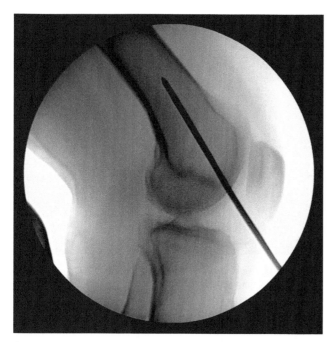

Figure 16-14 The starting point for a retrograde femoral nail is just anterior to the tip of Blumensaat's line on a lateral fluoroscopic image. A true lateral view of the knee (condyles superimposed) is critical to accurately determine the starting point.

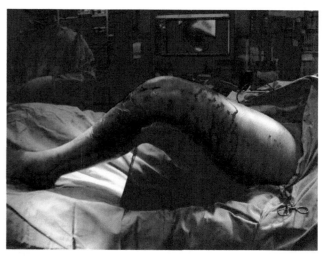

Figure 16-15 Note the use of a radiolucent triangle and several towels to act as a lever to help hold the position of the femoral shaft fracture and facilitate ease of entry into the femoral canal distally.

- This should be avoided for subtrochanteric femur fractures and peritrochanteric femur fractures.
  - The approach is helpful in obese patients.
- The starting point is just anterior to an extension of Blumensaat's line on the lateral view and in the center (or slightly medial to center) of the intercondylar notch on the AP view.
- A radiolucent triangle is used to flex the knee approximately 45 degrees, which helps to expose the starting point and facilitate fracture reduction; additional towel bumps may be used to facilitate reduction.

Technique

- For all approaches, steps for intramedullary nail placement, including reaming, nail insertion, and interlocking screw placement, are described in detail subsequently.

BRIEF SUMMARY OF SURGICAL STEPS

- Position the patient appropriately for the planned procedure
- Confirm that you can obtain and maintain an adequate reduction of the fracture with C-arm before prepping and draping
- Prep and drape the patient; ensure that a sterile field is present from at least the anterior superior iliac spine proximally and the tibial tubercle distally (prep the entire leg if on a Jackson table)
- Make incision (as described previously) and obtain a perfect starting point with a guidewire
- Drill over the guidewire with the appropriate cannulated entry reamer; drill to the appropriate entry depth, depending on manufacturer of nailing system
- Take care to use a soft tissue guide while reaming to protect the abductors
- Remove the entry guidewire
- Pass a long guidewire through the entry hole and across the fracture site
- A bend in the end of the guidewire may be helpful to facilitate passing of the wire across the fracture site
- A finger-type reducer may be helpful in passing guidewire in transverse fracture patterns, and subsequent advancement of the finger reducer across the fracture helps "set" reduction (Figs. 16-16 and 16-17, A)
- Sequentially ream with larger reamers (increase by 0.5 mm) over the guidewire until cortical "chatter" is heard
- Reaming typically begins with a 9-mm reamer
- Allow time between sequential reamings to allow intramedullary canal pressure to normalize to help avoid fat embolism
- Use the provided radiolucent ruler to measure the length of the nail
- The nail diameter should be 1 mm smaller than the diameter of the reamer used when one encounters chatter
- Take care to ensure that the guidewire is not inadvertently removed as the reamer is removed; one can use an obturator to block the exposed tip of the guidewire as the reamer is removed
- Once the desired nail diameter and length are confirmed, assemble the nail on the insertion handle on the back table; ensure that the drill guide for the proximal locking screw (typically a triple-sleeve construct) can fit through the handle with the tip of the guide aiming appropriately at the intended hole within the nail
- Pass the nail into the entry hole and across the fracture; typically the nail is inserted manually (no mallet) and rotated 90 degrees from its point of entry to the final orientation to match the bowl of the femur
- Manual pressure is used to push the nail as far distally as it will go, with care taken to use fluoroscopy to confirm the fracture is adequately reduced as the nail passes the fracture site; once resistance is reached, a mallet can be used to gently advance the nail down the canal
- Often, the nail helps to maintain alignment of the fracture itself
- Take care not to force the nail down the canal and risk blowing out one of the femoral cortices; consider rereaming if the nail does not progress down the canal
- Typically, nails are locked near the entry hole with a guide (proximal aiming device) on the insertion handle and at the opposite end with a freehand perfect circle technique

BRIEF SUMMARY OF SURGICAL STEPS—cont'd

- The vast majority of femoral nails are statically locked; dynamic locking may be used for transverse fracture patterns
  - Proximal screw insertion:
    - The drill sleeve is inserted through the aiming device to the skin, and a stab incision is made at this location through the skin and fascia
    - The drill sleeve is then advanced until it contacts the lateral cortex of the femur
    - Drill to the desired length, and measure the length off of the calibrated drill bit; then insert the appropriate length locking screw
    - Repeat previous steps for all proximal interlocking screws; verify placement via anteroposterior and lateral C-arm views to ensure the screws are through the interlocking holes in the nail
  - Distal interlocking screw insertion via freehand perfect circle technique:
    - Ensure fracture is adequately reduced, femoral rotation is appropriate, and nail is appropriately positioned
    - Magnify the C-arm image times two and localize the distal interlocking screw holes on the lateral view; these holes should be "perfect" circles; if the holes are oblong or slightly off-center, adjust the C-arm or the leg as needed
    - Use the tip of the scalpel to localize the center of the hole on the lateral view and make a stab incision; then use a hemostat to gently spread down to bone
    - Drill bicortical, taking care to ensure that the drill bit advances through the interlocking hole in the nail and not anterior or posterior to it (it is easy to skive off of cortex of the bone); if having trouble drilling on power, it can be helpful to drill unicortical down to the nail, remove the drill from the drill bit, and mallet the drill bit through the nail and through the second cortex
    - Measure the length of the screw either off of the drill bit, or with a depth gauge
    - Insert the screw manually, again taking care to ensure that the screw advances through the interlocking hole in the nail, in the path of the drill hole
    - Insert the second distal interlocking screw, repeating these steps
  - Backslap technique:
    - If one locks the distal segment first with interlocking screw (antegrade nail), a "backslap" technique can be used to pull the distal fragment proximal in retrograde fashion with a slotted mallet on the handle of the nail inserter
    - If one locks the proximal segment first (antegrade nail), traction can be released and the distal fragment can be pushed proximally with careful and gentle axial blows to the knee
- At end of every case, always check the imaging to rule out a femoral neck fracture; evaluate the knee for stability; and check alignment, rotation, and length

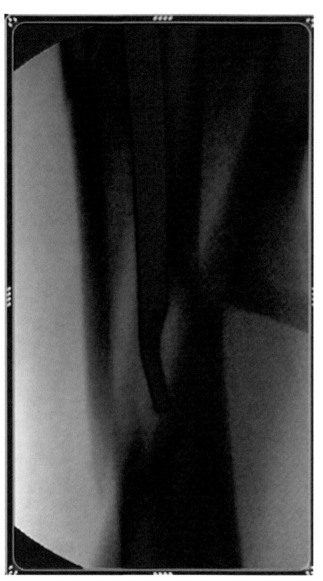

Figure 16-16 A reduction "finger" is passed across the fracture site; this cannulated instrument allows for a rigid reduction lever to reduce the proximal segment to the distal segment while passing across the fracture. A guidewire then may be introduced through the device (note that for retrograde nails, the distal segment is reduced to the proximal segment with the reduction finger).

REQUIRED EQUIPMENT

Appropriate table (Jackson table, fracture table, Hana table, etc.)

C-arm

Implant, including all available nail sizes, all interlocking screws, and preferably more than one set in case anything is dropped during the case

Sterile traction bow, sterile rope, and a traction assembly if using skeletal traction (especially with a Jackson table)

Electrocautery device and suction; be sure the base for the electrocautery device and the suction are on the opposite side of the table from where you are working to prevent them from being in the way or being knocked off during the case

Bone reduction forceps, ball-spike pusher, T-handle Chuck key, bone hooks, and Schanz pins should all be available in case an open reduction becomes necessary

Battery-powered drill and reamer, including a wire driver attachment and Chuck attachment (AO attachment and reaming adapters should be present in the vendors implant tray)

TECHNICAL PEARLS

- In bigger patients, use fluoroscopy to help identify the tip of the greater trochanter, then make the incision a handsbreadth proximal to that point
- Adduct the injured leg and move the upper body toward the opposite leg to provide for easier access to the tip of the trochanter and piriformis fossa
- Use a mallet to sink the guidewire slightly into bone when the starting point is obtained on one view; this prevents it from slipping off while you are trying to obtain the other view
- Ensure you can obtain good anteroposterior and lateral views of the injured extremity before draping and have the fluoroscopy technician memorize the positions of those views so they can be easily obtained again during the case
- All femoral nails need to be statically locked with at least one proximal and one distal interlocking screw
- Ensure that there is adequate bone-on-bone contact before interlocking; perform backslapping if necessary once the first set of interlocking screws is placed
- Always check for a femoral neck fracture before and after the case; there are usually pelvis and abdomen computed tomographic scans before surgery in trauma cases
  - Look carefully; at the end of a case, the authors recommend intraoperative fluoroscopy *and* a plain film

COMMON PITFALLS

(When to call for the attending physician)

- Accepting an inappropriate starting point, which leads to misalignment at the fracture site by forcing an anatomically shaped nail to take a nonanatomic path
- Reaming a fracture in an unreduced position: however the fracture looks while reamed it will look with the nail across it (see Fig. 16-17)
- Failure to obtain bone-on-bone contact

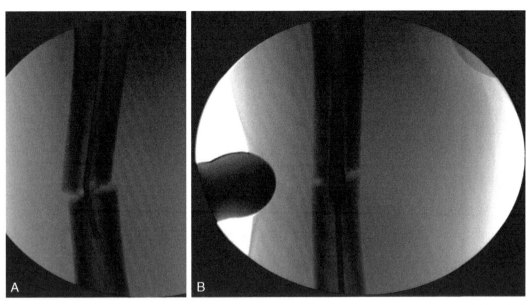

Figure 16-17 A, Reaming of a femur fracture in this position results in maintenance of this position when the nail is passed. Note the bend in the distal guidewire to facilitate directional changes of the guidewire to help with passing the nail across an angulated or displaced fracture. **B,** In this case, a padded mallet was used to provide a valgus force to correct the varus alignment, allowing for anatomic alignment while the reamer was passed across the fracture.

POSTOPERATIVE PROTOCOL

The weight-bearing status of the fractured femur is dependent on additional injuries. If the femoral shaft fracture is noncomminuted and has good cortical fit of nail, the patient can be weight-bearing as tolerated. The femur is the largest bone in the body, and weight bearing as tolerated (WBAT) without assistive devices is difficult initially. Let the patient know 2 to 4 weeks are needed to weight-bear without assistive devices.

For axially unstable fractures (i.e., comminuted, bone loss), there should be protected weight-bearing initially; full weight-bearing can commence with fracture healing at 3 months.

Patients should be instructed in physical therapy as follows: active range of motion (AROM) and active assist range of motion (AAROM) of hip, knee, and ankle. The patient should be instructed in strengthening as well. Goals given to the patient are always helpful, including: range of motion (ROM) 0 to 90 degrees at 2 weeks and ability to perform straight leg raises (SLR) within the first month. These goals can be accomplished with a home exercise program. Because of limits in physical therapy (PT) visits for each injury, formal therapy for gait training, proprioception, and increased strengthening should be reserved for when full weight-bearing and fracture is healing.

POSTOPERATIVE CLINIC VISIT PROTOCOL

The patient should return to clinic at 2 weeks for a wound and ROM check and for determination of whether limited PT is needed for supervision and advancement of a home exercise program. Additional visits for clinical evaluation and radiographs should be monthly for the first 3 months.

At the 3-month visit, full weight bearing (FWB) should begin if the patient has not been weight-bearing yet. A formal prescription for PT should be given to emphasize gait training; hip abductor, flexor, and extension strengthening; and quadriceps and hamstring strengthening. Additional exercises for proprioception are necessary.

After the 3-month visit, follow-up should occur at 18 weeks after injury to assess improvement with PT and appropriateness for return to recreational activity and work. There may still be limitations. Additional PT may be necessary.

A 6-month (24-week) visit is needed to assess advancement of activities, return to sports and work, and graduation from physical therapy. Depending on progress, a 9-month visit may be needed to assess progress.

The authors recommend a final visit at 1 year after surgery to ensure full return to function, work, or sport as before injury.

SUGGESTED READINGS

1. Moed BR, Watson JT. Intramedullary retrograde nailing of the femoral shaft. *J Am Acad Orthop Surg.* 1999;7(4):209-216.
2. Nork SE, Agel J, Russell GV, Mills WJ, Holt S, Routt ML. Mortality after reamed intramedullary nailing of bilateral femur fractures. *Clin Orthop Relat Res.* 2003;415:272-278.
3. Ostrum RF, Agarwal A, Lakatos R, Poka A. Prospective comparison of retrograde and antegrade femoral interamedullary nailing. *J Orthop Trauma.* 2000;14(7):496-501.
4. Ricci WM, Gallagher B, Haidukewych GJ. Intramedullary nailing of femoral shaft fractures. *Current Concepts.* 2009;17:296-305.
5. Stephen DJG, Kreder HJ, Schemitsch EH, Conlan LB, Wild L, McKee MD. Femoral intramedullary nailing: comparison of fracture-table and manual traction. A prospective randomized study. *J Bone Joint Surg Am.* 2002;84(9):1514-1521.

TIBIAL SHAFT FRACTURES
INTRAMEDULLARY NAILING

Matthew P. Sullivan | Samir Mehta

Tibial shaft fractures are the most common long bone fracture and the fourth most common lower extremity fracture, following proximal femur, metatarsal, and ankle fractures. They can generally be considered in the context of a low-energy mechanism that results in a torsional moment through the tibia or a high-energy mechanism that results in a direct blow to the tibia. The mechanism can give clues as to the fracture pattern. Low-energy torsional injuries often result in a spiral pattern with a fibula fracture at a different level than the tibial fracture. If the tibial shaft fracture is within the distal one third of the diaphysis and is spiral in nature, the chance of a concommitant ipsilateral posterior malleolus fracture is 39%. High-energy direct-impact injuries tend to be transverse or oblique with a fibula fracture at the same level. Likewise, high-energy tibial shaft fractures may be segmental, behaving like both a proximal one-third shaft fracture and a midshaft fracture. Often, these extremely high-energy injuries are appropriate to consider as soft tissue injuries with a broken bone underneath as the soft tissue envelope that overlies the anteromedial tibial is extremely thin and susceptible to massive insult. In these cases, it is prudent to involve a plastic surgeon early on because soft tissue coverage may be necessary to salvage the limb.

Management of tibial shaft fractures can be broadly divided into nonoperative and operative treatment. Nonoperative treatment generally requires immobilization of the knee and ankle for upward of 6 to 12 weeks. Historic criteria for nonoperative management of a tibial shaft fracture are a transverse or spiral fracture pattern with less than 5 degrees of varus/valgus and 10 degrees of flexion/extension angulation, less than 1 cm of shortening, and less than 10 degrees of malrotation. Oblique, segmental, or comminuted patterns should not be treated nonoperatively; these patterns have an extremely high likelihood of displacing. A wide array of operative management strategies exist, ranging from temporary monoplanar external fixation, to plate and screw constructs and intramedullary nailing, to thin-wire ring fixation; each has its own unique advantages and disadvantages. Reamed, locked intramedullary nailing has become the treatment of choice by most traumatologists for the majority of diaphyseal tibia fractures.

Intramedullary (IM) nailing of the tibia is appropriate for proximal one-third, midshaft, and distal one-third tibial shaft fractures. IM nailing may be combined with open reduction and internal fixation of tibial plateau fractures and tibial plafond fractures. As the fracture becomes more proximal or distal, involving the metadiaphysis or metaphysis, control of alignment and reduction becomes more challenging and the use of adjunct reduction techniques and tools may be necessary. Modern nailing systems allow a single nail design to be used for all patterns amenable to intramedullary fixation, in contrast to earlier generation nails with a long proximal (Herzog) bend. These older nails were not conducive to treatment of proximal one-third shaft fractures because the Herzog bend frequently sat at the same level as the fracture, resulting in excentuation of the apex-anterior deformity seen in proximal one-third shaft fractures. Much work has been published in the past several decades with study

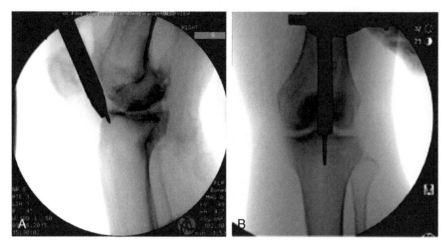

Figure 17-1 Lateral and anteroposterior fluoroscopic images of ideal tibial nail starting point. **A,** On the lateral image, note the entry point at the intersection of the articular surface and the anterior cortex. Also, note the trajectory in line with the anterior cortex of the tibia. **B,** On the anteroposterior image, note the perfect starting point in line with the medial slope of the lateral tibial spine.

of both the optimal entry point for tibial nail insertion and the various approaches available for nail insertion. Fracture pattern does not influence nail entry point. On the anteroposterior (AP) projection, the ideal entry point is on the medial slope of the lateral tibial spine. On the lateral projection, the ideal entry point is at the intersection between the anterior articular surface and the anterior shaft along the slope (Fig. 17-1).

Alhough these starting points are clearly defined, the appropriate fluoroscopic views in the operating room must be achieved with precision. At least two techniques are described for determination of the "perfect" AP projection of the proximal tibia. The fibular head bisector method uses the relationship of the proximal tibiofibular joint and the overlap of these two bones. According to this method, a perfect AP view is achieved when approximately 50% of the fibular head overlaps with the proximal tibia (Fig. 17-2). This can be problematic with a proximal tibia fracture or proximal tibiofibular joint disruption. The second method, known as the "twin peaks" view, uses the tibial spines for navigation; a perfect AP is achieved when the sharpest profile of the tibial spines is identified and found to be perpendicular to the tibial plateau. Traditionally, a perfect lateral is aquired by overlapping the medial and lateral femoral condyles on the lateral projection. For many anatomies, this method is sufficient; however, if any varus/valgus variation exists in the distal femur, this method is susceptible to error. Another method for the perfect lateral is the "flat plateau" method that relies on the proximal tibia for guidance. This technique depends on perfectly overlapping the medial and lateral plateau cortical surfaces on the lateral projection (Fig. 17-3). Regardless of the method used to determine the starting point, understanding the anatomy and having multiple checks serves the surgeon well in reproducibly locating the ideal tibial nail entry point.

Another important consideration for the surgeon is the exposure through which the nail is inserted. Essentially two broad categories of approaches can be used: traditional infrapatellar (flexed) nailing and semiextended nailing. Both allow for antegrade nailing with modern nailing systems. Infrapatellar nailing has been the classic tibial nailing technique since the advent of modern nailing; however, the introduction of semiextended nailing enhanced the the ability to treat proximal one-third shaft fractures in addition to paving the way to the next milestone in tibial nailing, the suprapatellar approach. Infrapatellar nailing typically uses a radiolucent triangle that is placed under the knee, which is flexed around 120 degrees. An infrapatellar incision is made, the patellar tendon is either split or mobilized in either direction (lateral or medial), and the nail is passed. This is in contrast to semiextended nailing, which is performed with the knee flexed approximately 15 to 20 degrees (Fig. 17-4).

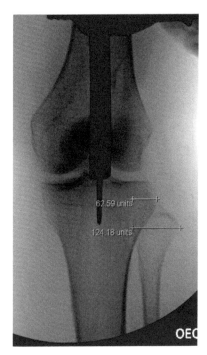

Figure 17-2 Perfect anteroposterior view of the proximal tibia with the fibular bisector method. Note the width of the proximal tibia (124 units) bisected by the lateral cortex of the proximal tibia (62 units).

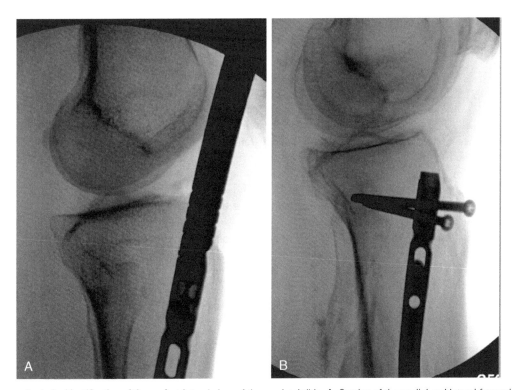

Figure 17-3 Two methods for identification of the perfect lateral view of the proximal tibia. **A,** Overlap of the medial and lateral femoral condyles is used in both rotation and varus/valgus. **B,** The flat plateau method is used in which the medial and lateral tibial plateaus are overlapped to produce a single sharp subchondral articular line.

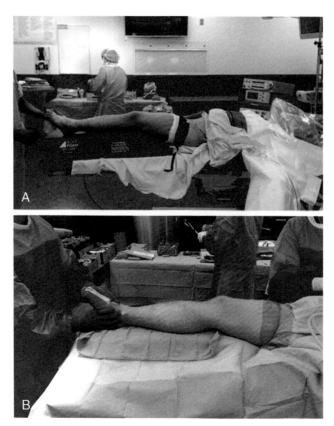

Figure 17-4 Clinical images of patient positioning for semiextended tibial nailing. **A,** Note that the patient is positioned with a bump under the ipsilateral hip and with a black foam ramp under the knee that allows for gentle flexion at the knee. **B,** The same patient is prepped and draped. The drapes are thoughtfully placed proximally, and the toes are covered. The entire leg and distal two thirds of the thigh are accessible if needed.

Semiextended nailing allows for a multitude of incision locations, including infrapatellar, paratendinous, parapatellar, and suprapatellar. The semiextended approach has two primary advantages. The first advantage is that it allows the surgeon to more easily control the deforming forces when the fracture is within the proximal one third of the shaft. Specifically, these fractures want to go into apex-anterior and valgus malalignment, with the deforming forces being the extensor mechanism and the medial hamstring muscles. Placement of the extremity in the semiextended position relaxes these forces, greatly aiding in fracture reduction. The second major advantage is the ease with which fluoroscopic images are obtained. With the tibia parallel to the floor, AP and lateral C-arm positioning becomes straightforward, with both images being taken orthogonal to the base of the machine and the floor. This is in contrast to flexed nailing, which requires a fair amount of technical skill on the part of the image intensifier operator to obtain excellent fluoroscopic images.

For the purposes of this technical chapter, the authors focus on semiextended tibial nailing through the suprapatellar approach.

SURGICAL TECHNIQUE

Room Set-Up

- The operating table is positioned slightly toward the ipsilateral side of the room as the injured extremity.

- An image intensifier is brought in from the contralateral side of the patient as the injured extremity.

Patient Positioning

- The patient is positioned supine, with the patient at the distal-most aspect of the bed (feet at edge of bed), and pulled over to the ipsilateral side of the bed.
- A small rolled blanket bolster (bump) is placed under the ipsilateral hip/flank.
- The ipsilateral arm is placed over the chest.
- The contralateral arm is out to the side.
- The contralateral leg is padded with egg crate and taped to the bed to prevent moving if the table is airplaned.
- A tourniquet is applied to the ipsilateral thigh as proximal as possible. *Do not inflate.*
- A radiolucent foam ramp is placed under the ipsilateral extremity (knee flexes to 15 to 20 degrees; tibia lies parallel to the floor).
- An impervious sticky U-drape is applied just distal to the tourniquet to ensure that the distal one half of the thigh is fully exposed and prepped into the surgical field.

Prepping and Draping

- Because of the instability of the limb when the tibia is fractured, two people are generally needed for sterile prep. One assistant is responsible for holding the extremity with sterile gloves, and the other assistant applies the nonsterile scrub followed by sterile prepping product of choice from tourniquet to toes.
- The limb should *not* be held up with a candy cane and stirrup from the toes. This set-up has the potential to further displace or comminute the fracture and cause soft tissue injury.
- Once sterile prep is completed, the limb may be rested on a sterile sheet while the surgeons scrub their hands.
- Once gowned and gloved, the surgeons should first cover the toes with an impervious draping material, such as a sterile incision drape or a stockinette. The toes harbor a unique array of microorganisms that are best kept away from the surgical site and may not be fully erradicated during the sterile prep.
- Next, a sterile U-shaped drape should be placed proximally, followed by an extremity drape (drape with hole cut out in it).
- The most superficial drape should be tightly sealed to the skin proximally with a strip of sterile incision tape.
- Finally, a side drape should be placed to assist in maintaining sterility during lateral fluoroscopic imaging.

Surgical Approach for Suprapatellar Nailing

- A straight skin incision should be marked out from the superior pole of the patella and extend proximally for approximately 3 cm.
- Sharply incise through skin and subcutaneous fat to, but not through, the quadiceps tendon epitendinous tissue.
- With a sponge, bluntly clear fat from the quadriceps tendon.
- The incision through the quadriceps tendon should be 2 to 3 cm in length and full thickness, in line with its fibers. This incision should be placed 3 to 4 mm medially off midline in the event that the approach is converted to a medial parapatellar approach.
- Once through tendon, bluntly dissect into the patellofemoral joint with a finger.
- Frequently, one encounters a synovial thickening that is tethering the superior-medial pole of the patella to the joint capsule. This may be released with heavy curved shears (Mayo scissors). Any additional synovial folds that appear to be limiting patella excursion may also be released.

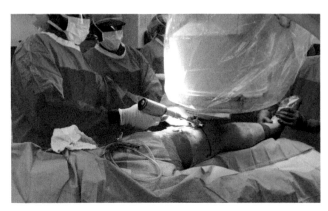

Figure 17-5 Clinical images of the reaming stage of suprapatellar nailing. Note that the surgeon's left hand is firmly holding the protective sleeve distally against the tibial plateau, protecting the patella articular cartilage from damage, and that the right hand is managing the reamer.

- For the instrumentation to safely be passed through the knee, the surgeon's index finger should fit into the patellofemoral joint. If the joint continues to remain very tight, the incision should be lengthened into a medial parapatellar approach.
- Understanding the instrumentation is critical for this procedure. Each manufacturer with suprapatellar instrumentation uses some variation of protection sleeve to keep patellofemoral joint cartilage uninjured during passage of reamers. The surgeon must remain vigilant throughout the procedure that the protection sleeve remains docked on the tibia as reamers are being passed in and out of the knee (Fig. 17-5).

Surgical Approach for Parapatellar Nailing

- Classically, the semiextended parapatellar approach as described by Tornetta and Collins uses a medial parapatellar incision. In the authors' experience, however, some knees are more amenable to a medial parapatellar approach, and others are more amenable to a lateral parapatellar approach. The patella should be evaluated before incision, and whichever side apprears to provide the most tension-free access to the entry point should be used.
  - Regardless of which side of the patella the incision is made, the dissection remains the same.
- The approach is intracapsular and extraarticular/extrasynovial. The joint should not be entered. A longitudinal, 2-cm to 3-cm skin incision should be placed about the distal two thirds of the patella. Blunt dissection is carried down to retinacular tissue, which is then cleared with a sponge.
- The retinacular tissue is sharply incised in line with the skin incision, with care taken not to violate the synovial layer that is adhered to its undersurface.
- Once through retinaculum, a tissue plane is developed between synovium and retinaculum with dissecting shears. This plane is carried distally into the infrapatellar pouch behind the patella tendon placing the surgeon directly onto the tibial plateau, while remaining extraarticular.

Nail Entry Point and Trajectory

- A detailed description of the nail entry point may be found in the introductory paragraphs (see Figs. 17-1, 17-2, and 17-3).
- After an optimal entry point is achieved, the trajectory of the nail's path is created. On the AP fluoroscopic view, the trajectory should be straight down the shaft, bisecting the intramedullary canal at the isthmus. On the lateral view, the trajectory should be nearly parallel or slightly posteriorly directed (no more that 5 to 10 degrees) relative to the anterior cortex of the tibia.

- Once the principles of the starting point and nail trajectory are understood, the cortex must be opened. Two basic ways exist to accomplish this task. The first is with an awl, which typically comes on the instrument tray for the nailing system. The second, which is the authors' preferred method, is through the use of a guidewire followed by an opening reamer.
- The guidewire is handheld and placed into the ideal entry point and trajectory. It is provisionally malleted into the cortex, then driven in to a depth of 4 cm with a power wire driver.
- Once the guidewire is sunk to its final depth, its correct position should be scrutinized with fluoroscopy. This is the last opportunity to adjust the entry point before creating a large cortical entry hole.
- The next step is to open ream the cortex. From this point and moving forward, one must ensure that the patellofemoral protection sleeve remains seated on the tibia to protect the articular cartilage.
- Care should be taken to meticulously guide the opening reamer through the metaphyseal bone. Changing the trajectory of the reamer is very easy, even with the guidewire in place. As such, this step should be performed with fluoroscopic assistance. Open reaming only needs to be applied to the proximal 4 to 5 cm of the tibia.

Fracture Reduction, Reaming, and Nail Insertion

- With the cortex now opened, the surgeon must pass a long ball-tip guidewire over which the nail will pass. This wire is placed into the medullary canal, across the fracture site, and seated into the distal tibia. It is not critical that the fracture be perfectly reduced to pass the ball-tip guidewire in isthmus fractures. However, in proximal or distal third fractures, where *canal-to-nail diameter mismatch* will occur, the fracture should be reduced before the guidewire is placed.
  - Distally, the ball-tip guidewire (and ultimately the nail) should sit in the center of the ankle in the coronal plain, which correlates to just slightly off-center laterally in the distal tibia. It should not be placed more distal than the physeal scar (Fig. 17-6).
  - Finally, once the wire is seated, it should be measured to determine the length of the ultimate nail.
- Many techniques exist for fracture reduction, but it should be appreciated that passage of the nail is not a reduction technique, particularly in nonisthmus fractures.
  - Several of the reduction techniques that the surgeon should be familiar with include manual traction, strategic placement of bumps and clamps, unicortical plating, use of cortical replacing screws (also known as Poller or blocking screws), and mechanical traction through an external fixator or commercially available distractor (i.e., large universal distractor).
- The importance of reducing the fracture before reaming cannot be overstated. Failure to do so may result in eccentric reaming at the fracture site and ultimately a malreduction, which may be very difficult to overcome on passage of the nail. Furthermore, the surgeon may choose to ream up to the fracture and push the reamer across as opposed to ream across the fracture. This technique may help to mitigate the risk of eccentrically reaming at the fracture.
- Reamer size may be increased sequentially until "chatter" is heard when the reamer encounters the canal at the isthmus. In general, the authors take 1 to 1.5 mm off the largest reamer that was passed to determine nail diameter.
- Once the dimensions of the nail are determined and the nail has been opened, the surgeon and scrub nurse should apply the jig together, and the slots should be checked to ensure that the jig and the interlocking holes line up perfectly.
- The nail then is placed over the guidewire and a mallet used to put into place. Use of fluoroscopic assistance is critical to pass the nail at three specific locations.

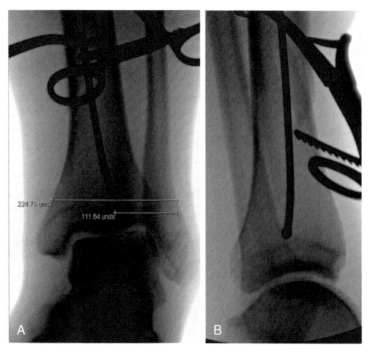

Figure 17-6 Appropriate guidewire placement is confirmed on the anteroposterior and lateral views of the ankle. **A,** Note that the tip of the guidewire is slightly off-center lateral in the distal tibia. This corresponds to the center of the ankle. **B,** On the lateral view, note that the guidewire is positioned centrally from anterior to posterior. In both views, the ball tip is seated down to the dense physeal scar.

- The first location is as the nail is crossing the fracture. Careless passage of the nail can significantly comminute or displace the fracture (Fig. 17-7).
  - The next is distally to ensure that the nail has not breached the tibial plafond and entered the ankle (Fig. 17-8).
  - Finally, a lateral image at the knee ensures that the nail is buried with the proximal tibia (Fig. 17-9).
- Interlocking the nail both proximally and distally is the final step. In general, the nail is first interlocked proximally, then distally; however, in certain situations, the surgeon may choose to interlock distally first.
  - A common example of this is when the fracture pattern is simple-transverse and the surgeon wishes to backslap the nail to compress across the fracture. In this situation, the nail is interlocked distally, and then a slap hammer is applied to the jig proximally, hammering cephalad and compressing at the fracture site.
- Most commercially available nails have between three and five holes proximally and three and four holes distally for interlocking bolts. The exact number of interlocking bolts for any particular fracture pattern has not been defined in the literature; however, in general, at least two bolts should be placed proximally and at least two bolts should be placed distally.
  - As many as three to five bolts should be placed proximally in proximal one-third shaft fractures. These tend to be very unstable injuries with strong deforming forces in an area of relatively poor quality bone. In addition, oblique or off-axis bolt placement may result in a stiffer construct; however, there is conflicting literature to support this.
- Interlocking bolt diameter plays an important role in load to failure. Whenever possible, 5.0-mm bolts should be used. Most nailing systems allow for the use of a 5.0-mm screw in nails over 8.5 or 9 mm in diameter. Larger diameter bolts allow for earlier weight-bearing.
- Proximal interlocking bolts are placed through the jig that was used to introduce the nail. Because of the vital neurovascular structures in the posterior knee, drilling for these bolts should be performed carefully. Distal interlocking bolts may be

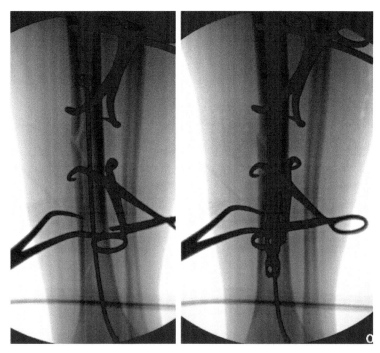

Figure 17-7 Imaging is performed as the nail passes across the fracture. This allows the surgeon to identify a nail-related malreduction.

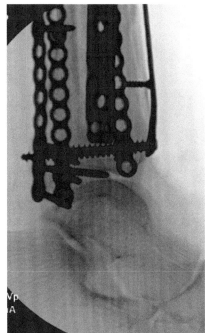

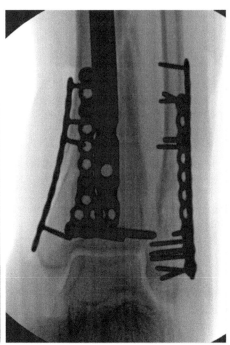

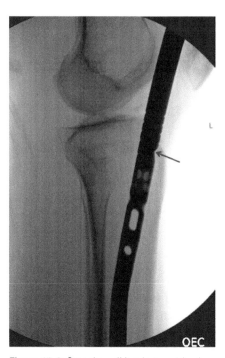

Figure 17-8 In this combined tibial plafond/tibial shaft fracture, magnified imaging of the ankle shows proper nail distalization to maximize nail working length before interlocking while at the same time ensuring that the nail has not breached the tibial plafond.

Figure 17-9 Once the nail has been put in place with a mallet, perfect imaging at the knee defines whether or not the nail remains proud or has been adequately sunk into tibia. Understanding the markings on the particular instrumentation that is being used is essential. In this system, the *arrow* points to the proximal end of the nail and thus an appropriately sunk nail.

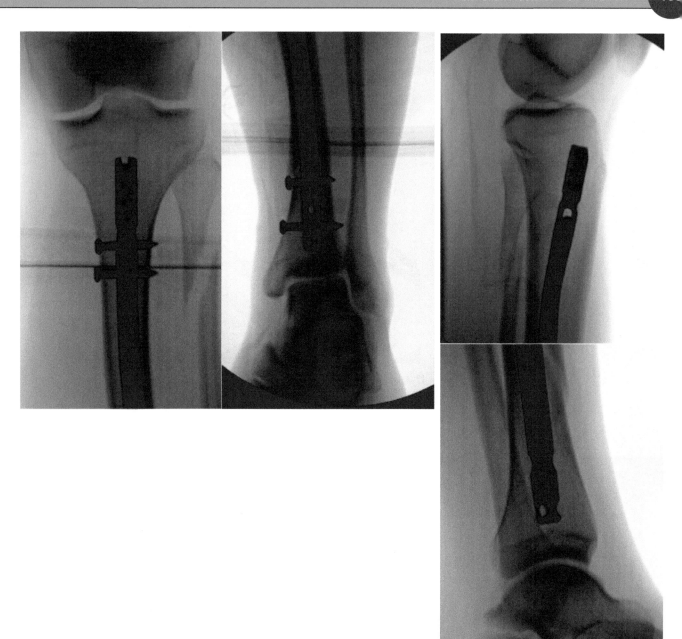

Figure 17-10 Final fluoroscopic imaging shows that two interlocking bolts have been placed both proximally and distally and that their positions are both bicortical and through their intended holes with in the nail.

placed freehand (perfect circle technique), with electromagnetic probe assistance (Trigen Sureshot, Smith and Nephew, Smith and Nephew Inc., Andover, MA) or an outrigger extension that some nail systems have available.

■ Once the nail has been interlocked both proximally and distally, final fluoroscopic images should be taken to confirm all bolts pass through the nail and have been seated appropriately (Fig. 17-10).

BRIEF SUMMARY OF SURGICAL STEPS

- Make suprapatellar incision and arthrotomy
- Introduce protection sleeve and place guidewire into nail entry point; confirm location with fluoroscopy
- Open the proximal tibial cortex with entry reamer
- Reduce the fracture
- Pass ball-tip guidewire into intermedullary canal across fracture and into the physeal scar of distal tibia
- Measure nail length over guidewire
- Ream canal while maintaining the fracture in a reduced position
- Place the nail and interlock proximally and distally

REQUIRED EQUIPMENT

Radiolucent table from waist to toes

Tibial nailing instruments and implants

Radiolucent ramp, towels or foam

Image intensfier

Tourniquet

Distractor or external fixator

Small fragment set

All-purpose fracture surgery instruments

TECHNICAL PEARLS

- The only absolute contraindication to suprapatellar nailing is a patellofemoral joint that is too tight to accept the specialized instruments. If a knee flexion contracture is noted before surgery, suprapatellar nailing should not be attempted. During surgery, if the surgeon's finger cannot slide into the patellofemoral joint, even after synovial fold releases, the incision should be carried medially for a medial parapatellar approach.
- Care should be taken to achieve perfect anteroposterior and lateral imaging based on the landmarks described previously. Without this, the surgeon cannot be confident in the entry point.
- The nail entry point is critical for this procedure. As such, extra time should be taken to ensure that it is optimal. This is particularly important for fractures proximal to the isthmus. A poorly placed entry point can result in a malreduction that requires advanced nailing techniques to correct.
- Trajectory is critical as well, and all attempts should be made to achieve a perfect trajectory with the guidewire; however, trajectory can be altered with the reamer once the cortex is opened.
- The protection sleeve must be maintained snuggly against the tibial cortex during reaming to protect the patellofemoral joint.
- An anatomic reduction of the fracture is impossible if the fracture is malreduced at the time of reaming. As such, care should be taken to (1) reduce and maintain a reduction during the entire reaming process and (2) push the reamer across the fracture (rather than ream across the fracture). Failure to do either of these results in eccentric reaming and a malreduction.
- The nail should be sunk below the cortical bone of the proximal tibia to prevent prominence into the joint.
- Fracture pattern and location dictate how many interlocking bolts to place proximally and distally. Whenever possible, 5.0-mm or greater diameter bolts should be used.

COMMON PITFALLS

(When to call for the attending physician)

- Unable to reduce the fracture manually before reaming
- Considering use of adjunctive/advanced reduction techniques: distractor, cortical replacing screws, unicortical plate
- Reaming has comminuted or displaced the fracture
- Nail passage has comminuted or displaced the fracture
- The nail has been incorrectly measured and is distracting the fracture
- After interlocking bolts have been placed and the limb clinically appears to be malrotated
- Violation of the proximal posterior cortex of the tibia
- Inability to easily pass the nail over the guidewire during insertion

POSTOPERATIVE PROTOCOL

Currently, there is inconclusive evidence to guide postoperative weight-bearing after tibial nailing. Femoral nailing studies suggest that immediate full weight-bearing is safe even in the setting of comminuted fractures when at least two distal interlocking bolts greater than 5.0 mm have been placed.

The tibial nailing data are more difficult to interpret. Specifically, when the risk of autodynamization (i.e., interlocking bolt breakage) is significant, immediate full weight-bearing may lead to increased adverse events; however, when the risk of auto-dynamization is low, full weight-bearing may greatly facilitate fracture union. The surgeon must always weigh the benefits of early mobilization in the traumatized patient with the risk of delayed union or malunion as a result of early mobilization. At the authors' institution, the default postoperative protocol after nailing of any kind is full weight-bearing, with exceptions made when severe bone loss is present.

Likewise, the use of chemical venous thromboembolism (VTE) prophylaxis is equally ill-guided by the literature. A reasonable amount of literature and specific guidelines support the use of chemical prophylaxis in polytrauma patients with pelvis fractures. In contrast, little to no primary literature support its use in isolated tibial shaft fractures. At the authors' institution, after tibial nailing, if patients are otherwise uninjured and will be allowed to bear weight, they are typically not managed with chemical VTE prophylaxis. Certainly, this is highly situation-specific and patient-specific, and the need for VTE chemoprophylaxis must be evaluated in the context of other injuries, comorbidities, and risk factors for VTE.

POSTOPERATIVE CLINIC VISIT PROTOCOL

Patients with isolated tibial shaft fractures that have been nailed are typically seen in the clinic first at 2 weeks for a wound check and suture removal. It is not the authors' practice to obtain radiographs at this time unless specific concern exists, such as obvious malalignment.

The patient is then typically seen again at 6 weeks after surgery to assess functional gains and obtain radiographs. At this point, there should be radiographic evidence of healing. If there is no evidence of healing, interventions may be made, such as vitamin supplementation, smoking cessation, nutrition counseling, and continued physiotherapy.

Once out of the 6-week window, if there is radiographic and clinical evidence of healing, the patient is seen back at 3 months, 6 months, and finally 1 year. Radiographs are obtained at each of those visits.

SUGGESTED READINGS

1. Bible JE, Choxi AA, Dhulipala SC, Evans JM, Mir HR. Tibia-based referencing for standard proximal tibial radiographs during intramedullary nailing. *Am J Orthop.* 2013;42(11):E95-E98.
2. Boraiah S, Gardner MJ, Helfet DL, Lorich DG. High association of posterior malleolus fractures with spiral distal tibial fractures. *Clin Orthop Relat Res.* 2008;466(7):1692-1698.
3. Brumback RJ, Toal TR, Murphy-Zane MS, Novak VP, Belkoff SM. Immediate weight-bearing after treatment of a comminuted fracture of the femoral shaft with a statically locked intramedullary nail. *J Bone Joint Surg Am.* 1999;81(11):1538-1544.
4. Chen AL, Tejwani NC, Joseph TN, Kummer FJ, Koval KJ. The effect of distal screw orientation on the intrinsic stability of a tibial intramedullary nail. *Bull Hosp Jt Dis.* 2001-2002;60(2):80-83.
5. Court-Brown CM, Caesar B. Epidemiology of adult fractures: a review. *Injury.* 2006;37(8):691-697.
6. Freeman AL, Craig MR, Schmidt AH. Biomechanical comparison of tibial nail stability in a proximal third fracture: do screw quantity and locked, interlocking screws make a difference? *J Orthop Trauma.* 2011;25(6):333-339.
7. Laflamme GY, Heimlich D, Stephen D, Kreder HJ, Whyne CM. Proximal tibial fracture stability with intramedullary nail fixation using oblique interlocking screws. *J Orthop Trauma.* 2003;17(7):496-502.
8. Rogers FB, Cipolle MD, Velmahos G, Rozycki G, Luchette FA. Practice management guidelines for the prevention of venous thromboembolism in trauma patients: the EAST practice management guidelines work group. *J Trauma.* 2002;53(1):142-164.
9. Schemitsch EH, Bhandari M, Guyatt G, et al. Prognostic factors for predicting outcomes after intramedullary nailing of the tibia. *J Bone Joint Surg Am.* 2012;94(19):1786-1793.
10. Walker RM, Zdero R, McKee MD, Waddell JP, Schemitsch EH. Ideal tibial intramedullary nail insertion point varies with tibial rotation. *J Orthop Trauma.* 2011;25(12):726-730.

PEDIATRIC TECHNIQUES
SUPRACONDYLAR HUMERUS FRACTURE PERCUTANEOUS FIXATION

Brandon M. Tauberg | Martin J. Herman | Scott M. Doroshow

CASE MINIMUM REQUIREMENTS

- N = 5 Supracondylar humerus percutaneously

COMMONLY USED CPT CODES

- CPT Code: 24538—Percutaneous skeletal fixation of supracondylar/transcondylar humerus fracture with or without intercondylar extension
- CPT Code: 24566—Percutaneous treatment of humeral epicondylar fracture, medial or lateral with manipulation
- CPT Code: 24582—Percutaneous treatment of humerus condylar fracture, medial or lateral with manipulation

COMMONLY USED ICD9 CODES

- 812.41—Supracondylar humerus fracture, closed
- 812.51—Supracondylar humerus fracture, open

COMMONLY USED ICD10 CODES

- S42.41—Simple supracondylar fracture without intercondylar fracture of humerus
- S42.42—Comminuted supracondylar fracture without intercondylar fracture of humerus

Supracondylar humerus fractures are the most common elbow fracture in children and account for 3% to 18% of all pediatric fractures. Children typically are between ages 5 and 7 years, and boys and girls are affected equally. The nondominant hand, usually the left hand, is more commonly injured. Extension-type fractures are more common, accounting for 98% of supracondylar fractures, and are typically caused by a fall onto an outstretched hand with the elbow in full extension (Fig. 18-1). Forceful extension of the elbow brings the tip of the olecranon into the olecranon fossa and leads to an extension force that causes the distal humerus to fail anteriorly in the supracondylar area, where a thin segment of bone separates the medial and lateral columns of the distal humerus (Fig. 18-2). Flexion-type fractures comprise the other 2% and are typically a result of a child falling directly onto the posterior aspect of the flexed elbow (Fig. 18-3).

The child with a supracondylar fracture typically presents with pain and swelling around the elbow, limited and painful active elbow motion, and a deformity of the arm if displacement has occurred. Because other ipsilateral fractures can occur, most commonly fractures of the distal radius, the entire extremity should be evaluated carefully, including the soft tissues for swelling, ecchymosis, and lacerations. Open supracondylar fractures are rare but must be considered when a wound is identified around the distal humerus and antecubital fossa. A thorough neurovascular examination should be performed because approximately 11% of patients with supracondylar fractures have a nerve injury. *Extension-type fractures* may have neuropraxia of the anterior interosseous (most common), median, radial, and ulnar (least common) nerves. The ulnar nerve is most commonly injured in *flexion-type fractures.* Vascular status is critical to assess as well with palpation of the radial pulse and determination that the hand and fingers are warm and well-perfused. Hand and finger perfusion are sometimes better indicators of vascular status than the presence of a pulse because the brachial artery may be in spasm or collaterals may provide distal circulation. All patients with abnormal vascular examination results (i.e., a pulseless, pink hand or dysvascular limb) need emergent surgery.

The decision to surgically explore the brachial artery in the patient with a supracondylar humerus fracture with a perfused hand but no palpable radial pulse is controversial. Certainly, pediatric supracondylar fractures with pulseless, poorly perfused limbs should undergo emergent operative reduction and fixation, and if the hand remains pulseless *and* poorly perfused after fixation, the artery should be explored and reconstructed if necessary. In the setting of a supracondylar fracture with a pulseless but well-perfused limb, the fracture should also undergo emergent operative reduction and fixation; however, if the limb remains pulseless but well-perfused, one can consider immediate vascular exploration or observation for 24 to 48 hours for return of pulse.

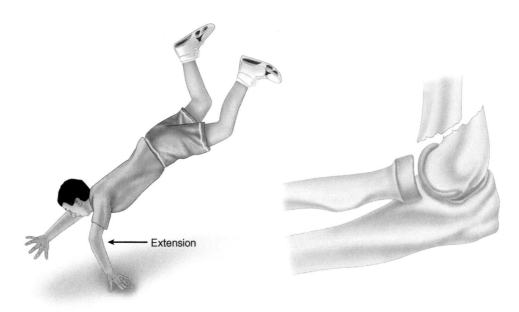

Figure 18-1 Supracondylar humerus fractures are most commonly extension-type, occuring when a child falls onto an oustretched arm with the elbow locked in extension.

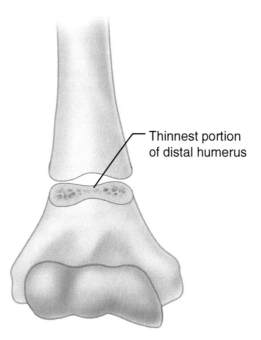

Thinnest portion of distal humerus

Figure 18-2 Supracondylar fractures occur in the thinnest part of the distal humerus, where the bone is most unstable.

The purpose of this chapter is to describe the surgical technique for closed reduction, percutaneous pinning of extension-type supracondylar humerus fractures in children.

Anteroposterior (AP) and lateral radiographic views of the elbow are used to diagnose and classify supracondylar fractures. The modified Gartland system is the most common radiographic classification system for supracondylar humerus fractures and management of fractures correlates with the fracture type (Table 18-1). Other radiographic findings are used to further define supracondylar humerus fractures. Initial images may be negative except for a posterior fat pad sign, a finding that correlates with a type 1 supracondylar fracture. On a true lateral radiograph, the anterior humeral line, drawn along the anterior humeral cortex and extended distally to the level of the capitellum, should cross the capitellum through the middle third in children older than 3 years of age; significant extension deformity is present when the capitellum is posterior to the anterior humeral line in an extension type fracture (Fig. 18-4). Baumann's angle is defined as the angle between the long axis at the humeral shaft and the physeal line of the lateral condyle. Typically, this angle is between 9 and 26 degrees, and as a general rule, any angle less than 10 degrees is considered to be a fracture in varus angulation (Fig. 18-5).

Before the wide viability of fluoroscopy and familiarity with closed pinning techniques, most displaced supracondylar fractures were treated with closed reduction and splinting or casting. In the modern era, nearly all displaced supracondylar humerus fractures are treated with closed reduction and percutaneous fixation with K-wires (Video 18-1). Although most fractures may be operated on the "next day" after injury (ideally within 8 to 12 hours from injury), important exceptions that demand emergency surgery include open fractures or those that are at risk for becoming open because of skin compromise, those associated with an ipsilateral fracture in the forearm or wrist, and those with abnormal vascular examination results. Open reduction is used when acceptable reduction cannot be achieved via closed techniques, for open fractures, and for injuries associated with nerve or vascular compromise that require exploration.

TABLE 18-1	THE GARTLAND CLASSIFICATION OF SUPRACONDYLAR HUMERUS FRACTURES	
CLASS	**EXAMINATION**	**TREATMENT**
Type I	Elbow pain/swelling Possible posterior fad pad sign	Nonoperative; 3 to 4 weeks of long-arm cast immobilization with the elbow flexed to 90 degrees and neutral forearm rotation
Type II	Hinged posteriorly On imaging, the anterior humeral line can be seen anterior to the capitellum	See subtype treatments below
Type IIA	Extended without rotational abnormality or fragment translation	Closed reduction and casting, with close observation for displacement
Type IIB	Some degree of rotational translation or displacement	Closed reduction and pinning
Type III	Completely displaced fracture without cortical contact	Closed reduction and pinning Can delay within 12 to 18 hours of injury
Type IV	Displaces into both flexion and extension, which is diagnosed with manipulation with imaging	Modified pinning technique that prevents the arm from being rotated

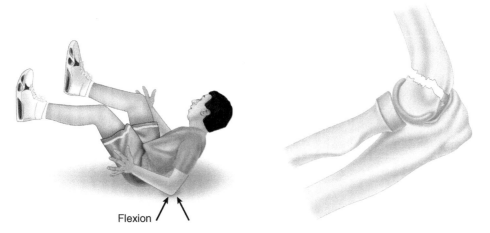

Flexion

Figure 18-3 Flexion-type supracondylar humerus fractures, although less common, occur when a child falls directly onto the apex of a flexed elbow.

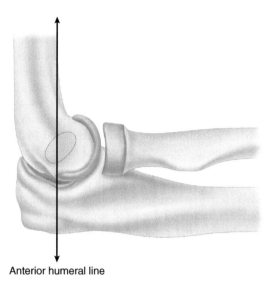

Figure 18-4 The anterior humeral line is a radiographic marker on the lateral radiograph that helps to determine the presence of a supracondylar humerus fracture.

Anterior humeral line

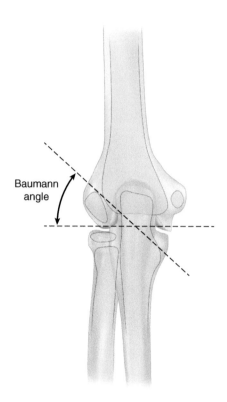

Baumann angle

Figure 18-5 Baumann's angle is a radiographic marker on the anteroposterior radiograph that helps to determine the presence of a supracondylar humerus fracture.

SURGICAL TECHNIQUE

Room Set-Up

- The bed is placed in the center of the room with appropriate access to anesthesia.
- A short radiolucent armboard is used (as an option, some surgeons use the sterile draped C-arm platform as the operating table).
- A fluoroscopy (C-arm) unit must be available.
- Stools are placed on either side of the armboard (or C-arm) for the surgeon and first assistant.
- The fluoroscopy monitor is positioned on the opposite side of the bed.

Patient Positioning

- The patient is positioned supine on the operating table, all the way to the side of the table.
- The arm must be distal enough on the armboard (or C-arm platform) that the elbow may be visualized with fluoroscopy; small children may need their entire shoulder/elbow on the board (Fig. 18-6).
- The monitor of the fluoroscopy unit is positioned so that the surgeon only has to look up from the surgical field without looking sideways or backwards.

Prepping and Draping

- Prophylactic intravenous antibiotics are administered before prepping.
- After induction of anesthesia, the patient's arm may be prepped and draped in sterile fashion, with all personnel gowned and the field fully draped.

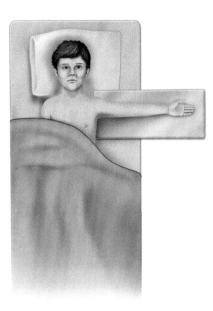

Figure 18-6 The child's elbow must be centered on the armboard to visualize the supracondylar area with fluoroscopy; sometimes the child's shoulder also needs to be on the board.

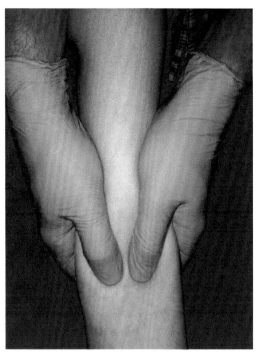

Figure 18-7 The "milking maneuver" may be used if the fracture fragment pierces the brachialis, "milking" the piece from proximal to distal to reduce it beneath the muscle.

- Alternatively, semisterile technique may be used because results are similar; the limb is prepped sterilely and the surgeon and assistant wear sterile gloves, but gowns and drapes of the entire field are not used.

Reduction

- Apply longitudinal traction with the elbow flexed to about 20 to 30 degrees while an assistant provides countertraction against the upper arm.
- The "milking maneuver" may be used if the proximal fragment has pierced the brachialis. The biceps is "milked" proximal to distal, past the proximal fragment until a palpable release of the humeral shaft posteriorly (Fig. 18-7).
- Correct varus/valgus angular alignment by moving the forearm. Direct movment of the distal fragment can be done with the surgeon's thumb to correct medial/lateral fracture translation. Correct malrotation by securing the humeral shaft while rotating the forearm and distal fracture fragment together. Slowly flex the elbow while applying anterior pressure with the thumb placed on the olcranon (Fig. 18-8).
- If the fracture cannot be reduced and a rubbery or no bone-on-bone feeling is experienced, the fracture likely needs an open reduction to remove the soft tissue or potentially the neurovascular structures (median nerve or brachial artery) from the fracture site.
  - Excessive manipulation greater than two to three attempts at closed reduction can lead to excessive swelling and increase the risk for development of a compartment syndrome.
- After reduction, hold the elbow flexed and the forearm pronated. Check the reduction with fluroscopy in the AP by shooting through the forearm (Jones view). The lateral view is obtained by rotating the humeral shaft, not the forearm, to ensure that reduction is not lost.
- Up to approximately 25% to 30% of translation of the distal fragment is acceptable in either plane, as is a mild-moderate amount of rotational malalignment. The anterior humeral line should intersect the capitellum.

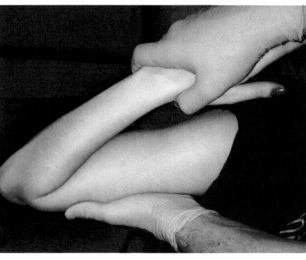

Figure 18-9 The elbow is kept hyperflexed after reduction to prevent its loss during pinning.

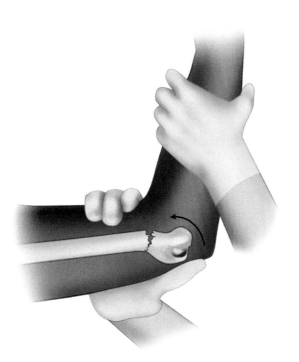

Reduction maneuver

Figure 18-8 Applying anterior pressure at the elbow with the thumb while slowly flexing the arm is a common maneuver used to reduce supracondylar fracture.

- After reduction, the elbow may be taped in a reduced position of elbow hyperflexion or be held by an assistant to prevent loss of the reduction during pinning (Fig. 18-9).

Pin Placement

- Position the elbow on a towel and palpate the lateral humeral condyle.
- A smooth K-wire (also called a pin), usually 0.062-inch in diameter, is held against the lateral condyle without piercing the skin, and placement is confirmed on AP fluoroscopy.
- If correctly positioned, the K-wire is placed through the skin into the cartilage of the distal lateral condyle, and the start point and trajectory are confirmed with fluoroscopy.
- The wire is advanced with a drill, engaging the distal fragment and then the medial cortex of the humerus proximal to the fracture site.
  - The feel of the wire advancing through the proximal cortex indicates that the wire has bicortical purchase, a key to stable fixation.
  - The pin may cross the olecranon fossa to increase the number of cortices captured by the pin, thus improving fixation, but the arm is not fully able to extend until the pin is removed.
- Typically, two lateral pins are used to stabilize type II fractures, and three lateral pins are used to stabilize type III fractures. In the coronal plane, the ideal pin configuration is one in which all wires are divergent and maximally spread across the fracture site, with at least one pin bridging the medial column of the distal humerus. In the sagittal plane, wires ideally pass through the capitellum starting in the anterior half of the bone but are directed 10 to 15 degrees posteriorly. Lateral pins are preferred because they decrease ulnar nerve injury, but medial pins may be needed if comminution is present or stability cannot be achieved with lateral pins only (Fig. 18-10).

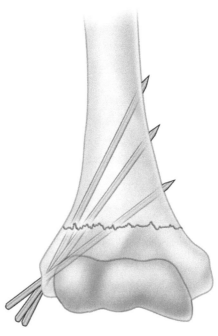

Divergent pinning

Figure 18-10 Proper pinning of a supracondylar humerus fracture in the anteroposterior plane, with maximal pin separating at the fracture site, engaging the medial and lateral column and engaging both sides of the fracture.

- Confirm reduction with AP, lateral, and oblique fluoroscopic views. If the pin configuration and reduction are acceptable, the fracture stability then is assessed by stressing the elbow with live fluoroscopy in valgus/varus and flexion/extension. Additional fixation or revision of fixation is done if the fracture is unstable.
- After reduction and fixation, recheck vascular status with the elbow extended.
  - For the arm that was dysvascular before reduction, emergent vascular exploration should be performed if no hand perfusion returns within 20 minutes after reduction and fixation (the time at which vascular spasm typically resolves).
  - If the hand is not well-perfused after reduction but the vascular status was normal before reduction, the brachial artery may be entrapped in the fracture site and requires exploration.
  - An extremity with a well-perfused hand, even without a palpable radial pulse, may be observed after surgery and does not require emergent exploration.
- Save reduction images that look the least reduced so that these images may be referred to if there is a concern for loss of reduction at follow-up.
- Bend the wires and cut them 1 to 2 cm off the skin.
- Place a sterile felt square or an antimicrobial disc with a slit cut into it around the wires where the skin is entered to protect the skin from the wires as the postoperative splint or cast is placed.

Splinting/Casting

- After surgery, immobilize the arm with a long-arm posterior splint that extends from the shoulder to the metacarpals heads, positioning the elbow at 60 to 80 degrees of flexion.
- Alternatively, a long arm cast that is bivalved may be applied in the operating room. This may then be overwrapped before discharge.
- A sling and swathe is sometimes applied to effectively immobilize children younger than 3 to 4 years of age.

BRIEF SUMMARY OF SURGICAL STEPS

- Room set-up
- Patient positioning
- Preparation and draping
- Imaging
- Reduction
- Imaging
- Pinning
- Imaging
- Splinting and casting

TECHNICAL PEARLS

- Lateral pins, although biomechanically slightly less stable than crossed pins, are preferred because of the decreased risk of ulnar nerve injury
- Stability of fracture fixation must be confirmed with live fluoroscopic examination of the elbow in varus/valgus and flexion/extension
- Generally, type II fractures require two pins and type III fractures require three pins to achieve stability
- Bridge the fracture site with wires that traverse both the medial and lateral columns
- Have a low threshold for use of additional lateral entry pins or a medial pin if there is concern about stability or location of the initial pins
- Separate pins as far as possible at the fracture site in both the coronal and the sagittal planes
- Cast elbow at 60 to 80 degrees of flexion to dimish the risk or worsening swelling or compartment syndrome; avoid wrapping cast padding or splint material circumferntially if swelling is severe after fixation

REQUIRED EQUIPMENT

0.062-inch K-wires (may be large or smaller depending on size of the child)
Wire driver
C-arm
Radiolucent armboard
Splinting or casting materials

COMMON PITFALLS

(When to call for the attending physician)

- Failure to engage both fragments with at least two pins
- Failure to gain bicortical fixation with at least two pins
- Failure to gain at least 2 mm of pin separation at the fracture site (Fig. 18-11)

POSTOPERATIVE PROTOCOL

With treatment of a fracture with closed reduction and pinning, if the patient has minimal swelling and is thought to be at minimal risk for compartment syndrome, the patient may be discharged home with appropriate postoperative instructions after several hours of observation. Most children, however, are admitted for overnight observation with vascular/compartment checks every 2 to 4 hours and discharged the next day. Acetaminophen or codeine are prescribed for pain control. The first postoperative visit should be scheduled for 1 week after discharge, and the guardian should be instructed to keep the extremity elevated and to monitor for fever, increasing pain, worsening swelling of the hand, and changes in neurovascular status.

POSTOPERATIVE CLINIC VISIT PROTOCOL

Patients return to clinic 5 to 7 days after surgery for radiographs to assess for maintenance of reduction. If maintained, the splint is overwrapped with fiberglass at that time, immobilizing the arm in 60 to 80 degrees of flexion. Some have proposed that clinical and radiographic evaluation can wait until the patient returns for pin removal. However, if there is any concern about stability after surgery, the patient should return for reevaluation in 5 days or less.

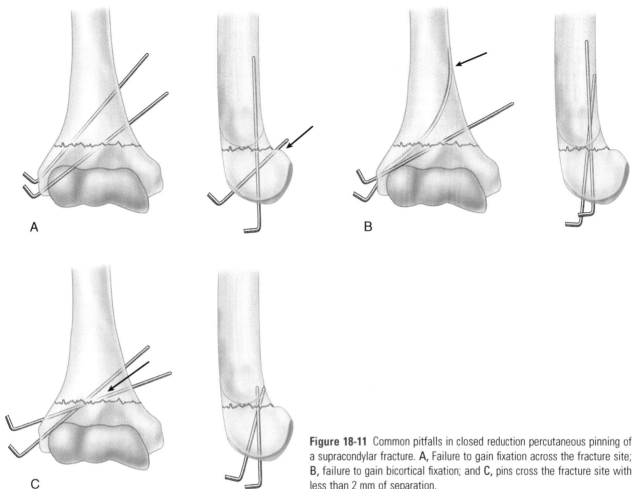

Figure 18-11 Common pitfalls in closed reduction percutaneous pinning of a supracondylar fracture. **A**, Failure to gain fixation across the fracture site; **B**, failure to gain bicortical fixation; and **C**, pins cross the fracture site with less than 2 mm of separation.

The cast and pins are removed at 3 to 4 weeks after surgery (often done in the clinic but can also be performed in the operating room), radiographs are obtained, and the arm is kept in a sling for the subsequent 1 to 2 weeks. Range-of-motion exercises are begun, with a focus on gentle flexion and extension and gradual progression, starting a few days after cast removal.

At 6 weeks after surgery, the patient may return for assessment of range of motion; no radiographs are necessary at that time.

SUGGESTED READINGS

1. Jobst CA, Sparkle C, King WF, Lopez M. Percutaneous pinning of pediatric supracondylar humerus fractures with the semi sterile technique: the Miami experience. *J Pediatr Orthop.* 2007;27(1):17-22.
2. Kocher MS, Kasser JR, Waters PM, et al. Lateral entry compared with medial and lateral entry pin fixation for completely displaced supracondylar humeral fractures in children. A randomized clinical trial. *J Bone Joint Surg Am.* 2007;89(4):706-712.
3. Kronner JM Jr, Legakis JE, Kovacevic N, et al. An evaluation of supracondylar humerus fractures: is there a correlation between postponing treatment and the need for open surgical intervention? *J Child Orthop.* 2013;7(2):131-137.
4. Lee YH, Lee SK, Kim BS, et al. Three lateral divergent or parallel pin fixations for the treatment of displaced supracondylar humerus fractures in children. *J Pediatr Orthop.* 2008;28(4):417-422.
5. Mitchelson AJ, Illingworth KD, Robinson BS, et al. Patient demographics and risk factors in pediatric distal humeral supracondylar fractures. *Orthopedics.* 2013;36(6):e700-e706.

6. Mulpuri K, Wilkins K. The treatment of displaced supracondylar humerus fractures: evidence-based guideline. *J Pediatr Orthop*. 2012;32(suppl 2):S143-S152.

7. Ponce BA, Hedequist DJ, Zurakowski D, et al. Complications and timing of follow-up after closed reduction and percutaneous pinning of supracondylar humerus fractures: follow-up after percutaneous pinning of supracondylar humerus fractures. *J Pediatr Orthop*. 2004;24(6):610-614.

8. Sankar WN, Hebela NM, Skaggs DL, et al. Loss of pin fixation in displaced supracondylar humeral fractures in children: causes and prevention. *J Bone Joint Surg Am*. 2007;89(4):713-717.

9. Shah AS, Waters PM, Bae DS. Treatment of the "pink pulseless hand" in pediatric supracondylar humerus fractures. *J Hand Surg [Am]*. 2013;38(7):1399-1403.

10. Skaggs DL, Cluck MW, Mostofi A, et al. Lateral-entry pin fixation in the management of supracondylar fractures in children. *J Bone Joint Surg Am*. 2004;86A(4):702-707.

PEDIATRIC TECHNIQUES
CLUBFOOT CASTING AND CLUBFOOT SURGICAL CORRECTION

Matthew B. Dobbs | Daniel K. Moon

CASE MINIMUM REQUIREMENTS

- Accurate diagnosis
- Full-term infant or older who is eating well and gaining weight

COMMONLY USED CPT CODES

- CPT Code: 28262—Capsulotomy, midfoot; extensive, including posterior talotibial capsulotomy and tendon(s) lengthening (e.g., resistant clubfoot deformity)
- CPT Code: 28261—Repair, revision, and/or reconstruction procedures on the foot and toes
- CPT Code: 28260—Repair, revision, and/or reconstruction procedures on the foot and toes

COMMONLY USED ICD9 CODES

- 754.51—Talipes equinovarus
- 754.50—Talipes varus
- 754.59—Talipes calcaneovarus

COMMONLY USED ICD10 CODES

- Q66.0—Congenital talipes equinovarus
- Q66.1—Congenital talipes calcaneovarus
- Q66.2—Congenital metatarsus (primus) varus

Clubfoot (talipes, congenital foot deformity) occurs in approximately 1 of every 1000 live births. The ratio of idiopathic clubfoot among males to females is 2:1 and is consistent across ethnic groups. Bilateral deformities occur in 50% of children. Approximately 80% of clubfeet are isolated (idiopathic) birth defects; the remaining 20% are associated with neuromuscular conditions and genetic syndromes.

Clubfoot has a distinct clinical appearance that is recognizable at birth, consisting of forefoot cavus and adduction and hindfoot equinus and varus (Fig. 19-1, A and B). It is often accompanied by internal tibial torsion, and the ankle, midtarsal, and subtalar joints all are involved in the pathologic process. Although the severity may differ from one clubfoot case to another, a common feature of all clubfeet is that the deformities cannot be fully corrected passively on initial examination.

The gold standard for clubfoot management is the Ponseti method, which consists of serial casting, a heel cord tenotomy, and foot abduction bracing. The goal of this minimally invasive method is to provide functional correction with less scar tissue and, as a result, more supple feet than results with more extensive surgery (Fig. 19-2).

SURGICAL TECHNIQUE

Room Set-Up

- Casting is done in the clinic setting, but it can be done in the operating room if combined with Achilles tenotomy.
- Necessary supplies include plaster, lukewarm water, cotton undercast padding, stockinette, and cast scissors.
- Toys may be needed for distraction, as well as a bottle of milk.
- The room should be quiet.
- Parents are needed for feeding, and another assistant should be present for entertaining the child.

Patient Positioning

- The patient is positioned supine.

Prepping and Draping

- No sterile field is required, unless the procedure is done in the operating room.

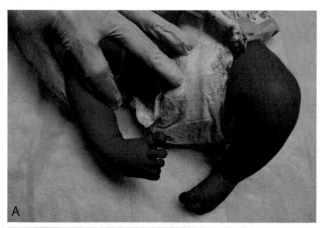

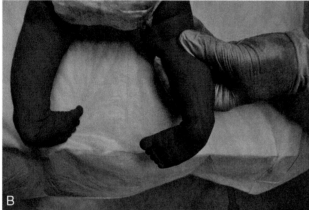

Figure 19-1 Pictures of an infant with right-sided clubfoot deformity show all components of the deformity with the patient positioned: **A**, supine; and **B**, prone.

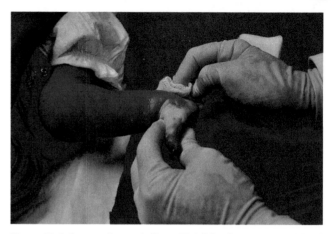

Figure 19-2 Same patient as in Figure 19-1 right after tenotomy with full correction.

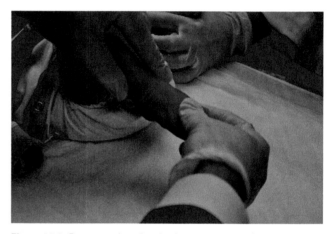

Figure 19-3 Demonstration of supination maneuver used to correct cavus in first cast.

CLUBFOOT CASTING PROCEDURE

- The cavus is corrected first by supinating the forefoot and dorsiflexing the first metatarsal (Fig. 19-3). Never pronate the forefoot because this worsens the cavus deformity. Supinating the forefoot achieves the first goal of correcting cavus by aligning the forefoot with the hindfoot. After stretching, the cast is applied.

- The next week, the cast is removed; at this stage, the varus and adduction are addressed by abducting the foot in supination while counterpressure is applied with the thumb on the head of the talus (Fig. 19-4). The calcaneus abducts by rotating and sliding under the talus while simultaneously extending and everting correcting heel varus. After manipulation, a long-leg cast is applied as described previously.

- The child returns the following week for repeat cast change. The same manipulation and casting described in step 2 is repeated. This is repeated weekly for a total of four to five casts to fully stretch the medial ligaments (Fig. 19-5). Never touch the calcaneus during manipulation because if it is held, the calcaneus is prevented from sliding from varus to valgus.

- Once the foot is externally rotated approximately 60 degrees and the hindfoot is in neutral to slight valgus, any residual equinus is corrected with a tenotomy of the Achilles tendon. This is done in the clinic with a local anesthetic for patients less than 1 year of age and in the operating room for those older than 1 year or those

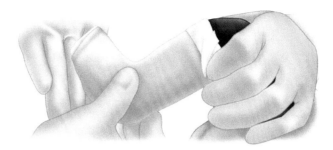

Figure 19-4 Example of cast molding with the thumb of the surgeon on the talus.

Clubfoot treatment over 4–6 weeks

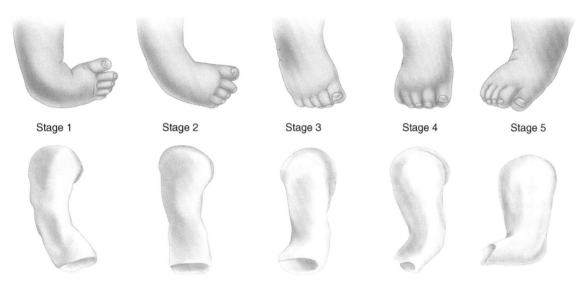

| Stage 1 | Stage 2 | Stage 3 | Stage 4 | Stage 5 |

Figure 19-5 Sequence of expected foot and ankle anatomy correction after 4 to 6 weeks of casting.

having a repeat tenotomy where the tendon is less easily palpated. The indication for tenotomy is for feet with less than 10 degrees of ankle dorsiflexion present. While an assistant holds the foot and leg, the surgeon performs a longitudinal stab incision just medial to the tendon and 1 cm above its insertion on the calcaneus. The tendon is cut completely from anterior to posterior (Fig. 19-6, *A*). A snap is felt and a sudden increase in ankle dorsiflexion (Fig. 19-6, *B*). The final cast is applied with the foot in 70 degrees of external rotation and 10 degrees of dorsiflexion. This cast is left on for 3 weeks to allow the tendon to heal. After removal, the child is placed in a foot abduction brace to prevent relapse (Video 19-1).

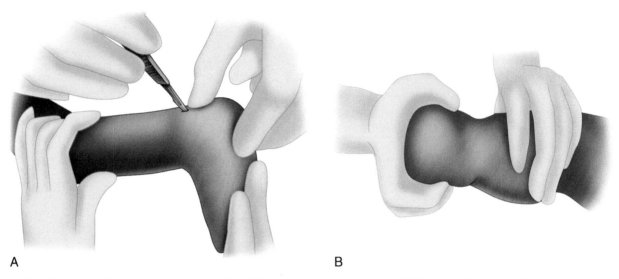

Figure 19-6 A, Longitudinal incision made along palpable Achilles tendon to perform tenotomy. **B,** Manual dorsiflexion of ankle to complete the release.

BRIEF SUMMARY OF SURGICAL STEPS

- Correct cavus first; supinate the forefoot and dorsiflex the first metatarsal (see Fig. 19-3)
- Take care not to pronate the forefoot
- Apply cast (stockinette, cotton undercast padding, plaster, mold)
- One week later, remove the cast
- Correct varus and adduction; abduct foot in supination while counterpressure is applied with the thumb on the head of the talus
- Abduct calcaneus by rotating and sliding under the talus while simultaneously extending and everting correcting heel varus (see Fig. 19-4)
- Apply cast (stockinette, cotton undercast padding, plaster, mold)
- One week later, remove the cast
- Repeat all previous actions in step 2 weekly for 4 to 5 weeks to fully stretch the medial ligaments
- Never touch the calcaneus during manipulation (as described previously)
- Once the foot is externally rotated approximately 60 degrees and the hindfoot is in neutral to slight valgus, any residual equinus is corrected with a tenotomy of the Achilles tendon
- Achilles tenotomy is done in the clinic with a local anesthetic for patients less than 1 year of age; otherwise, it is performed in the operating room
- Indication for tenotomy: less than 10 degrees of ankle dorsiflexion
- Assistant holds foot and leg
- Surgeon performs a longitudinal stab incision just medial to the tendon and 1 cm above its insertion on the calcaneus
  - The tendon is cut completely from anterior to posterior
  - A snap is felt and a sudden increase in ankle dorsiflexion
- The final cast is applied with the foot in 70 degrees of external rotation and 10 degrees of dorsiflexion
- This cast is left on for 3 weeks
- After removal, the child is placed in a foot abduction brace to prevent relapse

REQUIRED EQUIPMENT

Plaster
Cast padding
Cast scissors
Tenotomy blade
Bupivacaine
Syringe
Stockinette

TECHNICAL PEARLS

- Supination in first cast
- Never pronate in any cast
- Ability to palpate head of talus
- No dorsiflexion until tenotomy to avoid rocker-bottom
- 90-Degree bend at knee to avoid cast slipping
- Use long-leg casts
- Apply cast in stages
- Careful molding
- Expose tops of toes after cast dries but leave foot plate

COMMON PITFALLS

(When to call for the attending physician)

- Failure to supinate foot in first cast
- Externally rotating with the calcaneus rather than the head of talus as fulcrum
- Forceful and painful manipulations
- Poor molding that results in cast slipping
- Failure to use foot abduction brace

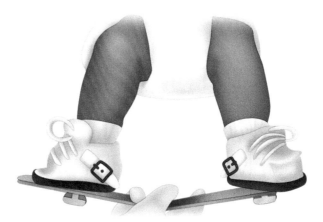

Figure 19-7 Example of Denis-Brown abduction shoes and bar to maintain correction after casting.

POSTOPERATIVE PROTOCOL

After the last cast is removed, the child is placed in the foot abduction brace (Fig. 19-7). The brace is essential to prevent relapse and is worn 23 hours a day for 3 months and then weaned slowly to night and naptime hours to be used for 2 to 4 years.

Perhaps the most difficult part of clubfoot management is recognizing and treating relapse. Most relapses can be corrected with repeat casting alone or casting followed by transfer of the tibialis anterior tendon to the third cuneiform. To help prevent relapse, patients are prescribed a foot abduction brace that parents are asked to use for up to 4 years. Not using the brace as prescribed is the most common reason given for relapse.

POSTOPERATIVE CLINIC VISIT PROTOCOL

Once bracing is initiated, patients follow-up at 1 month, then at another 2 months, and then at 3-month intervals until bracing is discontinued to watch for relapse. At each visit, a physical examination is done to ensure the feet are not relapsing and also to fit for new shoes and adjust the width of the bar as needed.

Once bracing is stopped, follow-up is at 6-month intervals for a year and then yearly for several years until risk of relapse has dissipated.

SUGGESTED READINGS

1. Cooper DM, Dietz FR. Treatment of idiopathic clubfoot. A thirty-year follow-up note. *J Bone Joint Surg Am.* 1995;77:1477-1489.
2. Dobbs MB, Nunley R, Schoenecker PL. Long-term follow-up of patients with clubfeet treated with extensive soft-tissue release. *J Bone Joint Surg Am.* 2006;88:986-996.
3. Ponseti IV. *Congenital Clubfoot: Fundamentals of Treatment.* 1st ed. Oxford University Press; 1996.
4. Boehm S, Limpaphayom N, Alaee F, Sinclair MF, Dobbs MB. Early results of the Ponseti method for the treatment of clubfoot in distal arthrogryposis. *J Bone Joint Surg Am.* 2008;90:1501-1507.
5. Gerlach DJ, Gurnett CA, Limpaphayom N, et al. Early results of the Ponseti method for the treatment of clubfoot associated with myelomeningocele. *J Bone Joint Surg Am.* 2009;91:1350-1359.
6. Gurnett CA, Boehm S, Connolly A, Reimschisel T, Dobbs MB. Impact of congenital talipes equinovarus etiology on treatment outcomes. *Dev Med Child Neurol.* 2008;50:498-502.
7. Garg SDM. Use of the Ponseti method for recurrent clubfoot following posteromedial release. *Indian J Orthop.* 2008;42:68-72.
8. Dobbs MB, Rudzki JR, Purcell DB, Walton T, Porter KR, Gurnett CA. Factors predictive of outcome after use of the Ponseti method for the treatment of idiopathic clubfeet. *J Bone Joint Surg Am.* 2004;86-A: 22-27.

CHAPTER 20

PEDIATRIC TECHNIQUES
PERCUTANEOUS PINNING FOR SLIPPED CAPITAL FEMORAL EPIPHYSIS

Nicole A. Friel | James W. Roach

Slipped capital femoral epiphysis (SCFE) is displacement of the femoral head relative to the neck and shaft. The term SCFE is actually a misnomer; the epiphysis (head) stays in the acetabulum, whereas the neck (usually) displaces anteriorly and externally rotates relative to the femoral head and acetabulum. The annual incidence rate of SCFE is 2 to 13 per 100,000, and the incidence is increasing. The single greatest risk factor for SCFE is obesity. The average age of children with SCFE is 12 ± 1.5 years for girls (range, 10 to 13 years) and 13.5 ± 1.7 years for boys (range, 12 to 15 years). The precise etiology of SCFE is unknown most of the time. The common pathway is a mechanical insufficiency of the proximal femoral physis to resist the load across it, whether there are physiologic loads across an abnormally weak physis or abnormally high loads across a normal physis. Several conditions weaken the physis, including endocrine abnormalities, systemic diseases such as renal osteodystrophy, and previous radiation therapy.

SCFE classically presents with pain at the hip, thigh, or knee. Patients often have decreased range of motion of the hip and may be obligated to externally rotate during hip flexion. The patient often walks with a limp. Anteroposterior (AP) and lateral (frog leg) radiographs of the pelvis should be carefully examined because a subtle slip can easily be overlooked. Although many classifications of SCFE have been described, the functional classification of SCFE, describing physeal stability, is most useful in predicting subsequent development of osteonecrosis. A patient has a stable SCFE if the individual is able to bear weight; an individual with an unstable SCFE is unable to bear weight, even with the aid of crutches. Stable SCFEs have a 0% risk of osteonecrosis, and unstable SCFEs have a reported 47% risk of osteonecrosis.

The goals of SCFE treatment are early detection, prevention of further slippage, and avoidance of complications. Although treatment options continue to evolve, the preferred initial treatment for most cases of SCFE is in situ screw fixation. Advantages include percutaneous placement with minimal soft tissue disruption, high success and patient satisfaction rates, and low incidence of slip progression, osteonecrosis, and chondrolysis.

Single screw fixation is usually adequate and supported by the literature, although two screws are occasionally used to increase the rotational stability in patients who are obese or unreliable. Prophylactic pinning of the contralateral hip, although controversial, may be beneficial to the long-term outcome in that setting. Prophylactic pinning is commonly performed in children with underlying endocrine disease, age less than 10 years at initial presentation, or previous pelvic radiation.

CASE MINIMUM REQUIREMENTS

- N = 0 Specific to slipped capital femoral epiphysis

COMMONLY USED CPT CODES

- CPT Code: 27175—Treatment of slipped capital femoral epiphysis; by traction, without reduction
- CPT Code: 27176—Treatment of slipped capital femoral epiphysis; by single or multiple pinning, in situ
- CPT Code: 27177—Open treatment of slipped capital femoral epiphysis; by single or multiple pinning or bone graft (includes obtaining graft)
- CPT Code: 27178—Open treatment of slipped capital femoral epiphysis; closed manipulation with single or multiple pinning
- CPT Code: 27181—Open treatment of slipped capital femoral epiphysis; osteotomy and internal fixation

COMMONLY USED ICD9 CODES

- 820.00—Closed unspecified intracapsular
- 820.01—Closed epiphyseal separation

SURGICAL TECHNIQUE

Room Set-Up

- A standard fracture table is positioned in the center of the room with appropriate access to the anesthesia team (Fig. 20-1).
- Alternatively, a radiolucent table may be used.
- When a fracture table is used, the C-arm is positioned at the foot of the bed with access between the legs.
- The C-arm monitor is positioned near the head of the bed on the side of the affected extremity.

Patient Positioning

- The patient is moved into a supine position on the fracture table.
- A well-padded perineal post is used.
- The affected leg is secured in the traction boot.
- The contralateral leg is flexed, externally rotated, and abducted on a leg holder.
- The arm on the unaffected side is extended out onto an armboard, and the arm on the affected side is secured over the chest (Fig. 20-2).
- The C-arm enters between the legs.
- Before prepping, ensure that AP and lateral images are attainable.
  - The entire proximal femoral epiphysis and hip joint space should be clearly visible on both views (Fig. 20-3).

Prepping and Draping

- The operative field is prepared with chlorhexidine or providone-iodine.
- Allow free access to the entire anterolateral surface of the thigh, from just below the iliac crest to just above the knee and from the pubis in the inguinal area to the midline posteriorly.
- A vertical isolation drape (shower curtain) is used to isolate the operative field (Fig. 20-4).

Determining the Course of the Guide Pin

- Hold the guide pin over the skin in the expected trajectory. Use the C-arm to obtain an AP image. Adjust the placement of the guide pin so that the pin points to the

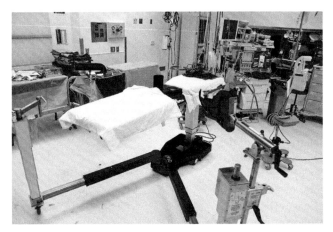

Figure 20-1 Room set-up with a fracture table for percutaneous pinning for slipped capital femoral epiphysis.

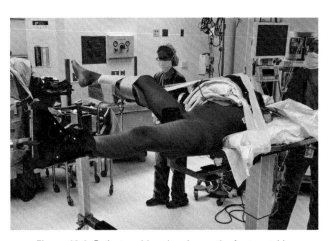

Figure 20-2 Patient positioned supine on the fracture table.

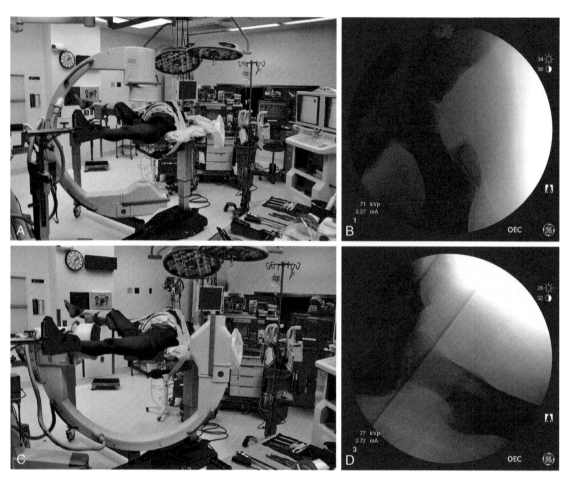

Figure 20-3 The C-arm enters between the legs. Adequate radiographs are obtained in both anteroposterior (**A** and **B**) and lateral positions (**C** and **D**) before draping.

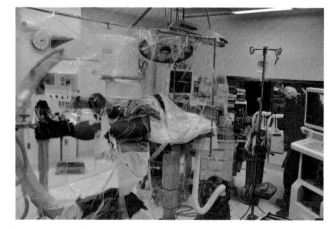

Figure 20-4 The operative field is prepped and draped with a vertical isolation drape (shower curtain).

center of the femoral head. A line is then drawn on the skin in the trajectory of the guide pin (Fig. 20-5).
- The C-arm then is moved to a lateral position, and the trajectory of the guide pin is again determined. The guide pin should point toward the center of the femoral head. Draw an additional line based on the lateral fluoroscopic images (Fig. 20-6).
- The intersection of the two lines gives the starting point of the guide pin.
  - Remember that the epiphysis is displaced posterior relative to the femoral neck; therefore, the trajectory for the guide pin must be from anterior to posterior

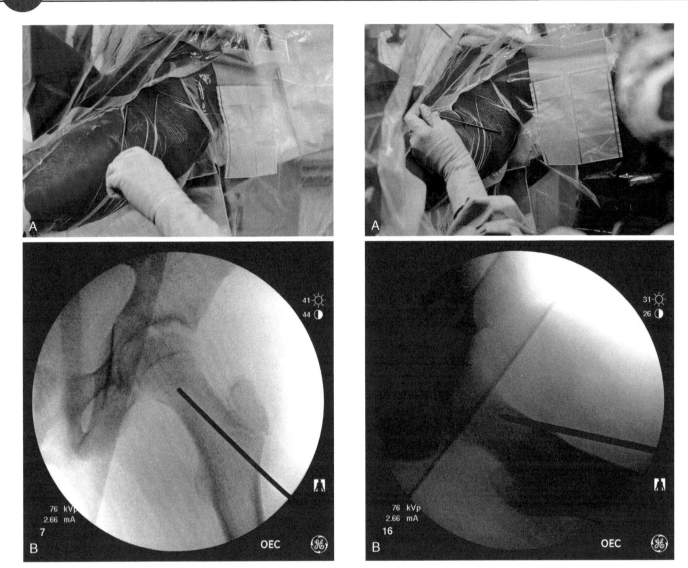

Figure 20-5 The trajectory of the guide pin is determined by holding the pin over the skin **(A)** and confirming the position with an anteroposterior image **(B)**. The guide pin should point toward the center of the femoral head.

Figure 20-6 The trajectory of the guide pin is then determined by holding the pin over the skin **(A)** and confirming the position with a lateral image **(B)**. The guide pin should point toward the center of the femoral head.

with the start point becoming more anterior on the femoral neck as the slip becomes more displaced.

- Therefore, the greater the degree of the slip, the more anterior the intersection to achieve a trajectory that centers in the femoral head (Fig. 20-7).

Guide Pin Placement

- Place a threaded pin through a small anterolateral puncture wound at the intersection of the two skin lines.
- Confirm both the start point placement of the pin and the trajectory on AP and lateral fluoroscopic images (Fig. 20-8).
- Use a mallet to engage the pin. Then, use the drill to insert the pin, monitoring proper alignment, position, and depth of insertion into the femoral head on fluoroscopic images as the pin is advanced (Fig. 20-9).
- The pin can be advanced to within 5 mm of the hip joint but should never penetrate the femoral head.
- Use a measuring device to determine the length of the screw.

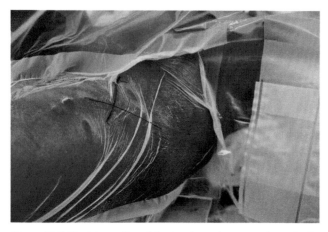

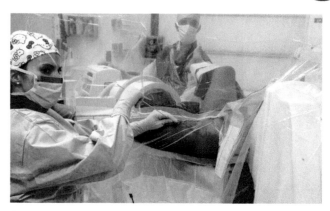

Figure 20-7 The intersection of the two lines gives a starting point for the guide pin.

Figure 20-8 A threaded guide pin is inserted through the skin down to the bone. The starting point again is confirmed with fluoroscopic images.

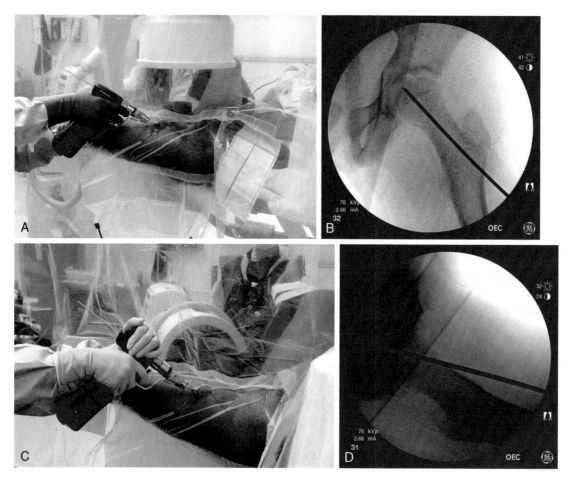

Figure 20-9 The guide pin is advanced into the bone toward the femoral head. The position is confirmed on both the anteroposterior (**A** and **B**) and lateral (**C** and **D**) images. The pin is advanced with fluoroscopic guidance.

Screw Insertion

- If planning to use a 6.5-mm screw, use a 5.0-mm drill bit to drill over the pin. Drill to, but not through, the subchondral bone in the femoral head.
- Insert a 6.5-mm cannulated, partially threaded (32-mm–long threads) stainless steel epiphysiodesis screw; the threads of the screws should traverse the physis.

Check Screw Position

- Check AP and lateral views to confirm screw position (Fig. 20-10).
- Take the affected leg out of traction. With continuous fluoroscopic viewing, internally and externally rotate the hip through an arc of motion.
  - This maneuver is helpful to ensure that there is no hardware penetration into the hip joint.
  - The tip of the screw should come not closer than 5 mm from the joint line.

Closure

- Close the incision with absorbable chromic sutures.
- Apply an impermeable dressing.

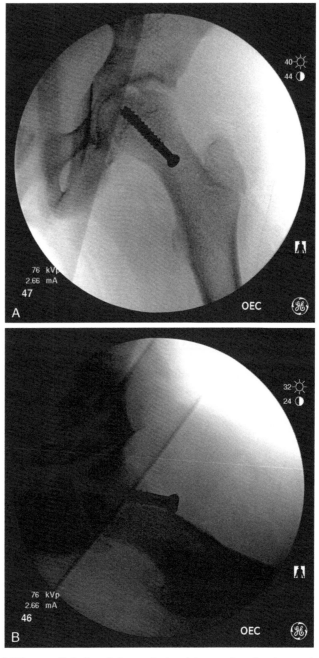

Figure 20-10 A 6.5-mm partially threaded screw is placed. Images show the placement of the screw in the anteroposterior (**A**) and lateral (**B**) images.

BRIEF SUMMARY OF SURGICAL STEPS

- Room set-up
- Patient positioning
- Prep and drape
- Determine the trajectory of the guide pin
- Insert the guide pin
- Ream lateral cortex
- Insert cannulated screw
- Ensure a safe distance between screw tip and joint surface
- Close

REQUIRED EQUIPMENT

Fracture table, or radiolucent table with traction device
C-arm
Guide pin
Wire driver
Cannulated drill and depth gauge
Cannulated screw
Screw driver

TECHNICAL PEARLS

- Confirm that the position of the guide pin and subsequent screw is centered in the femoral head to avoid penetration. Because there is only one central axis of the femoral head, placement of more than one screw increases the risk of femoral head penetration.
- Slipped capital femoral epiphysis most commonly involves anterior displacement of the femoral neck, which corresponds to the femoral head rotating posteriorly around the axis of the femoral neck. To achieve fixation that stays central in the femoral head, the starting point of the fixation is often in the femoral neck. In more severely displaced slips, the starting points are more anterior on the neck. In mild slips or when prophylactically pinning a contralateral slip, the starting point is more lateral.

COMMON PITFALLS

(When to call for the attending physician)

- Starting too lateral so the pin does not cross perpendicular to the physis or misses the center of the femoral head
- Placement of the fixation in the superior and anterior quadrant of the femoral head; the terminal branches of the lateral ascending cervical artery traverse this quadrant, and fixation into this area puts the patient at increased risk of osteonecrosis
- Penetration of the screw into the joint

POSTOPERATIVE PROTOCOL

Postoperative AP and lateral pelvis radiographs can be obtained in the recovery area (Fig. 20-11).

Patients can begin physical therapy later the same day.

Uncomplicated cases are often treated with outpatient surgery.

Touchdown weight-bearing with crutches is maintained for 2 to 3 weeks for stable slips and for 6 to 8 weeks with unstable slips.

If the contralateral hip is prophylactically pinned at the same time, the patient may be weight-bearing as tolerated on the prophylactically pinned hip.

Running, jumping, and other rigorous exercises should not begin until the physes have closed.

POSTOPERATIVE CLINIC VISIT PROTOCOL

After discharge from the hospital, patients are seen back in the office in 10 to 14 days to evaluate the incision, verify that the child is doing well with the prescribed weight-bearing, and address any concerns of the child or family members.

The patient is seen again in the office at 3 months after surgery.

At this time, new radiographs are obtained to evaluate the alignment, fixation, and status of the physis.

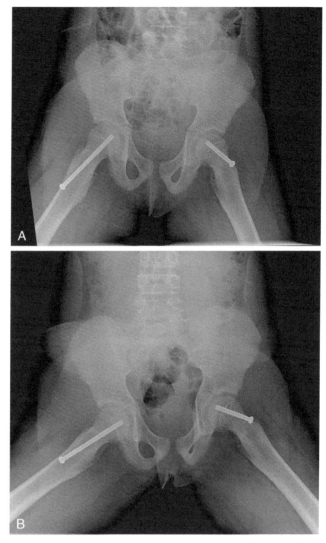

Figure 20-11 Postoperative anteroposterior (**A**) and frog lateral (**B**) pelvis radiographs can be obtained in the recovery area. Note that this patient underwent prophylactic pinning of the contralateral hip.

SUGGESTED READINGS

1. Blanco JS, Taylor B, Johnston CE 2nd. Comparison of single pin versus multiple pin fixation in treatment of slipped capital femoral epiphysis. *J Pediatr Orthop*. 1992;12(3):384-389.
2. Goodman WW, Johnson JT, Robertson WW Jr. Single screw fixation for acute and acute-on-chronic slipped capital femoral epiphysis. *Clin Orthop Relat Res*. 1996;(322):86-90.
3. Loder RT, Richards BS, Shapiro PS, Reznick LR, Aronson DD. Acute slipped capital femoral epiphysis: the importance of physeal stability. *J Bone Joint Surg Am*. 1993;75(8):1134-1140.
4. Schultz WR, Weinstein JN, Weinstein SL, Smith BG. Prophylactic pinning of the contralateral hip in slipped capital femoral epiphysis: evaluation of long-term outcome for the contralateral hip with use of decision analysis. *J Bone Joint Surg Am*. 2002;84-A(8):1305-1314.
5. Segal LS, Jacobson JA, Saunders MM. Biomechanical analysis of in situ single versus double screw fixation in a nonreduced slipped capital femoral epiphysis model. *J Pediatr Orthop*. 2006;26(4):479-485. doi:10.1097/01.bpo.0000226285.46943.ea.

CHAPTER 21

EPIPHYSIODESIS FOR LIMB LENGTH DISCREPANCY AND ANGULAR DEFORMITY

Yale A. Fillingham | Monica Kogan

Growth deformities are among the most common conditions to present in the pediatric orthopaedic clinic. The basic principles of exploiting growing bone to correct growth deformities have been used for centuries in the field of bone and joint surgery. Previously, osteotomy has been the surgical choice of care in children with limb length discrepancies or angular deformities of the knee; this method requires the child to be immobile and non–weight-bearing during recuperation. Corrections can now be achieved with newer, less traumatic techniques with lower risks and less need for revision (Fig. 21-1). Angular correction and length equalization can be attained through minimally invasive hemiepiphyseal arrest with devices such as Blount staples, transphyseal screws, and tension-band plates. Complications have been observed with the Blount staple method, including staple breakage, extrusion, changes in mechanical axis, and physis damage that causes permanent closure of the growth plate. Transphyseal screws were proposed as a method for temporary hemiepiphysiodesis, but the screws were found to violate the physis causing a higher risk of irreversible plate closure.

As a result of issues with the Blount staples and transphyseal screws, a novel device comprised of two screws and a two-hole plate was developed and marketed as the PediPlates® (OrthoPediatrics Corp, Warsaw, IN) and Eight-Plate® Guided Growth System (Orthofix, McKinney, TX). This innovation brought on the phrase "guided growth" in regards to minimally invasive temporary hemiepiphysiodesis to correct growth deformities in children who are still skeletally immature and have sufficient growth potential around the knee. These implants are designed as a tension band, which allows for a lower risk of physeal arrest by preventing compressive forces across the physis created by the staple. The rigid screws are more resistant to extrusion as opposed to the smooth staples, and the longer moment arm should lead to a faster correction. The development of the tension band plates has been among the promising advancements in the use of temporary hemiepiphysiodesis with promising results with high rates of success and minimal complications (Fig. 21-2).

The authors prefer the use of a tension band system to achieve either a permanent or a reversible epiphysiodesis for the management of angular deformity or limb length inequality in patients with open growth plates. In the clinical example used for the technique of epiphysiodesis, the patient was a 14-year-old boy with genu valgum of the right lower extremity (Fig. 21-3). Because the patient continued to have an open proximal tibia physis, he underwent epiphysiodesis with a two-hole tension band plate of the medial proximal tibia physis. Placement of the plates to achieve ephiphysiodesis is done based on the desired amount of length or angular correction, which commonly includes medial or lateral physis of the distal femur and proximal tibia.

CASE MINIMUM REQUIREMENTS

- N = 0

COMMONLY USED CPT CODES

- CPT Code: 27185—Epiphyseal arrest with epiphysiodesis or stapling, greater trochanter of femur
- CPT Code: 27475—Arrest, epiphyseal, any method (e.g., epiphysiodesis); distal femur
- CPT Code: 27477—Arrest, epiphyseal, any method (e.g., epiphysiodesis); tibia and fibula, proximal
- CPT Code: 27479—Arrest, epiphyseal, any method (e.g., epiphysiodesis); combined distal femur, proximal tibia and fibula
- CPT Code: 27485—Arrest, hemiepiphyseal, distal femur or proximal tibia or fibula (e.g., genu varus or valgus)
- CPT Code: 27730—Arrest, epiphyseal (epiphysiodesis), open; distal tibia
- CPT Code: 27732—Arrest, epiphyseal (epiphysiodesis), open; distal fibula
- CPT Code: 27734—Arrest, epiphyseal (epiphysiodesis), open; distal tibia and fibula
- CPT Code: 27740—Arrest, epiphyseal (epiphysiodesis), any method, combined, proximal and distal tibia and fibula
- CPT Code: 27742—Arrest, epiphyseal (epiphysiodesis), any method, combined, proximal and distal tibia and fibula; and distal femur

COMMONLY USED ICD9 CODES

- 736.41—Genu valgum (acquired)
- 736.42—Genu varum (acquired)
- 736.5—Genu recurvatum (acquired)
- 736.6—Other acquired deformities of knee
- 736.81—Unequal leg length (acquired)
- 736.89—Other acquired deformity of other parts of limb
- 736.9—Acquired deformity of limb, site unspecified

COMMONLY USED ICD10 CODES

- M21.06—Valgus deformity, not elsewhere classified, knee
- M21.16—Varus deformity, not elsewhere classified, knee
- M21.86—Other specified acquired deformities of lower leg
- M21.75—Unequal limb length (acquired), femur
- M21.96—Unspecified acquired deformity of lower leg

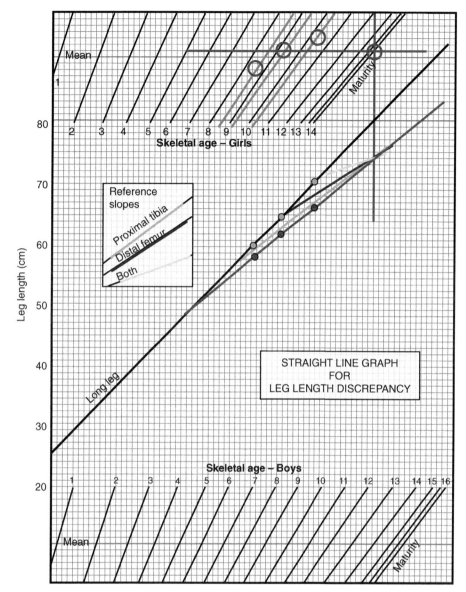

Figure 21-1 Moseley's straight line graph for leg-length discrepancies. (With permission from Moseley CF. A straight-line graph for leg-length discrepancies. *J Bone Joint Surg Am.* 1977;59:174-179.)

SURGICAL TECHNIQUE

Room Set-Up

- The operating bed is placed in the center of the room with appropriate access to the anesthesia staff.
- Use of fluoroscopy with the C-arm machine positioned to enter the operative field opposite from the surgeon and viewing monitors positioned for comfortable viewing by the surgeon should be anticipated before beginning the procedure.

Patient Positioning

- The patient is positioned supine on a radiolucent operating table.

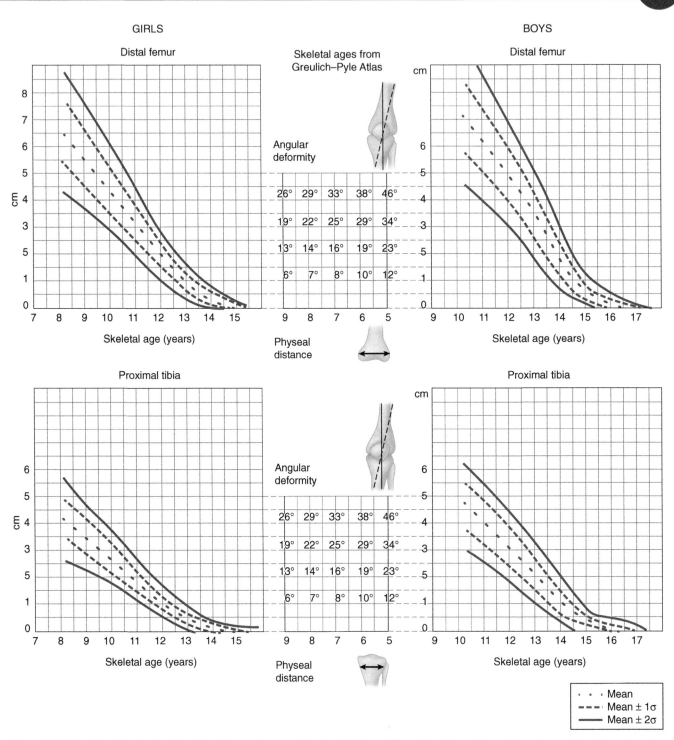

Figure 21-2 Chart for timing hemiepiphysiodesis for angular correction about the knee. The width of the physis and growth remaining is based on the Green-Anderson growth remaining chart. The physeal width is located on the central part of the chart, and the degree of angular deformity, anatomic tibiofemoral angle, on the corresponding vertical line is noted. A horizontal line is drawn from this point to the growth percentile on the appropriate Green-Anderson quadrant. A vertical line is extended downward from that percentile point to locate the age at which the epiphysiodesis should be performed. Quadrant used is according to gender and location of deformity. (With permission from Bowen JR, Leahey JL, Zhang ZH, MacEwen GD. Partial epiphysiodesis at the knee to correct angular deformity. *Clin Orthop Relat Res.* 1985;198:184-190.)

Prepping and Draping

- Apply a tourniquet located on the proximal thigh of the operative lower extremity with a clear U-drape as a barrier. With a candy cane stirrup leg holder, prepare the operative lower extremity with the desired antiseptic solution (Fig. 21-4).
- Drape the operative extremity with an impervious stockinette and Coban™ (3M Company, St. Paul, MN) over the distal aspect of the leg and standard lower extremity drape (Fig. 21-5).

Surgical Approach

- Identify the location of the desired physis with the assistance of fluoroscopy (Fig. 21-6, *A* and *B*). When identifying the distal femoral physis, the anatomic landmark is the midpatellar axis (Fig. 21-7, *A* and *B*).
- Mark the intended 1.5-cm to 2.5-cm incision centered over the desired physis. In the case of the distal femur, the incision should be on a slight angle in line with Langer's lines over the physis. For the proximal tibial incision, the authors prefer to angle the incision to accommodate Langer's lines (Fig. 21-8).
- The extremity is exsanguinated with an esmarch bandage and the tourniquet inflated. After the incision has been made, dissection is carried down to the periosteum (Video 21-1). The periosteum should not be violated in the dissection for concern of permanent damage to the underlying growth plate. Remember: If the tissue can be picked up, it is not the periosteum.

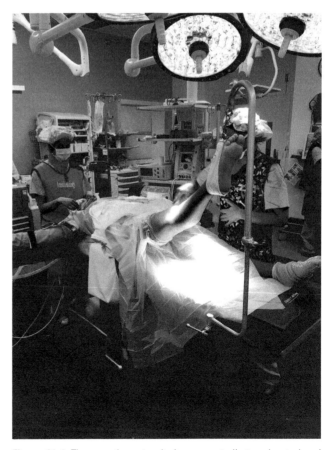

Figure 21-4 The operative extremity has an unsterile tourniquet placed proximally on the thigh followed by an unsterile clear plastic U-drape. With use of a candy cane stirrup, the extremity is prepared with an antiseptic solution.

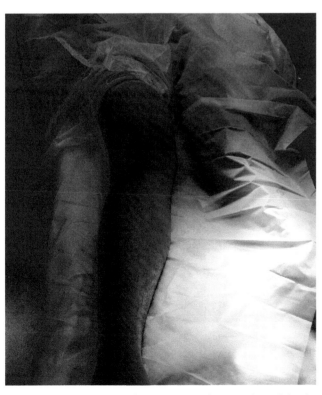

Figure 21-3 Clinical picture shows the patient's genu valgum deformity of the right lower extremity at the level of the knee.

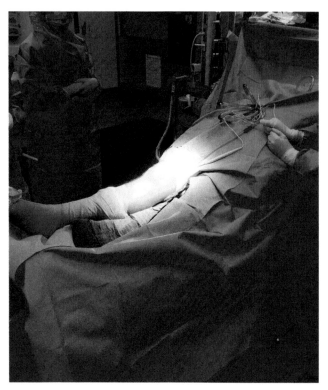

Figure 21-5 A standard lower extremity draping technique is used for the procedure.

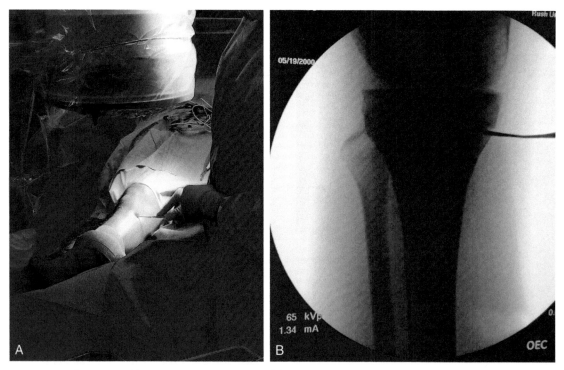

Figure 21-6 With use of a radiopaque object (**A**), the physis can be identified on fluoroscopy (**B**).

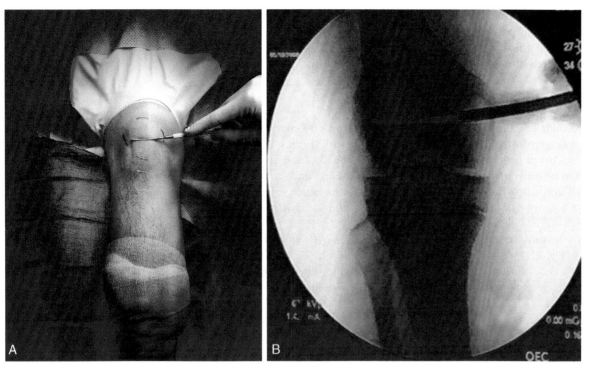

Figure 21-7 Marking the borders of the patella (**A**) to identify the midpatellar axis typically aligns with the distal femoral physis on fluoroscopy (**B**).

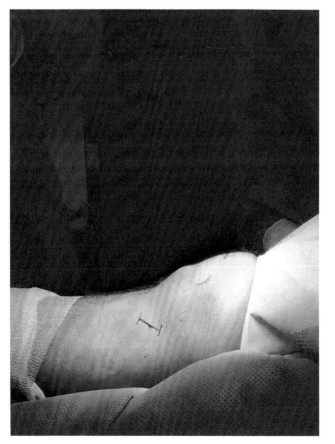

Figure 21-8 The incision should be 1.5 to 2.5 cm centered over the physis.

- Dissect down to but not through the periosteum because the plate should sit directly over the periosteum. The periosteum is adherent to the osseous surface, so it can be identified by the inability to use forceps to pick up the tissue (see Video 21-1). A leash of vessels may be overlying the periosteum.

Implantation

- The PediPlates® and Eight-Plate® Guided Growth systems contain all the implants and necessary instruments, other than the power drill (Fig. 21-9, *A* and *B*).
- With a curved hemostat, grasp the plate with the end of the instrument to allow for it to be easily placed against the bone (Fig. 21-10, *A* and *B*).
- After fluoroscopy has confirmed the position of the plate (Fig. 21-11), the plate is temporarily fixated with placement of a 1.60-mm guidewire in the center hole (Fig. 21-12, *A* and *B*; see Video 21-1).
- Verify the position of the plate on anteroposterior (AP) and lateral fluoroscopic views (Fig. 21-13, *A* and *B*).
- Insert a 1.60-mm guidewire into the center of the superior and inferior holes of the plate with the self-centering ball-tip double-drill guide (Fig. 21-14; see Video 21-1).
- Validate depth and position of the guidewires on AP and lateral fluoroscopic views (Fig. 21-15, *A* and *B*) and measure the screw length (Fig. 21-16).
- With the hand-driven screwdriver, insert the screws over the guidewire. After AP and lateral views have confirmed the final plate and screw position, the guidewires are removed (Fig. 21-17, *A* and *B*).

Closure

- The wound is copiously irrigated, followed by standard closure of the deep fascia over the plate and subsequent layers.
- The patient then is dressed with a sterile dressing, followed by a compressive wrap bandage (Fig. 21-18).

Text continued on p. 207

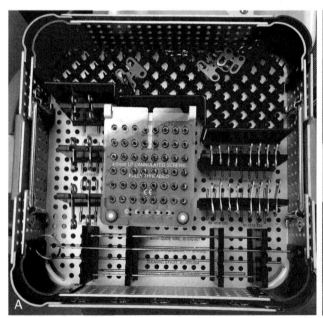
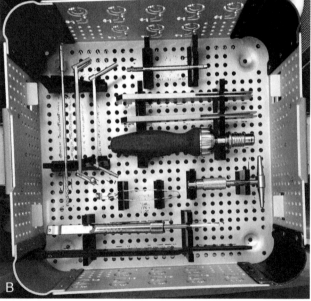

Figure 21-9 The PediPlates® System Tray (OrthoPediatrics Corp, Warsaw, IN) has two layers, with the top layer **(A)** containing guidewires, plates, and screws. The bottom layer **(B)** has the instruments for implantation that include the self-centering ball-tip guide, measuring device, 3.5-hex screwdriver head, and handle.

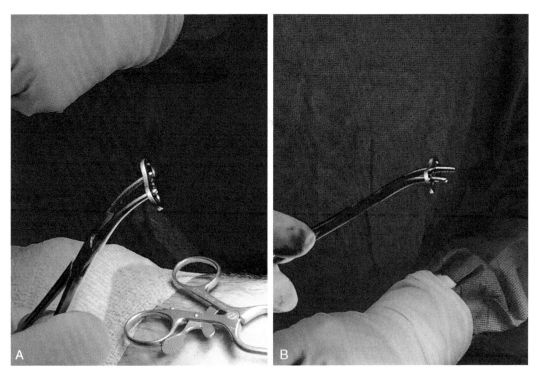

Figure 21-10 Use of a curved hemostat to hold the plate allows for the ability to hold the plate and insert the temporary guidewire. Placement of the plate at the end of the hemostat (**A**) allows for more accurate placement directly on the periosteum as opposed to holding the plate farther from the ends of the hemostat (**B**).

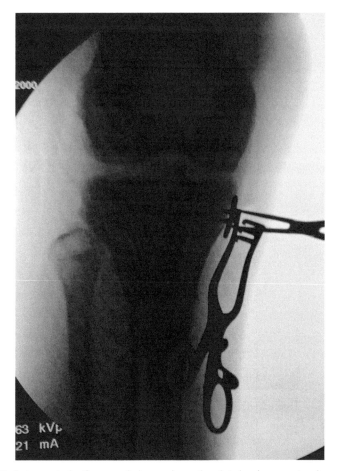

Figure 21-11 Anteroposterior fluoroscopic image shows the plate has been centered over the medial physis of the proximal tibia.

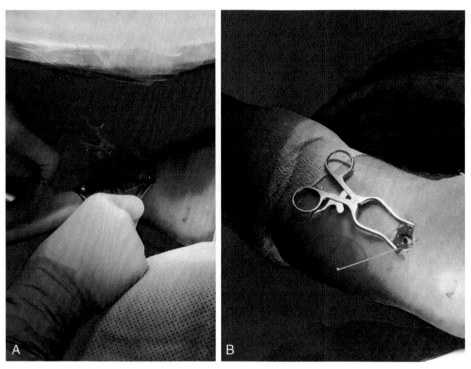

Figure 21-12 The 1.6-mm guidewire is inserted into the center hole of the plate while the plate is stabilized with the opposite hand and curved hemostat (**A**), and the plate is temporarily secured in place (**B**).

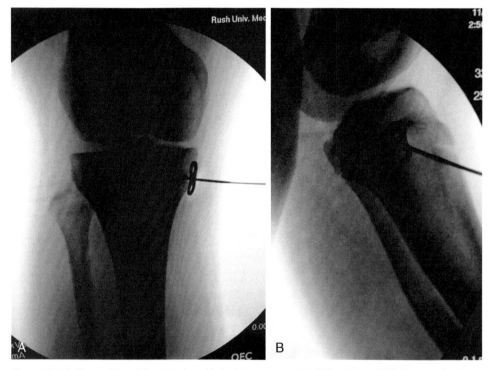

Figure 21-13 The position of the plate is verified with anteroposterior (**A**) and lateral (**B**) fluoroscopic views.

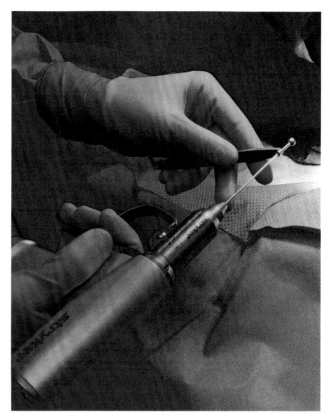

Figure 21-14 The guidewires for the cannulated screws need to be placed in the center of the holes. Use of the self-centering ball-tip guide helps obtain the desired position.

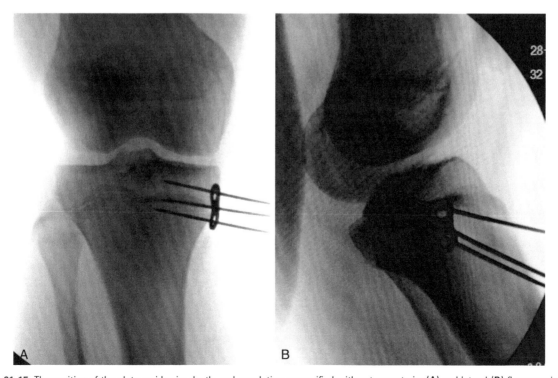

Figure 21-15 The position of the plate, guidewire depth, and angulation are verified with anteroposterior (**A**) and lateral (**B**) fluoroscopic views.

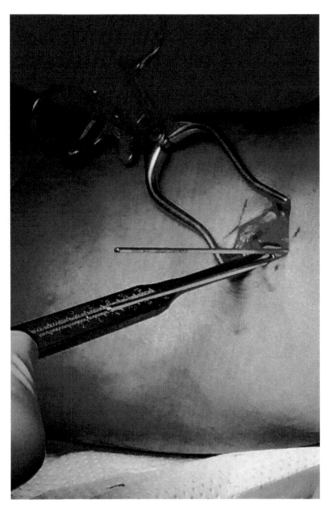

Figure 21-16 With use of the supplied measuring device, the screw lengths can easily be determined based on the guidewires.

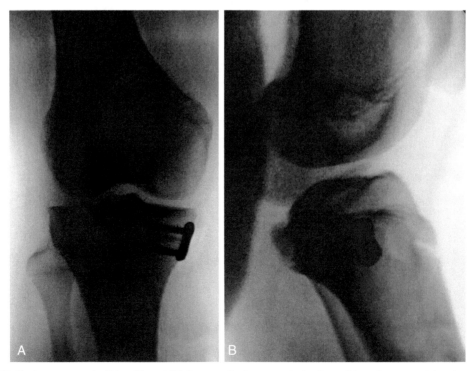

Figure 21-17 Final anteroposterior (**A**) and lateral (**B**) fluoroscopic views are obtained to validate placement of the plate and screws.

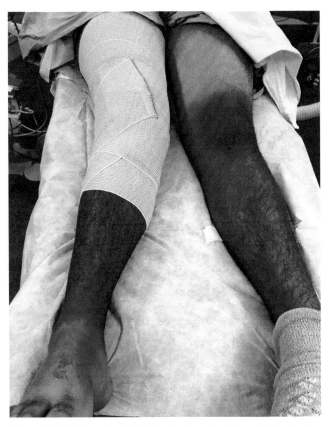

Figure 21-18 The patient's incision is dressed with a sterile dressing covered with a compressive wrap bandage. As expected, no correction was obtained during surgery. However, patients sometimes expect a correction immediately after surgery, so remind the patients that the correction happens over the subsequent weeks and months.

BRIEF SUMMARY OF SURGICAL STEPS

- Room set-up
- Position patient
- Prepare and drape
- Identify the physis with fluoroscopy
- Dissect to the level of periosteum
- Identify position of the plate and temporarily fixate it
- Measure and insert screws
- Closure and dressing application

REQUIRED EQUIPMENT

Minor orthopaedic ray

PediPlates® System Tray (OrthoPediatrics Corp, Warsaw, IN)

Standard power drill set

Desired suture for closure

TECHNICAL PEARLS

- When operating on the medial aspect of the knee, use a bump on the operative field so the nonoperative extremity does not interfere with the procedure
- As long you are able to grasp the tissue with the forceps, it is not periosteum and can be cut
- The guidewires used for the cannulated screws must be located in the center of the screw holes to allow for the screw heads to completely be seated into the plate
- Ensure that the plate is sitting flush on the periosteum while inserting the screws
- Obtain a true lateral by rotating the C-arm around the table, not by outwardly rotating the knee
- A leash of vessels may be found over the periosteum; when you see the vessels, do not dissect deeper

COMMON PITFALLS

(When to call for the attending physician)

- Violation of the periosteum on dissection
- Misplacement of the guidewire intraarticularly into the knee joint
- Having the screws too close to the posterior cortex
- Plates lying too anterior or posterior, resulting in either recurvatum or procurvatum
- Not placing the wire directly in the center of the circle, resulting in impingement of the screw against the plate on insertion; if you hear squeaking, check the placement of the screw
- Not being collinear with the wire on insertion of the screw, resulting in wire breakage
- Do not minimize how much pain the patients may be in for at least 1 week

POSTOPERATIVE PROTOCOL

After surgery, patients are provided crutches strictly for comfort measures but are instructed to be full weight-bearing with encouragement to return to normal activity as tolerated on the affected lower extremity, with the only restriction of no contact sports for 2 weeks, and to discontinue use of crutches as they can tolerate. On the basis of the authors' published findings in a retrospective review, a short course of postoperative physical therapy is prescribed to assist with improved pain control, discontinued use of crutches, and range of motion at the initial 2-week postoperative follow-up visit, especially for patients over 11 years of age who appear to have a substantial amount of pain.

POSTOPERATIVE CLINIC VISIT PROTOCOL

After discharge from the hospital on an outpatient basis, patients are followed in the clinic at 2 weeks and then at intervals of 3 months to document progression and identify timing of hardware removal. The follow-up intervals are altered at the surgeon's discretion as a result of variable growth rates and variable levels of correction required. Each routine follow-up visit in the clinic should include assessment of strength, range of motion, functional status, and radiographic investigation to evaluate for correction of growth deformity and hardware position.

SUGGESTED READINGS

1. Ballal MS, Bruce CE, Nayagam S. Correcting genu varum and genu valgum in children by guided growth: temporary hemiepiphysiodesis using tension band plates. *J Bone Joint Surg Br.* 2010;92(2): 273-276.
2. Boero S, Michelis MB, Riganti S. Use of the eight-plate for angular correction of knee deformities due to idiopathic and pathologic physis: initiating treatment according to etiology. *J Child Orthop.* 2011;5(3):209-216.
3. Burghardt RD, Herzenberg JE. Temporary hemiepiphysiodesis with the eight-plate for angular deformities: mid-term results. *J Orthop Sci.* 2010;15(5):699-704.
4. Eastwood DM, Sanghrajka AP. Guided growth: recent advances in a deep-rooted concept. *J Bone Joint Surg Br.* 2011;93(1):12-18.
5. Fillingham YA, Kroin E, Frank RM, Erickson B, Hellman M, Kogan M. Post-operative delay in return of function following guided growth tension plating and use of corrective physical therapy. *J Child Orthop.* 2014;8(3):265-271.
6. Gorman TM, Vanderwerff R, Pond M, MacWilliams B, Santora SD. Mechanical axis following staple epiphysiodesis for limb-length inequality. *J Bone Joint Surg Am.* 2009;91(10):2430-2439.
7. Saran N, Rathjen KE. Guided growth for the correction of pediatric lower limb angular deformity. *J Am Acad Orthop Surg.* 2010;18(9):528-536.
8. Stevens PM, Klatt JB. Guided growth for pathological physes: radiographic improvement during realignment. *J Pediatr Orthop.* 2008;28(6):632-639.
9. Stevens PM. Guided growth for angular correction: a preliminary series using a tension band plate. *J Pediatr Orthop.* 2007;27(3):253-259.
10. Wiemann JM 4th, Tryon C, Szalay EA. Physeal stapling versus 8-plate hemiepiphysiodesis for guided correction of angular deformity about the knee. *J Pediatr Orthop.* 2009;29(5):481-485.

ONCOLOGY TECHNIQUES
BIOPSY PRINCIPLES AND TECHNIQUES

Peter Chimenti | Emily E. Carmody

CASE MINIMUM REQUIREMENTS

- Adequate preoperative evaluation, including history, physical examination, laboratory studies (comprehensive metabolic panel [CMP], complete blood count [CBC], erythrocyte sedimentation rate [ESR], c-reactive protein [CRP], alkaline phosphatase [AlkPhos], lactate dehydrogenase [LDH], serum protein electrophoresis [SPEP], urine protein electrophoresis [UPEP], beta-2-microglobulin), depending on clinical suspicion
- Local staging studies should be completed before any biopsy
- An experienced musculoskeletal pathologist or the ability to send the pathology specimen to a treatment center familiar with orthopaedic oncology

The two main categories of biopsy are open biopsy and needle biopsy; this chapter addresses only the open biopsy and its indications, risks, and procedures. An open biopsy may *not* be required in several clinical scenarios, including benign bony lesions, such as nonossifying fibroma, simple bone cysts, enchondromas, and osteochondromas. Soft tissue lesions that have classic imaging characteristics, such as a lipoma or a ganglion cyst, may also be followed with observation without a biopsy. Many lesions, especially soft tissue tumors, are amenable to needle biopsy, either with or without image guidance. Bony lesions that demonstrate periosteal reaction, cortical destruction, or change in size on serial imaging and soft tissue lesions that are larger than roughly 5 cm, deep to the muscle fascia, painful, or growing in size should be considered for a biopsy.

Thorough preoperative assessment is critical in performing a successful biopsy with minimal risk to the patient. In general, local staging studies should be completed before the biopsy to eliminate postprocedural artifact or reactive edema from the biopsy itself. In addition, this allows the biopsy to be interpreted in the context of the imaging and laboratory data. Studies have shown that lesions suspected of being malignant are best managed by an experienced orthopaedic oncologist in a specialized center; unacceptably high rates of unnecessary amputations or complex reconstructive procedures are found when biopsies are performed outside of referral centers. The surgeon undertaking the biopsy should be prepared to perform the definitive limb-salvage procedure or amputation depending on the results of the biopsy; otherwise the patient is best served by referral to an orthopaedic oncologist for care. Poorly placed or inadequately performed biopsies can significantly alter the treatment plan for a patient and adversely affect morbidity and functional outcome for patients.

Open biopsy can be categorized as either incisional (the tumor capsule is intentionally violated as part of the procedure, and a portion of the mass or lesion is removed) or excisional (the entire tumor is removed). Incisional biopsy is generally recommended for suspected benign lesions that can be treated definitively at the time of biopsy or in cases where greater volumes of tissue may be required to perform special staining or molecular diagnostics than can be obtained with a needle biopsy (Video 22-1). Incisional biopsies are also often performed when a needle biopsy result is nondiagnostic. For incisional biopsies, the incision and dissection tract are planned such that they can be excised during the definitive limb-salvage procedure. Excisional biopsy may be performed through the reactive zone that surrounds the tumor, in which case it is termed marginal excision, or with a cuff of healthy tissue, in which case it is considered a primary wide excision. Excisional biopsy in general carries major risk if the pathology shows a malignant lesion, given that significantly more contamination is incurred from the larger incision and more extensive dissection. Therefore, this method is indicated in lesions with benign imaging characteristics and in smaller superficial lesions where a primary wide excision does not significantly increase morbidity for the patient. If the surgeon performing the biopsy is not comfortable performing definitive treatment or if the lesion or mass is indeed a sarcoma, the patient should be referred to an experienced orthopaedic oncologist.

SURGICAL TECHNIQUE

Room Set-Up

- Specific room set-up requirements are dictated by the exact site and the type of biopsy being performed. For bony lesions undergoing incisional biopsy, use of fluoroscopy can be helpful for localization.
- Radiolucent tables are used for bone biopsies.
- At the authors' institution, an "orthopaedic oncology" pan of instruments is used, which includes a set of osteotomes, curettes, pituitary rongeurs, and standard dissection scissors (Fig. 22-1).

Patient Positioning

- The patient is positioned as needed for the location of the biopsy to be performed.
  - For lower extremity tumors, the patient can be positioned supine.
  - For pelvic and thorax tumors, the patient can be positioned lateral on a bean bag.
  - For upper extremity tumors, the patient can be positioned either lateral or in a beach chair position, depending on location.

Prepping and Draping

- Prepping and draping is performed as dictated by the location and type of biopsy performed.
  - When biopsies are performed below the knee or below the elbow, a tourniquet and an extremity drape can be used.
  - When biopsies are performed above the knee or elbow, split sheets should be used for draping.
- The authors' preferred technique for prepping is alcohol followed by chlordexidine gluconate + isopropyl alcohol.

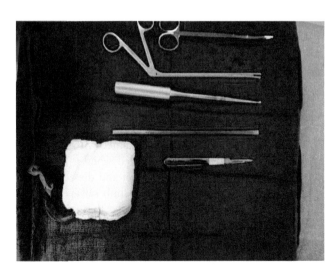

Figure 22-1 Required equipment for performing bone or soft tissue biopsy. From *top* to *bottom:* Dissecting scissors, pituitary rongeur, small curette, small osteotome, #15 blade scalpel, sponge. Note all instruments are pointed in the same direction to minimize cross contamination caused by handling of the instruments.

COMMONLY USED CPT CODES

- CPT Code: 20220/20225—Biopsy, bone, trocar, or needle; superficial/deep
- CPT Code: 38220/38221—Bone marrow biopsy, aspiration only/needle core
- CPT Code: 20240/20245—Biopsy, bone, open; superficial/deep
- CPT Code: 20200/20205—Biopsy, muscle; superficial/deep
- CPT Code: 23065/23066—Biopsy soft tissue shoulder; superficial/deep
- CPT Code: 24065/24066—Biopsy soft tissue arm or elbow; superficial/deep
- CPT Code: 25065/25066—Biopsy soft tissue forearm or wrist; superficial/deep
- CPT Code: 27040/27041—Biopsy soft tissue pelvis; superficial/deep
- CPT Code: 27323/27324—Biopsy soft tissue thigh or knee; superficial/deep
- CPT Code: 27613/27614—Biopsy soft tissue leg or ankle; superficial/deep

COMMONLY USED ICD9 CODES

- 238.0—Neoplasm of uncertain behavior of bone and articular cartilage
- 238.1—Neoplasm of uncertain behavior of connective and other soft tissue
- 239.2—Neoplasm of unspecified nature
- 198.5—Secondary malignant neoplasm of bone and bone marrow

COMMONLY USED ICD10 CODES

- D48.0—Neoplasm of uncertain behavior of bone and articular cartilage
- D48.1—Neoplasm of uncertain behavior of connective and other soft tissue
- D49.2—Neoplasm of unspecified behavior of bone, soft tissue, and skin
- C79.51—Secondary malignant neoplasm of bone

Incisional Biopsy Technique

- Longitudinal or expansile incisions should be used; transverse skin incisions are to be avoided.
- Incisions should be kept as small as possible and placed in locations that account for future reconstructive or salvage procedures.
- Dissection should proceed through a single muscle compartment rather than between fascial planes to limit soft tissue contamination.
- Meticulous hemostasis is critical in limiting contamination of surrounding tissue; therefore, if a tourniquet is used, it should be deflated before closure to ensure good hemostasis. Exsanguination should not be used before tourniquet inflation because of the risk of introducing tumor cells into the systemic circulation during exsanguination.
- The biopsy site is considered contaminated; all instruments or sponges in contact with the wound are similarly contaminated. To reduce the risk of reintroducing tumor cells into the wound, the surgeon should avoid placing fingers directly into the wound, all instruments should be pointed in the same direction on the mayo stand, and all sponges should be removed from the field with minimal handling.
- Once the lesion is encountered, specimens are obtained and sent for frozen section. This ensures that an adequate specimen has been obtained for pathologic diagnosis.
- Whenever a tissue biopsy is obtained, cultures should be sent concurrently with the frozen section specimens. Antibiotics are often held until cultures are obtained, especially if infection is considered a likely diagnosis.
- Permanent section specimens then are obtained. These should be sent as fresh tissue, *not* in formalin.
- If bone must be sampled during the biopsy, round or oval windows are preferred over sharp edges to reduce the stress riser created at the biopsy site.
- Cortical windows for bone biopsies are often plugged with cement.
- If a drain is used, it should exit in line with the incision in a longitudinal fashion as close as possible to the end of the incision because this tract will be excised during definitive treatment (Fig. 22-2).
- The wound is closed tightly in layers after hemostasis is achieved.

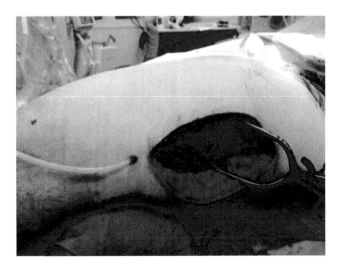

Figure 22-2 Correct placement of the drain exit site is shown. Note that the drain exits in line with the incision and immediately adjacent to its end. This tract will be excised during definitive management with wide excision.

Excisional Biopsy Technique

- Excisional biopsy follows the same principles as outlined previously, including avoidance of exsanguination, creation of longitudinally oriented incisions, and holding of antibiotics until samples can be obtained for culture, if infection is considered likely.
- If a primary wide excision is to be performed, then dissection should proceed circumferentially around the lesion through healthy tissue without violating the reactive zone of the lesion to minimize local contamination.
- Once the lesion is removed, it should be marked for orientation before being sent to the pathologist.
- Before closure, specimens from the superficial and deep margins should also be sent for frozen section analysis to confirm adequate margins have been obtained.
- Meticulous hemostasis must be obtained before closure to reduce the risk of contamination.

Common Biopsy Errors

- Transverse or nonexpansile incisions. These make definitive reconstructive procedures more challenging and increase the likelihood of needing soft tissue coverage to manage the defect created by excising a transverse incision (Fig. 22-3).
- Hematoma. Thorough hemostasis is important in preventing complications related to increased soft tissue contamination (Fig. 22-4).
  - Hematoma can be decreased with use of bone wax or cement to fill bony defects created during the biopsy, with deflating the tourniquet before closure, and with application of a compressive dressing after surgery.
- Lack of preoperative planning or imaging. This can lead to an unplanned excision of a malignant lesion, which then may require wider reexcision and increased morbidity to the patient.
- Implantation. This occurs when multiple surgical sites are exposed during the biopsy procedure, such as obtaining iliac crest bone graft to place into a bony lesion.

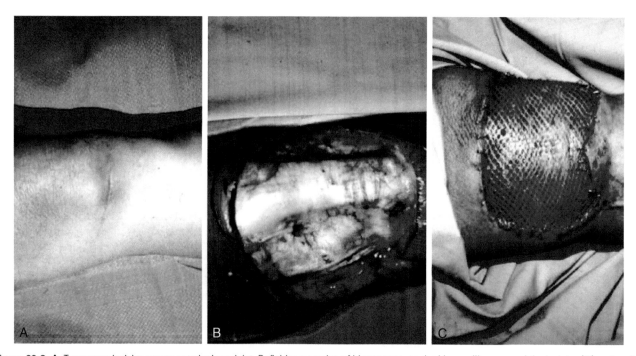

Figure 22-3 A, Transverse incision across anterior knee joint. Definitive resection of biopsy tract required large ellipse around the incision **(B)** and medial gastrocnemius flap coverage of the resulting defect **(C)**. (Photographs courtesy of Mark T. Scarborough, University of Florida.)

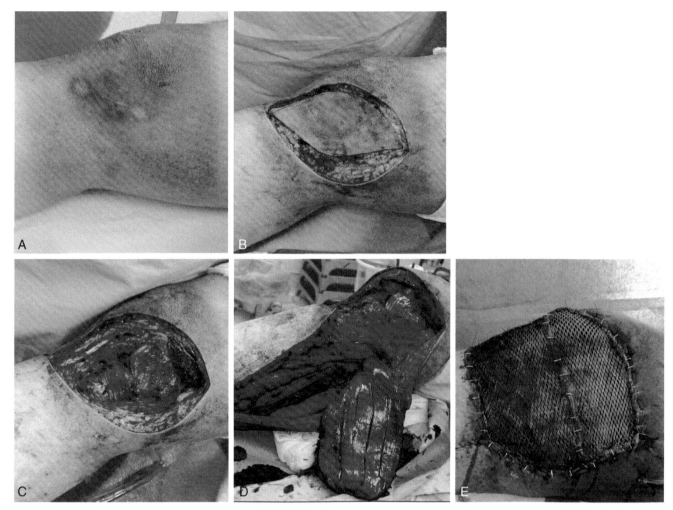

Figure 22-4 Hematoma formation after biopsy. **A,** Tourniquet was deflated after skin closure, resulting in contamination. **B,** Incision for wide margin around contaminated area. **C,** Definitive resection. **D,** Medial gastrocnemius flap raised for wound coverage. **E,** Final intraoperative appearance after skin grafting. (Photos courtesy of Mark T. Scarborough, University of Florida.)

Meticulous attention to contamination of instruments and surgical fields must be maintained to avoid implanting tumor cells into a distant site (Fig. 22-5).

- Presumed metastatic disease. A history of cancer elsewhere does not mean that the lesion is metastatic, and if it is the first metastasis for that patient, then a tissue diagnosis is required before treatment. Sending reamings during surgery for a pathologic fracture is inadequate for adequate pathologic diagnosis and has already contaminated the entire bone with tumor cells as a result of reamer passage. A small open incisional biopsy should be performed at the level of the lesion with frozen sections before treatment with an intramedullary device because the diagnosis of primary bone sarcoma would dramatically alter the treatment plan (Fig. 22-6).

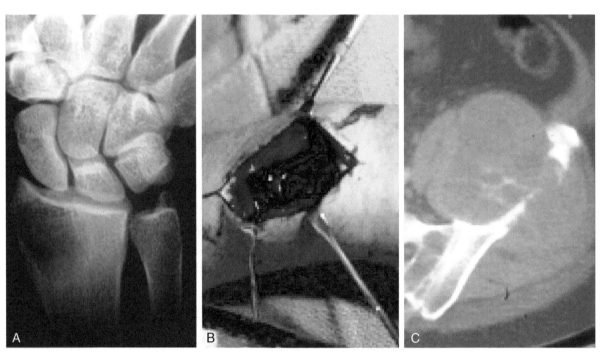

Figure 22-5 Distant implantation of giant cell tumor in a 25-year-old woman with distal radius giant cell tumor. **A,** Radiograph shows lytic lesion in the metaphysis of the distal radius. **B,** Open curettage and bone grafting; graft was taken from iliac crest. **C,** At 16 months after surgery, patient had development of distant giant cell tumor of the iliac crest from implantation as a result of cross contamination of instrumentation.

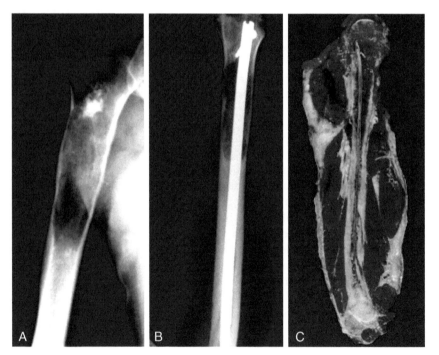

Figure 22-6 Presumed metastatic disease in a 60-year-old man with arm pain and remote history of carcinoma, treated as metastatic carcinoma. **A,** Radiographs show lytic lesion in the proximal humeral metadiaphysis; stipled calcifications appear to be present. **B,** Postoperative radiograph after intramedullary nailing for impending pathologic fracture. **C,** Biopsy at time of nailing confirmed chondrosarcoma; the patient subsequently needed forequarter amputation for definitive management. Gross specimen shown. (Photographs courtesy of Mark T. Scarborough, University of Florida.)

BRIEF SUMMARY OF SURGICAL STEPS

- Plan biopsy with laboratory and staging studies
- Hold antibiotics until sample obtained for culture
- Apply tourniquet if desired, but do not exsanguinate
- Incisional biopsy: Smallest possible longitudinal incision, single compartment dissection, tight closure
- Excisional biopsy: Longitudinal incision, raise flaps only as necessary, avoid penetrating tumor capsule
- Await frozen section analysis before closure
- Sample margin tissue for excisional biopsy
- Tight layered closure; drain if needed, exiting in line with incision

TECHNICAL PEARLS

- Always plan biopsy incision in line with definitive resection
- Longitudinal or expansile incisions
- Smallest incision possible to obtain adequate tissue
- Single muscle compartment dissection, avoiding raising flaps when possible
- Meticulous hemostasis, gelfoam and thrombin, bone wax, and bone cement can be used
- Await frozen section results before closure
- When sending tissue for pathology, also always send cultures
- If not comfortable with definitive management, refer to an experienced orthopaedic oncologist

REQUIRED EQUIPMENT

#15 Blade scaplel
Cushing forceps
Metzenbaum or Stevens tenotomy scissors
Set of osteotomes
Set of curettes
Set of pituitary rongeurs
Drain
Nylon sutures for closure

COMMON PITFALLS

(When to call for the attending physician)

- Transverse or inappropriate incisions
- Hematoma formation
- Presumed metastatic disease
- Inappropriate or no preoperative imaging
- Distant drain site placement
- Contamination or distant implantation

POSTOPERATIVE PROTOCOL

The postoperative protocol is dictated by the location and type of biopsy that was performed. No specific rehabilitation is generally required unless lesion excision included surrounding healthy muscle tissue (i.e., the quadriceps). In this case, therapy can be guided by the physical therapist to the tolerance of the patient as there are no specific limitations from an oncologic standpoint.

The most important aspect of the postoperative protocol is correctly interpreting and managing the results of the biopsy. Benign lesions that were treated with primary wide or marginal excision can be considered to be cured but may be followed with clinical examination with or without imaging to monitor for local recurrence. Patients undergoing incisional biopsies that are confirmed to be malignant should be managed by an experienced orthopaedic oncologist for definitive treatment.

POSTOPERATIVE CLINIC VISIT PROTOCOL

In general, sutures are removed at the 10-day to 14-day postoperative visit. Follow-up visits vary depending on the diagnosis. Wide excision of malignant lesions that have confirmed negative margins are followed with serial computed tomographic scans of the lungs to evaluate for distant metastasis and with magnetic resonance imaging evaluation of the tumor bed to evaluate for local recurrence. The schedule for this follow-up at the authors' institution is as follows: every 3 months for years 1 and 2, every 4 months during year 3, every 6 months from years 4 and 5, and then yearly. Advanced imaging may not be necessary beyond 5 years but is done based on physician preference.

SUGGESTED READINGS

1. Biermann JS, Holt GE, Lewis VO, Schwartz HS, Yaszemski MJ. Metastatic bone disease: diagnosis, evaluation, and treatment. *J Bone Joint Surg Am.* 2009;91(6):1518-1530.
2. Mankin HJ, Lange TA, Spanier SS. The hazards of biopsy in patients with malignant primary bone and soft tissue tumors. *J Bone Joint Surg Am.* 1982;64:1121-1127.
3. Mankin HJ, Mankin CJ, Simon MA. The hazards of biopsy, revisited. *J Bone Joint Surg Am.* 1996;78:656-663.

OPEN REDUCTION AND INTERNAL FIXATION OF A PATHOLOGIC HUMERAL SHAFT FRACTURE

Cara A. Cipriano | Andrew Park

CASE MINIMUM REQUIREMENTS

- No minimum requirement

COMMONLY USED CPT CODES

- 24515—Open treatment of humeral shaft fracture with plate/screws, with or without cerclage
- 24516—Treatment of humeral shaft fracture, with insertion of intramedullary implant, with or without cerclage and/or locking screws
- 24430—Repair of nonunion or malunion, humerus; without graft (e.g., compression technique
- 24435—Repair of nonunion or malunion, humerus; with iliac or other autograft (includes obtaining graft)
- 23150—Osteophyte resection—humerus

COMMONLY USED ICD9 CODES

- 733.11— Pathologic fracture of humerus

COMMONLY USED ICD10 CODES

- M84—Disorder of continuity of bone
- M84.42—Pathological fracture, unspecified humerus

A 64-year-old right-hand–dominant woman with metastatic breast cancer presented with several days of pain in her right arm without any antecedent trauma. Plain x-ray results showed permeative, osteoblastic, and osteolytic lesions throughout the right humerus and a nondisplaced pathologic humeral shaft fracture (Fig. 23-1). She also had numerous small lesions in the glenoid and humeral head, but her shoulder joint was intact with no radiographic evidence of arthritis or impending humeral head fracture. She was neurovascularly intact.

Three months before this presentation, the patient underwent intramedullary nailing of both femurs for pathologic midshaft femur fractures. Tissue obtained from the femoral lesions was sent to pathology at that time, and histologic analysis revealed metastatic adenocarcinoma consistent with a breast primary. Given her multifocal osseous disease and prior confirmation of metastatic breast cancer, no preoperative biopsy of the humeral shaft lesions was indicated. However, had this been a solitary bone lesion, a biopsy would have been necessary to establish the diagnosis before surgical fixation.

Because metastases were present throughout the humerus, treatment options for this patient included chemotherapy and local radiation combined with either nonoperative treatment in a Sarmiento brace, open reduction and internal fixation (ORIF) with cement and plates spanning the entire humerus, or total humerus endoprosthetic replacement. Nonoperative management with radiation alone is associated with prolonged time to healing and unreliable outcomes; total humerus endoprosthesis results in limited function from detachment of the rotator cuff and other soft tissue insertions. Because the objectives of treatment were pain relief, function, and local tumor control, the authors elected to perform cemented ORIF to provide immediate stability.

SURGICAL TECHNIQUE

Room Set-Up

- Use a standard operating room table with radiolucent hand table attached.
- Turn the bed 90 degrees to maximize the working space around the operative extremity.
- Position the C-arm at the head and the monitor at the foot.
- The electrocautery device is set at approximately 30/45 Hz, pending surgeon preference.

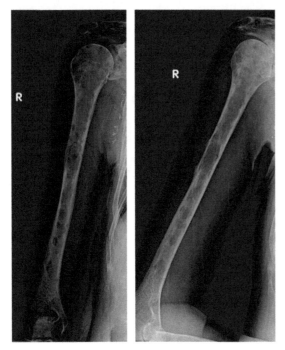

Figure 23-1 Anteroposterior and lateral radiographs show predominantly osteolytic lesions throughout the humerus and a nondisplaced midshaft fracture. (Photo credit: Ed Linn, Department of Orthopaedic Surgery Photographer, Washington University in St. Louis.)

Patient Positioning

- Position the patient supine on the operating room table.
- Angle the torso to bring the operative extremity onto the arm table.
- Place a bump under the scapula on the operative side.
- Apply sequential compression devices to both legs.

Prepping and Draping

- Administer preoperative antibiotics.
- Prep the entire arm past the shoulder to the base of the neck.
- Drape with split sheets to allow access to the subclavian vasculature.
- Cover the hand with a stockinette and cohesive bandage wrapping.

Surgical Approach

- Mark the coracoid process, deltopectoral groove, lateral bicipital sulcus, and distal biceps tendon with a marking pen (Fig. 23-2).
- Make a longitudinal incision that begins 1 cm lateral to the coracoid process, extends along the lateral border of the biceps, and ends 1 cm lateral to the biceps tendon at the level of the elbow.
- Proximally, dissect through the subcutaneous fat and develop the deltopectoral interval along the course of the cephalic vein between the deltoid (axillary nerve) and the pectoralis major (medial and lateral pectoral nerves). The cephalic vein can be taken either medially or laterally (Fig. 23-3). At the distal aspect of the deltopectoral interval, release the anterior fibers of the deltoid insertion to gain full exposure to the humeral shaft.
- Over the humeral diaphysis, extend the deltopectoral interval to the anterolateral approach to the arm. Retract the biceps (musculocutaneous nerve) medially to expose the brachialis overlying the humerus (Fig. 23-4). Split the brachialis between its medial (musculocutaneous nerve) and lateral (radial nerve) halves to allow access to the length of the shaft (Fig. 23-5).

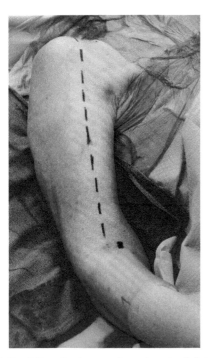

Figure 23-2 The deltopectoral approach can be extended distally to the anterolateral approach to the humerus. The incision begins 1 cm lateral to the coracoid process, extends along the lateral border of the biceps, and ends 1 cm lateral to the biceps tendon at the level of the elbow. (Photo credit: Ed Linn, Department of Orthopaedic Surgery Photographer, Washington University in St. Louis.)

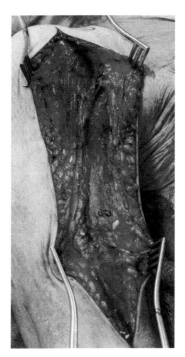

Figure 23-3 The cephalic vein is visible and delineates the deltopectoral interval. (Photo credit: Ed Linn, Department of Orthopaedic Surgery Photographer, Washington University in St. Louis.)

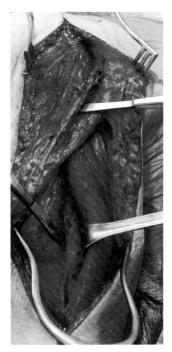

Figure 23-4 The proximal forceps show the deltopectoral interval with the cephalic vein taken laterally. Distally, the biceps is being retracted medially, and the distal forceps show the middle of the brachialis. (Photo credit: Ed Linn, Department of Orthopaedic Surgery Photographer, Washington University in St. Louis.)

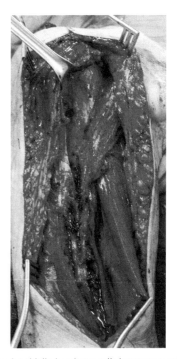

Figure 23-5 The brachialis has been split between portions innervated by the musculocutaneous and radial nerves, providing access to the humeral shaft. (Photo credit: Ed Linn, Department of Orthopaedic Surgery Photographer, Washington University in St. Louis.)

- Distally, the brachioradialis (radial nerve) can be retracted laterally and the brachialis medially to expose the lateral aspect of the distal humeral metadiaphysis. The radial nerve lies in this interval after it pierces the lateral intermuscular septum.

Curettage

- Deliver the fracture ends into the wound with a Cobb elevator.
- If the procedure is being performed to stabilize an impending rather than completed pathologic fracture, create a long trench in the anterior cortex with a 4-mm burr to access the tumor.
- Remove all intramedullary tumor with a combination of straight, curved, and (if available) uterine curettes. All gross tumors should be debrided in this fashion.
- Ensure that the instruments have been passed far enough into the canal to access and evacuate all metastatic foci (Fig. 23-6). If any uncertainty exists, this should be confirmed with fluoroscopy.

Cementing and Internal Fixation

- Provisionally reduce the fracture and select a plate that will bridge all metastatic lesions, allowing for adequate fixation proximally and distally. If no single plate is long enough, two plates should be placed with several overlapping screw holes to reduce strain at the junction (Figs. 23-7, 23-8, and 23-9).
- Use plate benders to contour the plate if needed. This is necessary most often around the distal metaphyseal flare.
- Provisionally fix the plate to either the proximal or distal fragment with a unicortical pin or screw to allow easy reduction of the fracture against the plate after cement insertion.

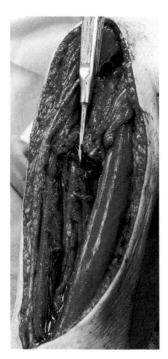

Figure 23-6 The distal fracture fragment has been delivered into the wound and a curette has been placed deep into the canal to remove the gross tumor. (Photo credit: Ed Linn, Department of Orthopaedic Surgery Photographer, Washington University in St. Louis.)

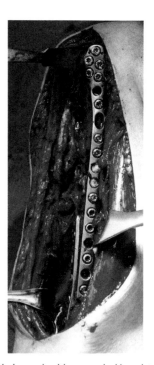

Figure 23-7 A 13-hole proximal humerus locking plate has been placed on the anterior aspect of the humerus, and a slightly contoured six-hole 3.5-mm large fragment plate has been placed distal and lateral. Note that the area of missing cortex at the fracture site has been filled with cement and screws have not been placed at this level. (Photo credit: Ed Linn, Department of Orthopaedic Surgery Photographer, Washington University in St. Louis.)

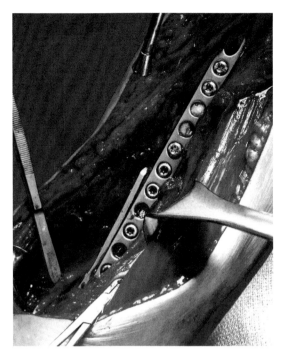

Figure 23-8 The forceps in the *bottom left* are pointing to the radial nerve, which was dissected free and protected. The musculocutaneous nerve can be found deep to the biceps, as shown here overlying the medial instrument. (Photo credit: Ed Linn, Department of Orthopaedic Surgery Photographer, Washington University in St. Louis.)

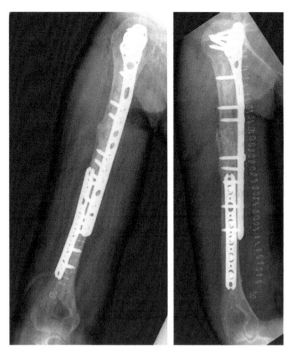

Figure 23-9 Postoperative anteroposterior and lateral radiographs of the humerus show cement and plate fixation of the pathologic humeral shaft fracture. (Photo credit: Ed Linn, Department of Orthopaedic Surgery Photographer, Washington University in St. Louis.)

- Irrigate, suction, and pack the canal in both directions.
- With a narrow-nozzled cement gun, insert low-viscosity cement into the canal proximally and distally. Pass the nozzle as far as possible into the canal and withdraw slowly while expressing cement to avoid formation of air pockets. Cement can also be used to fill any cortical defects at the site of the fracture.
- Hold the fracture reduced against the plate until the cement dries.
- Once the cement has fully hardened, fix the plates to the bone with multiple screws according the principles of fracture stabilization. Avoid placing screws into the most bone-deficient segments, which weakens the cement without strengthening the construct; instead, bridge these areas and place the screws where they have cortical purchase (Fig. 23-7).

Closure

- Irrigate the wound with saline solution.
- Establish hemostasis and place a drain if indicated.
- Repair the brachialis over the plate.
- Close the fascia, subcutaneous layer, and skin.
- Dress the wound, gently wrap the extremity from hand to axilla, and place the arm in a sling.

BRIEF SUMMARY OF SURGICAL STEPS

- Develop the deltopectoral interval and mobilize the biceps medially
- Split the brachialis and elevate it off the humerus
- Deliver the ends of the fracture into the wound and remove the tumor with curettes
- Irrigate and pack the canal to prepare for cementation
- Insert cement in the canal under pressure and reduce the fracture while the cement hardens
- Span the involved bone with plates then fix them in place with screws
- Place a drain if indicated
- Repair the brachialis over the plate
- Close the skin

REQUIRED EQUIPMENT

Radiolucent hand table
Curettes
Pulsatile irrigator
Narrow-nozzled cement gun
Low-viscosity polymethylmethacrylate cement
Large fragment set (or small fragment set in select cases)
Proximal humerus locking plates
Plate benders
Extra drill bits

TECHNICAL PEARLS

- Fluoroscopy is typically not necessary for screw placement but should be considered for plate selection; because the location and extent of the lesions are not visible during surgery, the length needed tends to be underestimated
- If a proximal humerus plate is indicated, selection of one designed to fit on the anterior rather than the lateral cortex allows easier screw insertion through this approach by minimizing the need for deltoid retraction
- Before mixing cement, measure the distance the nozzle of the cement gun will pass into the canal distally and proximally, then cut the nozzle to the longer of these two lengths; this allows for easier expression of the cement, which can otherwise be difficult through the long, narrow nozzle; when cementing, bury the nozzle to the hilt to ensure that you have inserted it as far as possible
- Begin cementing the canal when the cement is very wet to ease the process of insertion and to maximize fill and interdigitation; if significant cortical defects are present at the fracture site, wait a few minutes for the cement to become more viscous before filling these areas
- Drilling through cement is technically challenging because the canal has been filled; therefore, the tactile and auditory cues that you have reached the second cortex are absent. Be patient and take care not to plunge
- Clean the drill bit often when drilling through cement, and replace it if it becomes dull over the course of the case
- Because the friction from drilling focally melts the cement, the drill hole can become occluded by cement particles that reharden; therefore, if the depth gauge does not pass easily, a second, light application of the drill should easily resolve the problem

COMMON PITFALLS

(When to call for the attending physician)

- If you notice unexpected extension, displacement, or comminution of the fracture, call the attending
- If there is difficulty obtaining bicortical purchase while inserting screws, which is most likely due to the inherently poor bone quality, call the attending
- If there is any difficulty with cementing the canal, call the attending immediately
- Of note, the radial and musculocutaneous nerves can be injured during fracture manipulation as well as during cementing (radial nerve especially); call the attending if there is any concern for neurovascular injury

POSTOPERATIVE PROTOCOL

Place a sling on the patient before leaving the operating room; this is solely for comfort and can be discontinued as initial postoperative pain subsides. The patient can bear weight as tolerated through the operative arm. Occupational therapy should begin immediately with elbow, wrist, and hand range of motion and pendulum exercises for the shoulder. Outpatient occupational therapy is typically not required, and full strength and range of motion are expected to return within 4 to 6 weeks.

POSTOPERATIVE CLINIC VISIT PROTOCOL

The patient should follow up in 2 weeks for a wound check and staple removal. Of critical importance, the patient must receive radiation to the entire bone to prevent progression of the metastases and loss of fixation. The patient should be referred to a radiation oncologist immediately after surgery, and treatment itself should commence approximately 2 weeks after surgery, once initial healing has taken place and staples have been removed. The patient should follow up 6 weeks after surgery for a final visit.

SUGGESTED READINGS

1. Dijkstra S, Stapert J, Boxma H, et al. Treatment of pathological fractures of the humeral shaft due to bone metastases: a comparison of intramedullary locking nail and plate osteosynthesis with adjunctive bone cement. *Eur J Surg Oncol*. 1996;22:621-626.
2. Sarahrudi K, Wolf H, Funovics P, et al. Surgical treatment of pathological fractures of the shaft of the humerus. *J Trauma*. 2009;66:789-794.
3. Weber KL. Evaluation of the adult patient (aged >40 years) with a destructive bone lesion. *J Am Acad Orthop Surg*. 2010;18(3):169-179.
4. Al-Jahwari A, Schemitsch EH, Wunder JS, et al. The biomechanical effect of torsion on humeral shaft repair techniques for completed pathological fractures. *J Biomech Eng*. 2012;134(2):024501.
5. Ouyang H, Xiong J, Xiang P, et al. Plate versus intramedullary nail fixation in the treatment of humeral shaft fractures: an updated meta-analysis. *J Shoulder Elbow Surg*. 2013;22:387-395.

CHAPTER 24

PRINCIPLES OF FRACTURE FIXATION

PLATES/SCREWS AND INTRAMEDULLARY NAILS

Arvind von Keudell | Michael Collins | Jesse B. Jupiter

U nderstanding of bone healing and the biomechanics of fracture fixation is an important part of daily practice. Orthopaedic surgeons must properly reduce and repair fractured or diseased bone to restore function. Methods of doing so have evolved greatly over time. The Egyptians were known to use wooden splints in 300 BC, and plaster was used in Arabia as early as 800 AD. The method of internal fixation is a more elaborate and modern art. Tension wire use in fracture care was recorded in the 18th century. Intramedullary nailing started with Aztec physicians in the 16th century with wooden rods and later ivory. Robert Danis (1880-1962), known as the father of modern osteosynthesis, described compression plating in a 1938 paper.

We have advanced on the work of these past physicians as we continue to learn and refine orthopaedic care every day. Many of the principles that helped Danis and others discover early fracture care are the same ones we use today. This chapter presents basic engineering and biomechanical principles regarding bone fractures and characteristics of the materials used for repair of the musculoskeletal system.

BONE REGENERATION

- The goal of bone regeneration after the occurrence of a fracture is to restore stiffness and strength to provide the necessary physiologic load-bearing integrity of bone.
- Fracture healing is a complex interplay between biologic and mechanical mechanisms and occurs in four different tissue types: namely, cortical bone, intramedullary bone, periosteum, and surrounding soft tissues.
- Bone healing is thought to occur in three phases: inflammation, repair, and remodeling.
- Direct, primary bone healing occurs with direct cortical apposition under compression and minimal interfragmentary movement (rigid immobilization and anatomic reduction with a compression device; Fig. 24-1).
- Indirect, secondary bone healing occurs in less biomechanical rigid environments (load-sharing devices such as intramedullary nails, external fixators, or bridging plates). In contrast to primary bone healing, periosteum and surrounding tissues help with bone restoration integrating endochondral and intramembranous ossification (Fig. 24-2).
- *Clinical union* is defined as progressively increasing stiffness and strength, which is provided by the mineralization process to obtain a stable and pain-free fracture site. *Radiographic union* is defined as radiographic evidence of bone trabeculae or cortical bone crossing a fracture site.

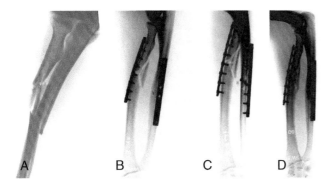

Figure 24-1 Radiographs show a complex radius fracture. **A,** Before surgery; **B,** immediately after surgery; **C,** at 6 weeks; and **D,** at 4 months after fixation yielded absolute stability. (With permission from Browner BD, et al, eds. *Skeletal Trauma*. 4th ed. Philadelphia: Elsevier; 2008. Figure 41-13, A-D.)

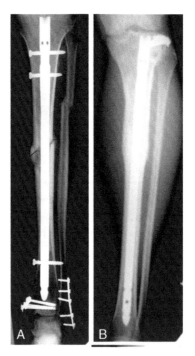

Figure 24-2 Proximal tibial fracture. **A,** Anteroposterior and **B,** lateral radiograph at 18 months after intramedullary nailing, demonstrating fracture healing achieved with relative stability. (With permission from Browner BD, et al, eds. *Skeletal Trauma*. 4th ed. Philadelphia: Elsevier; 2008. Figures 58-32, C and 58-31, F.)

BIOMECHANICS OF SURGICAL TREATMENT OF FRACTURED BONE

- The numerous fixation options for fracture treatment depend on location, fracture pattern, and surrounding soft tissue. The ultimate goal for all modalities is to provide sufficient stability to allow fracture healing to occur. The Association for Osteosynthesis (AO) principles have underscored the importance of anatomic reduction, stable fixation, preservation of blood supply, and early mobilization to accomplish the goal.
- **Stress** is defined by the intensity of the force per unit area of the tissue. Several types of stresses occur, such as tensile, compressive, shear, bending, torsional, and combined stress. **Strain** is the observed deformation of the tissue relative of the initial condition. Bone is an anisotropic material, which means it exhibits different stress-strain relationships depending on the direction of the applied stress.
- The stress-strain curve provides information about characteristics of tissue with four regions: elastic region, plastic region, yield point, and failure point. The **elastic modulus** or **stiffness** is defined as the elastic region and can be tensile or compressive, which ends at the yield point (Fig. 24-3).
- The strain theory is commonly used to explain fracture healing. **Fracture gap strain** is defined as the relative change in the fracture gap divided by the original fracture gap. The magnitude of interfragmentary strain is thought to determine the subsequent differentiation of fracture gap tissue, with high strain (>10%) leading to fibrous tissue, mild strains (2%-10%) to cartilaginous tissue, and minimal strain (<2%) to direct bone formation (Fig. 24-4).

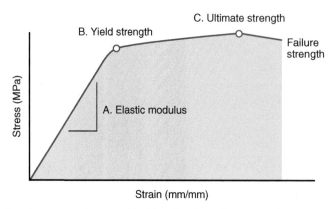

Figure 24-3 Sample stress-strain curve with *A* denoting slope, *B* yield, and *C* ultimate strength; energy is *shaded*. (With permission from Browner BD, et al, eds. *Skeletal Trauma*. 5th ed. Philadelphia: Elsevier; 2015. Figure 5-8.)

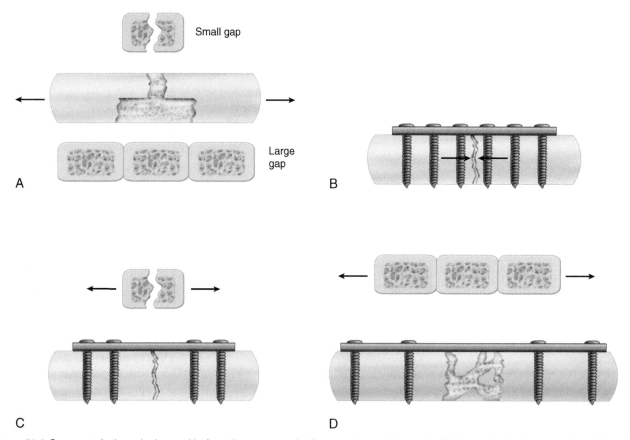

Figure 24-4 Perrens strain theory is shown with: **A,** motion represented at fracture site producing strain; **B,** fracture fixed with compression plating minimizing motion and strain; **C,** bridging plate exposing the fracture to high strain; and **D,** bridge plating a large complex fracture, which produces low strain despite motion. (Redrawn with permission from Wilber JH, Baumgaertel F. Bridge plating. In: Rüedi TP, Buckley RE, Moran CG, eds. *AO Principles of Fracture Management*. Stuttgart/New York: Thieme Verlag; 2007.)

OSTEOSYNTHESIS: PLATE AND SCREWS FIXATION

- Screws are mechanical devices that convert torsional into compressive forces (Fig. 24-5).
- The basic screw design depends on different variables, such as the outer diameter, the core diameter (both determine the bending and shear strength), and the screw pitch (distance between the threads or the distance the screw travels for each 360-degree turn).

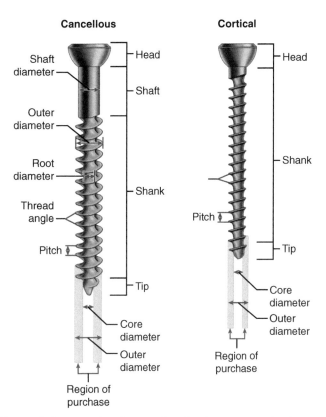

Figure 24-5 Diagram depicts properties of a screw that allow it to convert torsional energy into compression. (With permission from Browner BD, et al, eds. *Skeletal Trauma*. 5th ed. Philadelphia: Elsevier; 2015. Figure 8-7.)

- The various kinds of screws can be classified depending on their function (lag screw versus compression screw versus positional screw), their configuration (self-tapping versus non–self-tapping), their application (cortex, cancellous, pelvic cortex, malleolar), and thread length (partially threaded versus fully threaded).

SELF-TAPPING VERSUS NON–SELF-TAPPING SCREWS

- Self-tapping screws are inserted into the bone after a drill hole has been made without a prior use of a tap. The cutting flutes or trocar design aid in creating a screw hole; however, these screws have lower pullout strength than non–self-tapping screws.

CORTICAL SCREWS, CANCELLOUS SCREWS, MALLEOLAR SCREWS

- Cortical screws come in different sizes and can function either as a positional screw or as a lag screw for interfragmentary compression.
- Cancellous screws consist of a thicker inner diameter with thinner threads that provide more purchase in cancellous bone, usually in the metaphyseal area.
- The malleolar screw is a special form of cancellous screw. These screws are partially threaded with a self-tapping trephine tip to act as an interfragmentary screw fixation type, sometimes augmented with a plastic or metal washer.

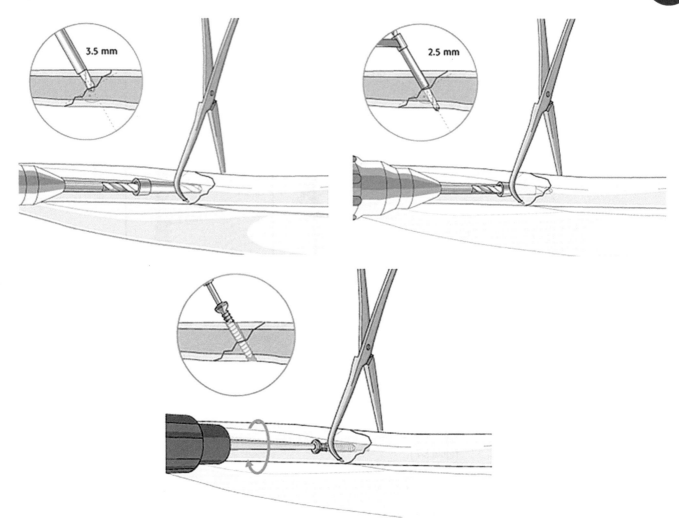

Figure 24-6 Diagram depicts proper placement of a lag screw crossing the fracture fragment and perpendicularly compressing the two fragments. (With permission from Browner BD, et al, eds. *Skeletal Trauma*. 5th ed. Philadelphia: Elsevier; 2015. Figure 8-21.)

LAG SCREW FIXATION TECHNIQUE

- Lag screw technique relies on the fact the screw thread catches only the far cortex and thereby produces interfragmentary compression. This can be achieved with overdrilling of the near cortex. The compression obtained with this technique can be used for various types of fractures, except horizontal or short oblique patterns, which have to be augmented with a combined screw and plate fixation or another form of internal fixation (Fig. 24-6).

HOW MANY SCREWS IN A PLATE AND SCREW CONSTRUCT?

- Retrospective reviews of fracture fixations have led to the generally recommended number of cortices on each side of a fracture: seven in the femur, six in the tibia or humerus, and five in the radius or ulna (Fig. 24-7).
- Every screw placed in a plate screw construct reduces stress by increasing surface area between plate and bone; however, these screws can also act as a stress riser that may cause failure at the interface.
- Empty drill holes are a source for stress concentration and should be avoided.

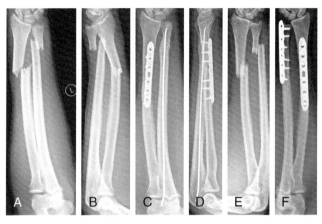

Figure 24-7 **A** and **B** show a preoperative bone fracture of the forearm. **C** through **F** are after fixation with six cortical contacts on each side of the fracture line. (With permission from Browner BD, et al, eds. *Skeletal Trauma*. 5th ed. Philadelphia: Elsevier; 2015. Figure 45-22.)

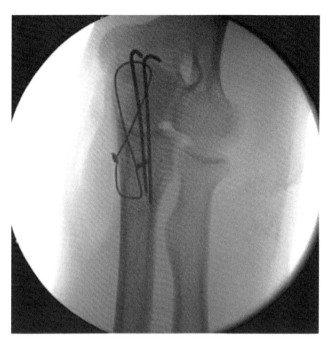

Figure 24-8 Intraoperative fluoroscopic picture of tension band use for an olecranon fracture. (With permission from Browner BD, et al, eds. *Skeletal Trauma*. 5th ed. Philadelphia: Elsevier; 2015. Figure 46-7, A.)

PLATE AND SCREW CONSTRUCT

- The plate and screw fixation stems from early research of the tension band principles (i.e., application of a screw wire fixation technique on the tension side of the bone [convex] to accomplish compression).
- Danis was the first to describe true compression plating, which was subsequently further developed by the AO group in Switzerland in 1961 to revolutionize fracture management. The plate provides load-bearing characteristics from the two fracture ends; this must be protected from premature weight-bearing.
- Several plate categories now exist, such as the neutralization plate, compression plate, buttress plate, and bridge plate.

TENSION BAND TECHNIQUE

- The tension band is placed along the tension/convex site and thereby produces compressive forces. The principle remains one of the cornerstones of plate designs (Fig. 24-8).

BRIDGING PLATES

- Comminuted fracture and unstable fracture patterns are amenable for bridge plating. Those span the defect and do not attempt to provide rigid stability, but rather maintain length and alignment (Fig. 24-9).
- Limited dissection is recommended to avoid the impairment of biologic repair capabilities.
- A wave plate design is similar but leaves more space between the cortex of the bone and the plate to maximize the biologic repair, especially in the treatments of nonunions that require bone grafting.

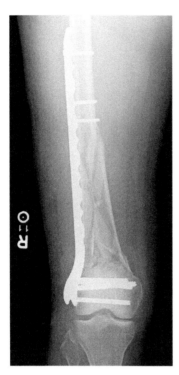

Figure 24-9 Comminuted fracture of the femur fixed with a bridge plate. (With permission from Browner BD, et al, eds. *Skeletal Trauma*. 5th ed. Philadelphia: Elsevier; 2015. Figure 8-50, B.)

NEUTRALIZATION PLATE

- Neutralization plates are used in combination with interfragmentary (lag) screw fixation to neutralize torsional, bending, and shear forces (Fig. 24-10).
- This method is the traditional and effective way to obtain rigid fixation of simple diaphyseal fractures.
- Lag screws should be used wherever possible because this construct has been shown to provide the highest amount of strength.

BUTTRESS PLATE

- Buttress or antiglide plates are used in epiphyseal or metaphyseal fractures, especially in tibial plateau or pilon fractures, because of the thin cortical bone and brittle spongiosa (Fig. 24-11).
- The plate screw construct negates shear and compression forces and is frequently used in association with lag screw techniques to augment stability.
- Contouring and rigid fixation to the supporting fracture fragment is mandatory, and special attention should be observed for support of the shoulder of the plate screw construct to prevent axial deformation with loading. Screw insertion should be in a manner to prevent gliding of the plate (i.e., buttress mode).

COMPRESSION PLATES

- Horizontal or short oblique fracture patterns that are not amenable for interfragmentary screw fixation are a good indication for compression plating.
- Compression through a plate device can be achieved with an articulating tension device, with overbending of the plate, or with eccentric positioning of screws.

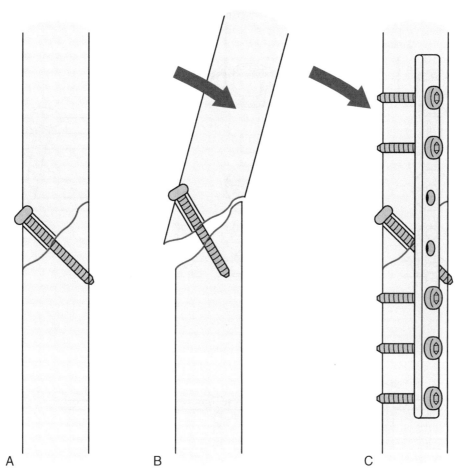

Figure 24-10 Diagram depicts a fracture fixated with: **A-B,** a lag screw; and **C,** a neutralization plate. (With permission from Browner BD, et al, eds. *Skeletal Trauma.* 5th ed. Philadelphia: Elsevier; 2015. Figure 8-43.)

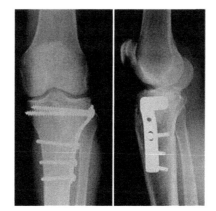

Figure 24-11 Radiographs depict a tibial plateau fracture held together with a lateral buttress plate. (With permission from Browner BD, et al, eds. *Skeletal Trauma.* 5th ed. Philadelphia: Elsevier; 2015. Figure 62-48, B.)

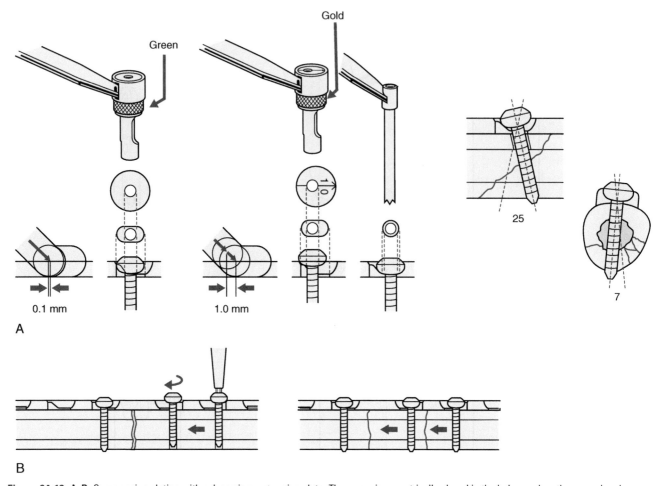

Figure 24-12 A-B, Compression plating with a dynamic compression plate. The screw is eccentrically placed in the hole so when the screw head engages the plate, a perpendicular displacement occurs, compressing the fracture. (With permission from Browner BD, et al, eds. *Skeletal Trauma.* 5th ed. Philadelphia: Elsevier; 2015. Figure 8-45.)

- Various plates have been designed and modified, such as the first AO self-compression plate (semitubular, one-third tubular, or quarter tubular plates) or the dynamic compression plates (DCP), which evolved into limited contact dynamic compression plates (LC-DCP) to help with promoting in biologic healing (Fig. 24-12).

RECONSTRUCTION PLATE

- Reconstruction plates have the advantage of being able to be contoured in any plane because of their design with notches in its side.
- This mainstay of fracture treatment in the pelvis, however, is also used in the fixation of distal humerus fractures and can be also used in a compression mode (Fig. 24-13).

LOCKING PLATES

- Locking plates had its origin in the 1970s in Poland. The Zespol system was similar to a combination of an external fixator and locked plate screw design.

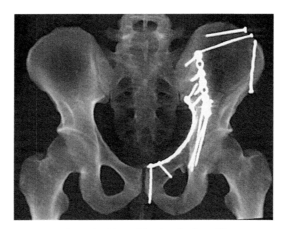

Figure 24-13 Anteroposterior radiograph of the pelvis after fixation with a reconstruction plate contoured to fit along the cortex of the pelvis. (With permission from Browner BD, et al, eds. *Skeletal Trauma.* 5th ed. Philadelphia: Elsevier; 2015. Figure 41-6, O.)

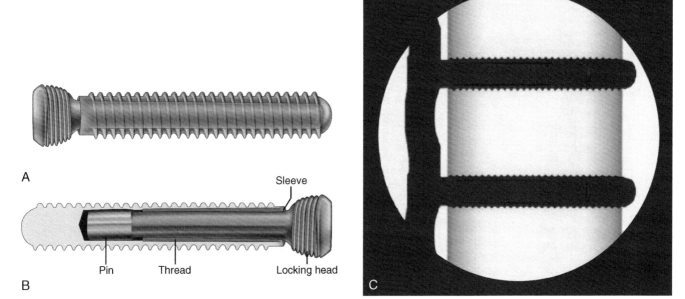

Figure 24-14 Diagram depicts a locking plate. Note the threaded screw head, which when engaged into the plate creates a fixed angle device. (With permission from Browner BD, et al, eds. *Skeletal Trauma.* 5th ed. Philadelphia: Elsevier; 2015. Figure 69-11.)

- The discovery of impaired periosteal blood flow as a result of compression plates in combination with the rise of minimally invasive techniques with indirect reduction techniques and the recognition of the difficulties of treatment of osteoporotic fracture have finally led to the development of fixed angle devices.
- The Schuhli nut (Synthes, Paoli, PA) was the first attempt to lock screws into the plate. The idea was further nurtured and produced the point contact fixator, which jammed the screw into the plate and created a fixed angle device (Fig. 24-14).
- Locking compression plates and less invasive stabilization systems now are used for specific fracture patterns and bone biology. The latest development of polyaxial locking head screws can potentially help to address fractures with consideration of specific location and individual bone quality (Fig. 24-15).

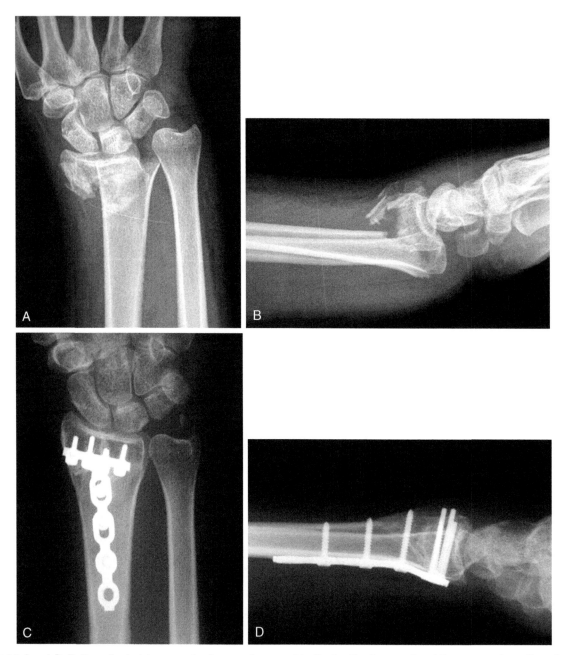

Figure 24-15 **A** and **B,** Radiographs depict preoperative images of an unstable distal radius fracture; **C** and **D,** postoperative radiographs following fracture fixation utilizing a volar locking plate. (With permission from Browner BD, et al, eds. *Skeletal Trauma.* 5th ed. Philadelphia: Elsevier; 2015. Figure 44-13.)

ANGLED PLATES

- The enormous stress that occurs at the proximal and distal femur traditionally has been addressed with either a 130-degree blade plate or a 95-degree condylar blade plate.
- Those plates are characterized to have a thicker shaft than the blade to withstand higher amount of forces (e.g., in the subtrochanteric region).
- The precise placement and small room for error have caused a decrease in usage despite their good reported outcomes, with the sliding hip screw or trochanteric femoral nails taking over (Fig. 24-16).

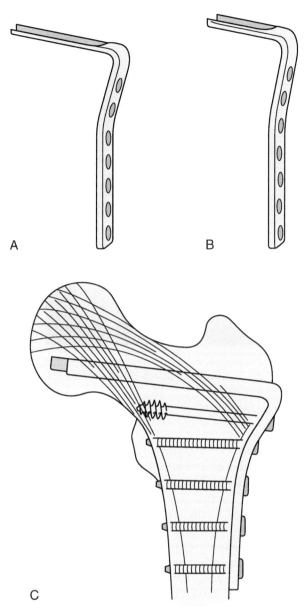

Figure 24-16 A-B, Diagram depicts a 95-degree angled blade plate and its use in a femoral fracture (**C**). (With permission from Browner BD, et al, eds. *Skeletal Trauma.* 5th ed. Philadelphia: Elsevier; 2015. Figure 8-36.)

SLIDING HIP SCREW AND COMPRESSION PLATES

- Sliding hip devices use the combined force vector to allow for optimal impaction of the two fracture fragments.
- Compression across the fracture site is obtained by placing the lag screw and the barrel across the fracture site and by providing a distance for the lag screw to slide through the barrel to close the fracture gap.
- Those two basic principles must be applied to achieve fracture healing.
- An extension plate is used in cases in which the lateral femoral wall is not intact (Fig. 24-17).

INTRAMEDULLARY NAILING

- Intramedullary rods act as an internal splint to fractures, most commonly used in diaphyseal long bone.

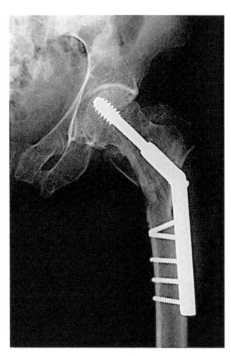

Figure 24-17 Postoperative radiograph shows an intertrochanteric femur fracture fixed with a sliding hip screw. (With permission from Browner BD, et al, eds. *Skeletal Trauma.* 5th ed. Philadelphia: Elsevier; 2015. Figure 55-6, B.)

- They were introduced in 1939 and provide a load-sharing characteristic that appears to create a biomechanical environment that results in high rates of unions.
- Cross-sectional geometry, rod length, the presence of a longitudinal slot, and the elastic modulus of the material play a significant role in determining the rigidity of the construct. This specifically applies in the characteristic of an intramedullary device.
- The rigidity of an intramedullary nail is proportional to the fourth power of the rod radius but is also dependent on the wall thickness. Longitudinal slots had the benefit to expand like a spring according to the diameter of the intramedullary canal but demonstrated a dramatic reduction in torsional rigidity and thus were discontinued.
- The working length of a fracture is defined as the distance between the proximal and distal end of the fracture.
- Bending and torsional forces that act on the bone-rod construct alter the amount interfragmentary motion when the working length is changed.
- Although bending forces occur at four different points along the bone implant construct, torsional forces exert most motion at the mechanical interlocking screw fixation points. Application of an interlocking mechanism at either proximal or distal site can increase forces transmitted through the fracture, whereas locking at both sites helps with reduction of axial displacement and increases torsional rigidity (Fig. 24-18).

UNLOCKED INTRAMEDULLARY NAILS VERSUS LOCKED INTRAMEDULLARY NAILS

- Unlocked intramedullary nails have been used but lack the longitudinal and rotational stability and therefore need an external stabilizer. Unlocked intramedullary nails obtain their stability from their three-point curvature mismatch, whereas locked intramedullary nails, be it in either dynamic, static, or double-locked mode, control stability with insertion of a screw through the nail.

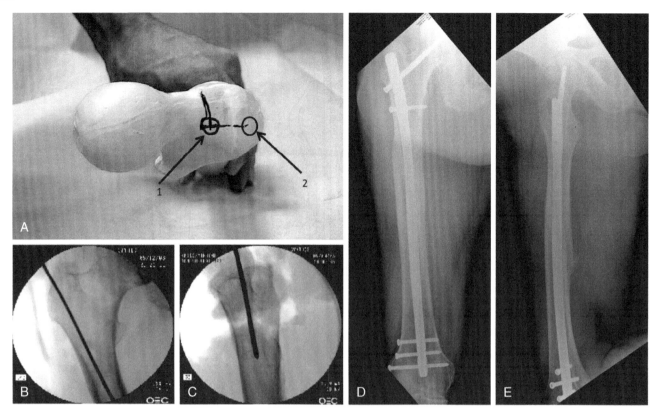

Figure 24-18 **A,** Piriformis (1) and trochanteric (2) entry points for an intramedullary femoral nail are shown. **B** and **C** show fluoroscopic images. **D** and **E,** Radiographs after anterograde intramedullary nailing of the femur. (With permission from Browner BD, et al, eds. *Skeletal Trauma.* 5th ed. Philadelphia: Elsevier; 2015. Figure 58-20.)

REAMING VERSUS NONREAMING

- Reaming of the intramedullary cavity has been shown to cause significant disruption of the endosteal blood system and potential altering of the infection rate. However, the benefits of a larger radius and tight-fitting nail appear to negate the potential downside of disrupting the biology and the negative effect on the pulmonary system, especially in the polytrauma case. However, this approach cannot be generalized, and the individual fracture pattern, fracture biology, and patient have to be taken into account (Fig. 24-19).

EXTERNAL FIXATOR

- The external fixator is now commonly used for the treatment of open fracture, especially of the lower extremity.
- Multiple pins are introduced into the bone and are interconnected with external rods.
- Various factors influence the amount of desired stability of the external fixator, most importantly, the size of the inserted pins followed by the contact of the fracture ends, the number of pins, pins in different planes, increased size of the rods, increased spacing between pins, and decreased bone-to-rod distance.
- The Ilizarov external fixator is a circular external fixator that can be applied for a multitude of fractures; however, most applications are in the treatment of nonunions and deformities (Fig. 24-20).

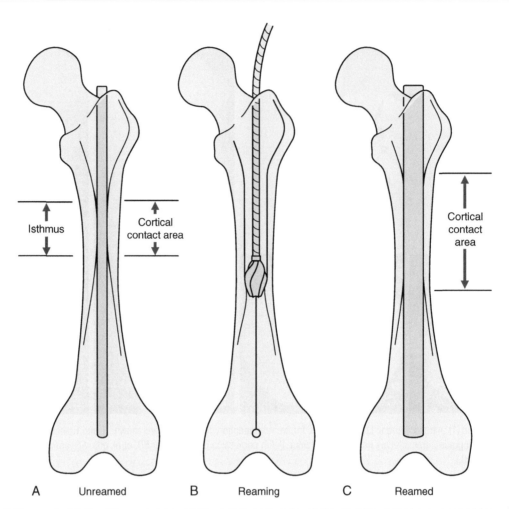

Figure 24-19 A-C, Diagram depicts the difference in intramedullary nail diameter and cortical contact in a reamed and unreamed femur. (With permission from Browner BD, et al, eds. *Skeletal Trauma.* 5th ed. Philadelphia: Elsevier; 2015. Figure 8-58.)

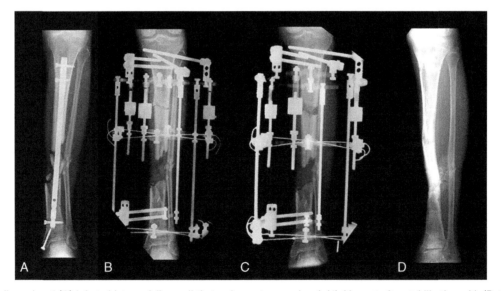

Figure 24-20 Radiographs of **(A)** infected intramedullary nail that underwent removal and débridement after stabilization with **(B, C,** and **D)** Ilizarov external fixator. (With permission from Browner BD, et al, eds. *Skeletal Trauma.* 4th ed. Philadelphia: Elsevier, 2008. Figure 11-34BC.)

SUGGESTED READINGS

1. The classic. The aims of internal fixation. *Clin Orthop Relat Res.* 1979;(138):23-25.
2. Einhorn TA, Gerstenfeld LC. Fracture healing: mechanisms and interventions. *Nat Rev Rheumatol.* 2015;11(1):45-54.
3. Pauwels F. *Biomechanics of the Locomotor Apparatus.* Berlin/Heidelberg/New York: Springer Verlag; 1980.
4. Küntscher G. *Praxis der Marknagelung.* Stuttgart: Schattauer; 1962.
5. Kempf I, Grosse A, Beck G. Closed locked intramedullary nailing. Its application to comminuted fractures of the femur. *J Bone Joint Surg Am.* 1985;67(5):709-720.
6. Miclau T, Martin RE. The evolution of modern plate osteosynthesis. *Injury.* 1997;28(suppl 1):A3-A6.
7. Mueller ME, Schneider R, et al. *Manual of Internal Fixation: Techniques Recommended by the AO-ASIF Group.* 3rd ed. Berlin: Springer Verlag; 1990.
8. Perren SM, Cordey J, Enzler M, Matter P, Rahn BA, Schlapfer F. [Mechanics of bone screw with internal fixation plates (author's transl)]. *Unfallheilkunde.* 1978;81(4):201-218.

CHAPTER 25

SKELETAL TRACTION PIN PLACEMENT

FEMORAL, TIBIAL, AND CALCANEAL

Amar Arun Patel | Stephen M. Quinnan

A key principle of fracture management is early alignment and stabilization of broken bones to minimize ongoing soft tissue injury and decrease pain. This is also important to relieve pressure and deformity of nerves and blood vessels in the extremity. Many long bone fractures are adequately controlled with splints; however, more unstable fractures often necessitate constant, controlled force for initial stabilization. In some situations, skin or bucks traction may be considered, but only limited amounts of weight can be applied without a high risk of skin complications. Skeletal traction is a powerful and generally preferred alternative for temporary stabilization of long bone and acetabular fractures until operative treatment can be performed.

Proximal tibial traction pins are indicated for femoral shaft fractures and high-energy proximal femur fractures. These pins should not be placed in cases with ipsilateral knee ligament injury. Distal femoral traction is the method of choice for acetabular fractures, vertical shear pelvis fractures, and unstable hip dislocations. Calcaneal traction pins currently are integrated in ankle-spanning external fixators (i.e., for distal tibia or pilon fractures) and are used very infrequently at this time. As a rule, traction pins should never be inserted through a fracture, lytic lesion, or large wound.

In general, two types of traction set-ups are commonly used. The first uses centrally threaded Steinmann pins with sizes of either 4.5-mm or 5.0-mm diameter recommended for adults. Smaller threaded pins are recommended for distal femoral traction in pediatric patients with femur fractures. The second type of traction uses a smooth wire 1.6 to 2.5 mm in diameter under high tension with a Kirschner bow. This type of traction can be used for all fractures but is especially helpful for avoiding prostheses or implants.

CASE MINIMUM REQUIREMENTS

- None

COMMONLY USED CPT CODES

- CPT Code: 20690—Application of a uniplane (pins or wires in one plane), unilateral, external fixation system
- CPT Code: 27193—Closed treatment of pelvic ring fracture, dislocation, diastasis or subluxation; without manipulation
- CPT Code: 27222—Closed treatment of acetabulum (hip socket) fracture(s); with manipulation, with or without skeletal traction
- CPT Code: 27232—Closed treatment of intertrochanteric, peritrochanteric, or subtrochanteric femoral fracture; with manipulation, with or without skin or skeletal traction
- CPT Code: 27501—Closed treatment of supracondylar or transcondylar femoral fracture with or without intercondylar extension, without manipulation
- CPT Code: 27502—Closed treatment of femoral shaft fracture, with manipulation, with or without skin or skeletal traction

SURGICAL TECHNIQUE

Room Set-Up

- Informed consent must be obtained before the procedure.
- Orthogonal radiographs of the fracture and site of traction pin insertion should be obtained before pin insertion.
- If possible, bedside sedation or anesthesia should be administered.
- The patient shoud be in the center of the room on a stretcher or an operating room table.
- Sterile equipment should be placed on the surgeon's side, and a nonsterile assistant should be on the contralateral side.

Patient Positioning

- The patient is positioned supine.

Prepping and Draping

- Draping should allow for palpation of marked bony landmarks.
- Chlorhexidine or iodine-based solution should be applied to the skin.
- Draping should consist of sterile sheets placed around the sterile field.
- An assistant should be nonsterile and should maintain proper limb alignment (i.e., patella facing anterior) during the procedure.

Proximal Tibial Traction Pin

- Landmarks are the tibial tubercle, fibular head, patella, and knee joint line.
- The entry point is at 2 cm posterior and 1 cm distal to the tibial tubercle (Fig. 25-1; Video 25-1).
- The direction should be lateral to medial.
- Dangers include the peroneal nerve with distal placement and weaker cancellous bone with proximal placement.
- After the entry point is determined, infiltrate the overlying skin and periosteum with a topical anesthetic (i.e., lidocaine). Infiltrate the projected exit point in a similar fashion.
- Make a 1-cm stab incision at the entry point. Spread the deep tissues with a hemostat to stay out of the anterior compartment.
- With the Steinmann pin, palpate the anterior and posterior edge of the tibia, and engage the tip at the midpoint. With a battery-powered or hand drill, spin the Steinmann pin in a clockwise fashion.
- As the pin engages, ensure that it is traveling parallel to the floor and parallel to the joint line. It is helpful to have the assistant verify this for you. To prevent skiving, start drilling the pin at an oblique angle to engage the bone and then change the position of the pin before drilling further.
- Once the pin is drilled throught the far cortex and is abutting the skin, make an incision at the projected exit point. Continue spinning the pin until there is approximaly 5 cm remaining on the near side.

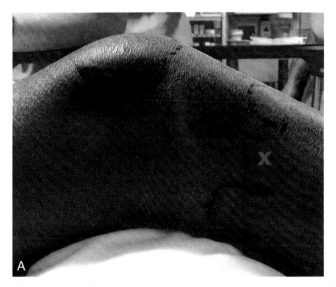
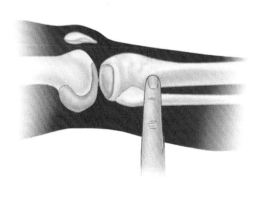

A   B

Figure 25-1 **A**, Clinical photograph; **B**, schematic demonstrating intended location of pin insertion on the tibia. Bony landmarks for proximal tibial traction pin, placed from lateral to medial along the proximal aspect of tibia. The entry point is 2 cm posterior and 1 cm distal to the tibial tubercle. (Part B redrawn from Tibial skeletal traction. In: Thompson SR, Zlotolow DA, eds. *Handbook of Splinting and Casting*. Philadelphia: Elsevier; 2012. Figure 16-5.)

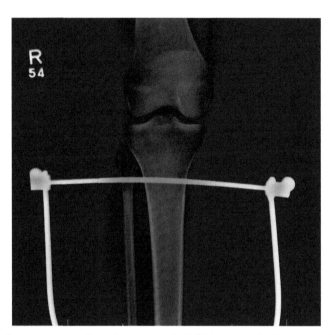

Figure 25-2 Anteroposterior radiograph shows proximal tibial traction pin placement within the tibial metaphysis and parallel to the knee joint line.

- Once the pin is seated, manually pull the pin back and forth in the axial plane to ensure that it is within bone.
- Radiographs should be taken to verify the pin placement (Fig. 25-2).

Distal Femoral Traction Pin

- The landmarks are the patella, knee joint line, and adductor tubercle.
- The entry point is at the adductor tubercle (proximal to medial epicondyle), which also correlates with the level of the superior pole of the patella on the medial femur (Fig. 25-3; Video 25-2).
- The direction should be medial to lateral.
- Dangers include the femoral artery in Hunter's canal with proximal placement.
- Place a small stack of towels under the distal femur to allow clearance of the contralateral extremity.
- Insert the pin with the same principles outlined previously.
- Ensure that the pin is placed parallel to the joint line and not perpendicular to the femoral shaft.
- Radiographs should be taken to verify the pin placement (Fig. 25-4).

Calcaneal Traction Pin

- The landmarks are the medial malleolus, lateral malleolus, and calcaneal tuberosity.
- The entry point is at 2.5 cm inferior and 2.5 cm posterior to the inferior edge of the medial malleolus (Fig. 25-5; Video 25-3).
- The direction should be medial to lateral.
- Dangers include the posterior tibial neurovascular bundle.
- Insert the pin with the same principles outlined previously.
- Ensure the pin is parallel to the floor and parallel to the talus (roughly parallel to the transmalleolar axis).
- Calcaneal traction pins are usually performed in conjunction with an ankle-spanning external fixator with fluoroscopy available.
- Radiographs should be taken to verify the pin placement (Fig. 25-6).

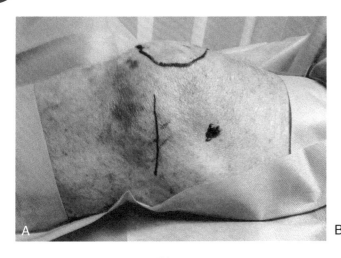

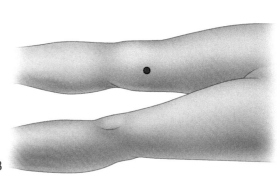

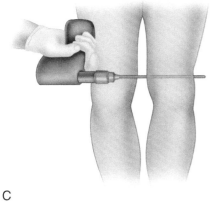

Figure 25-3 **A,** Bony landmarks for distal femoral traction pin, placed from medial to lateral, along the distal aspect of the femur. **B-C,** The entry point is at the adductor tubercle (proximal to medial epicondyle) and approximately at the level of the superior pole of the patella on the medial femur *(purple dot).* (Parts B and C redrawn from Femoral skeletal traction. In: Thompson SR, Zlotolow DA, eds. *Handbook of Splinting and Casting.* Philadelphia: Elsevier; 2012. Figures 15-7 and 15-8.)

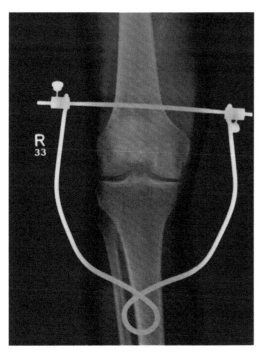

Figure 25-4 Anteroposterior radiograph shows distal femoral traction pin placement within femoral metaphysis and parallel to the knee joint line.

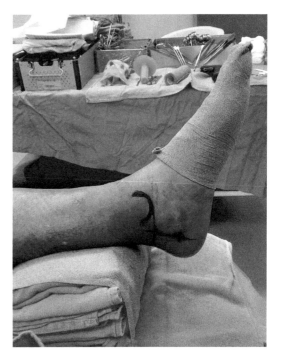

Figure 25-5 Bony landmarks for calcaneal traction pin, which is placed from medial to lateral in the calcaneal tuberosity. The entry point is 2.5 cm inferior and 2.5 cm posterior to the tip of the medial malleolus.

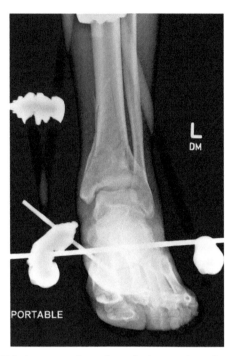

Figure 25-6 Anteroposterior radiograph shows calcaneal traction pin parallel to talar dome.

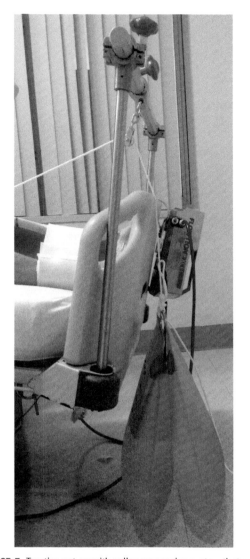

Figure 25-7 Traction set-up with pulley suspension system that connects traction bow to water bags holding appropriate weight.

Traction Set-Up

- Cut the sharp ends of the pin with a bolt cutter, leaving approximately 5 mm free. Endcaps should be applied to the cut ends.
- Apply petrolatum gauze followed by rolled gauze around the pin on either side. Bend the traction bow and fasten it securely to the pin. Overwrap the entire set-up with a gauze roll.
- Set up a bed frame at the foot of the bed with or without a pulley (Fig. 25-7).
- Shuttle a rope through the pulley and secure it through the loop of the traction bow with a surgeon's knot. Secure the free end with a slipknot to the traction bag.
- Fill the traction bag with 15% of the patient's body weight. More of the patient's body weight (15% to 20%) is generally acceptable for pelvic and acetabular fractures. Less weight (10% to 15%) should be used when 90-90 traction is set up for pediatric patients.
- Ensure that the patient is comfortable in the current traction set-up.

BRIEF SUMMARY OF SURGICAL STEPS

- Informed consent and proper sedation administered
- Mark bony landmarks and entry point before prepping
- Infiltrate entry and exit points with anesthetic
- Make 1 cm incision and identify bone
- Drill Steinmann pin parallel to joint line and floor
- Verify pin position manually or with fluoroscopy
- Cut and cap pins
- Apply traction up to 20% of body weight

REQUIRED EQUIPMENT

Threaded Steinmann pin set
Battery-powered or hand drill
Scalpel
Hemostat
Traction bow
Gauze and petrolatum gauze
Traction board (pulley optional)
Traction bag

TECHNICAL PEARLS

- Mark bony landmarks before incision
- Start pin in an oblique position to engage bone before drilling further
- Pay attention to the pin in relation to the floor and joint line during insertion
- Cut sharp ends off of the pin after insertion for safety
- Test the stability of the pin within bone with manual axial force
- Traction should be up to 20% of body weight
- Check radiographs before and after traction
- Continue daily pin site care until definite surgery

COMMON PITFALLS

(When to call for the attending physician)

- In the case of brisk arterial bleeding, remove the pin, apply pressure, and ask for assistance in exploring the wound
- If the pin is suspected to be entering the joint, remove the pin and obtain radiographs; consider administering empiric antibiotics for an iatrogenic open joint
- Always perform and document neurovascular status before and after the procedure

POSTOPERATIVE PROTOCOL

A neurovascular examination should be completed after the traction set-up is complete. Radiographs immediately after traction and serially until surgery should be performed to assess for alignment. Patients in traction should have daily pin site care with normal saline solution and hydrogen peroxide or chlorhexidine. Traction pins should not be reused after their removal.

SUGGESTED READINGS

1. Althausen PL, Hak DJ. Lower extremity traction pins: indications, technique, and complications. *Am J Orthop (Belle Mead NJ)*. 2002;31(1):43-47.
2. Bumpass DB, Ricci WM, McAndrew CM, Gardner MJ. A prospective study of pain reduction and knee dysfunction comparing femoral skeletal traction and splinting in adult trauma patients. *J Orthop Trauma*. 2015;29(2):112-118.
3. Casey D, McConnell T, Parekh S, Tornetta P 3rd. Percutaneous pin placement in the medial calcaneus: is anywhere safe? *J Orthop Trauma*. 2002;16(1):26-29.
4. Moskovich R. Proximal tibial transfixion for skeletal traction. An anatomic study of neurovascular structures. *Clin Orthop Relat Res*. 1987;(214):264-268.
5. Scannell BP, Waldrop NE, Sasser HC, Sing RF, Bosse MJ. Skeletal traction versus external fixation in the initial temporization of femoral shaft fractures in severely injured patients. *J Trauma*. 2010;68(3):633-640.

CHAPTER 26

JOINT ASPIRATION AND INJECTION

SHOULDER, ELBOW, WRIST, HIP, KNEE, AND ANKLE

Brandon J. Erickson | Nikhil N. Verma

Joint aspirations and injections are some of the most frequently performed procedures by orthopaedic surgeons, both in the operating room and in the clinic setting. Joint aspirations can be performed to obtain a diagnosis, relieve pain, or assist with range of motion; although injections are more frequently performed therapeutically, they can also serve a diagnostic purpose.

Joint aspirations most commonly are performed to diagnose a swollen, painful joint. Typically, the purpose is to rule out entities such as septic arthritis, gout, and so on. Aspiration can also serve a potential therapeutic purpose to alleviate pain and improve motion, commonly in the postoperative or acutely traumatic setting, and in cases of joint effusion from underlying intrinsic joint pathology.

Joint injections differ from aspirations in that these are frequently administered for therapeutic reasons but can also be used to aid in diagnosis. Joints can be injected with a variety of substances including platelet rich plasma (PRP), hyaluronic acid, or more frequently, a mixture of a local anesthetic and steroid to alleviate pain from arthritis, cartilage lesions, or other intraarticular pathologies. On the diagnostic side, an intraarticular injection can be helpful to identify the joint itself as the source of pain (e.g., a diagnostic acromioclavicular joint injection). If the pain completely resolves with the injection, the source is likely only the joint. However, if the pain decreases only slightly or not at all, the joint is unlikely to be the primary cause of the pain. Lastly, joints can be injected with contrast material in the setting of arthrograms (either computed tomography or magnetic resonance) to aid in diagnosis of various intraarticular pathologies (e.g., labral tears in the hip and shoulder).

SURGICAL TECHNIQUE

Room Set-Up

- The room set-up is variable for each type of aspiration or injection.
- All materials should be obtained before beginning, and the risks and benefits of the procedure should be clearly explained to the patient.
- If a hip aspiration or injection is being performed, the patient should be brought to a fluoroscopy suite, and a mini C-arm can be used for the wrist.

Patient Positioning

- Patient positioning varies by the targeted joint. All aspirations and injections except the shoulder and inferolateral or medial approach to the knee should be done with the patient positioned supine.
- The patient should be made as comfortable as possible to avoid active contraction of the muscles around the targeted joint during aspiration or injection.

CASE MINIMUM REQUIREMENTS

- No minimum requirements for aspirations and injections of these joints
- Common procedures with which every resident must be facile

COMMONLY USED CPT CODES

- CPT Code: 20610—Arthrocentesis, aspiration, and/or injection; major joint or bursa (e.g., shoulder, hip, knee joint, subacromial bursa)
- CPT Code: 20605—Arthrocentesis, aspiration, and/or injection; intermediate joint or bursa (e.g., acromioclavicular, wrist, elbow, ankle, olecranon bursa)

COMMONLY USED ICD9 CODES

- 711.0—Septic arthritis
- 719.0—Joint effusion
- 274.0—Gouty arthropathy

COMMONLY USED ICD10 CODES

- M00—Pyogenic arthritis
- M25.40—Effusion, unspecified joint
- M10.00—Idiopathic gout, unspecified site

Prepping and Draping

- These aspirations and injections should all be performed with a sterile technique.
- When any aspiration or injection is performed, use a providone-iodine swab stick twice to clean the entry site, followed by either an alcohol pad twice or chlordexidine gluconate+isopropyl alcohol; this technique is standard for all injections and aspirations in this chapter and is referred to as the standard sterile technique from hereafter.
- Sterile gloves should be worn during all aspirations and injections.

Knee Aspiration and Injection

- Superolateral and superomedial (Videos 26-1 and 26-2):
  - The patient is positioned supine with the knee flexed 20 degrees and a towel or pillow under the knee to ensure the knee is relaxed.
  - The patient must be relaxed in this setting because contraction of the quadriceps engages the patella and minimizes the space to insert the needle.
  - Feel and mark the superior, medial, and lateral borders of the patella.
  - For superolateral aspiration or injection, slide just posterior to where the superior and lateral lines meet (Fig. 26-1, A).
  - A soft spot is felt just anterior to the iliotibial (IT) band where the needle can be inserted.
  - Mark the soft spot with a marking pen.
  - Clean the entry site with the standard sterile technique.
  - The authors use an 18-gauge needle for aspirations and a 22-gauge needle for injections.
  - Insert the needle with a slight downward angle in the sagittal plane at a 45-degree angle toward the foot in the coronal plane, gliding under the patella to avoid damaging the cartilage (Fig. 26-1, B).
  - A pop is felt as the needle penetrates the joint and aspirates or injects.
  - Adjust the position of the needle if no fluid is aspirated or if bone is encountered.
  - The medial side of the knee can be pushed to milk any fluid toward the syringe.
  - Carefully remove the needle and place a bandage at the entry site.
  - The same technique can be repeated on the medial side.
- Inferolateral and inferomedial (Videos 26-3 and 26-4):
  - The patient should be sitting up with the knee freely hanging over the edge of the table and flexed at 90 degrees.
  - Feel and mark the inferior pole of the patella and the medial and lateral borders of the patellar tendon (see Fig. 26-1, A).
  - A soft spot is felt just medial or lateral to the edge of the patellar tendon, approximately 0.5 to 1.0 cm distal to the inferior pole of the patella.
  - Mark the entry site with a marking pen and clean with the standard sterile technique.
  - Insert the needle and aim for the intercondylar notch, parallel to floor in the coronal plane (Fig. 26-1, C). Free fluid flow should be achieved with minimal resistance to confirm entry into the joint. If excessive pressure is returned, or if the patient experiences significant pain, the needle may be engaged in the retropatellar fat pad and should be advanced.
  - Carefully remove the needle and place a bandage at the entry site.

Ankle Aspiration

- Anteromedial (Video 26-5):
  - With the patient supine and the ankle plantarflexed, mark out the medial malleolus, tibialis anterior tendon, and dorsalis pedis pulse (Fig. 26-2, A).

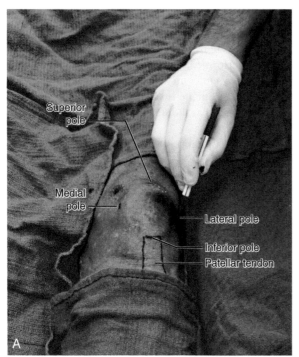

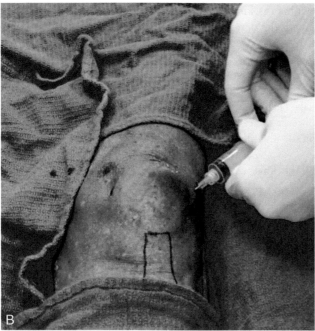

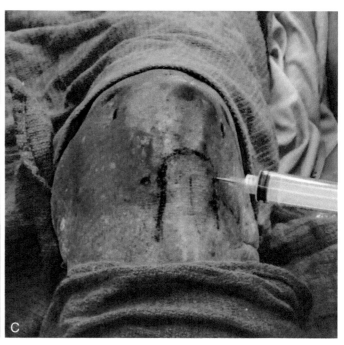

Figure 26-1 A, Superior, inferior, medial, and lateral pole of the patella and the patellar tendon marked out. **B**, Needle entry site and trajectory for superolateral injection or aspiration. **C**, Needle entry site and trajectory for inferolateral injection or aspiration.

- Take a thumb and feel the soft spot between the tibials anterior tendon and the medial malleolus.
- Once in the soft spot, place the thumb on the distal tibia.
- Dorsiflex and plantarflex the foot while moving the thumb distally until the space between the distal tibia and talus is felt.
- Mark this entry site and clean the skin using the "standard sterile technique."
- Use an 18-gauge needle for aspirations or 22-gauge needle for injections.
- The ankle is held in plantarflexion to open the joint space while the needle is inserted parallel to the distal tibia, aiming slightly lateral from the entry site (Fig. 26-2, *B*).

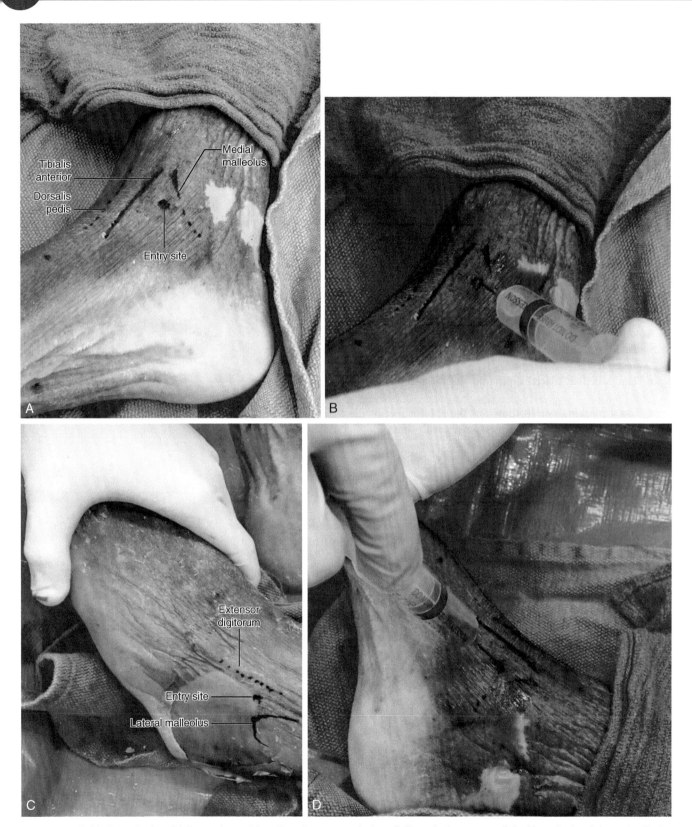

Figure 26-2 A, Medial malleolus, tibialis anterior, and dorsalis pedis artery marked out. **B,** Entry site for anteromedial ankle aspiration. **C,** Lateral malleolus and extensor digitorum marked out. **D,** Entry site for anterolateral ankle aspiration.

- A pop is felt once the joint is entered.
- If bone is felt, plantarflex and dorsiflex the ankle.
- If the needle moves, it is too distal in the talus; if it does not move, it is too proximal in the tibia.
- Adjust the trajectory accordingly, and once intraarticular, inject or aspirate.
- Carefully remove the needle and place a bandage at the entry site.
- Anterolateral (Video 26-6):
  - With the same positioning as in the anteromedial technique, mark out the lateral malleolus and extensor digitorum tendon (Fig. 26-2, C).
  - Feel the soft spot between these two structures, and dorsiflex and plantarflex the foot while moving the thumb distally, starting on the tibia until the joint space is felt.
  - Plantarflex the foot and insert the needle parallel to the distal tibia, aiming slightly medial (Fig. 26-2, D).
- Aspirate or inject
  - Carefully remove the needle and place a bandage at the entry site.

Hip Aspiration

- Anterolateral (Video 26-7):
  - This is a difficult joint to aspirate or inject, and fluoroscopic guidance is often necessary.
  - The patient is placed supine on the fluoroscopy table with the hip and groin exposed.
  - Use a marking pen to draw out the anterosuperior iliac spine (ASIS), greater trochanter, angle of the femoral neck with fluoroscopic guidance, and femoral pulse (Fig. 26-3, A).
  - It is essential to stay lateral to the femoral pulse.
  - The needle entry site is approximately 2 to 3 cm below the level of the ASIS, depending on the patient's anatomy and body habitus, in the crease of the groin.
  - Alternatively, one can draw a line medially from the superior edge of the greater trochanter and distally from the ASIS; where the two points meet is the entry site.
  - The medial to lateral aspect of the entry site varies based on the weight of the patient. Starting too lateral in an obese patient may preclude the needle from reaching the joint.
  - Once the entry site is marked, clean the skin in the standard sterile technique.
  - The authors use an 18-gauge spinal needle for aspirations and a 22-gauge spinal needle for injections.
  - The needle trajectory should be at approximately a 45-degree angle to the floor, aiming for the femoral head/neck junction (Fig. 26-3, B).
  - The stylet is left in the spinal needle until the needle is intraarticular to prevent introducing skin and bacteria into the joint. The stylet is removed and the syringe attached once the needle is thought to be in the hip joint.
  - Check the trajectory of the needle with fluoroscopy and adjust accordingly to ensure the needle is heading for the head/neck junction.
  - Continue to advance the needle with fluoroscopic guidance.
  - In a patient with a total hip arthroplasty (THA), the needle can be felt to hit metal; verify it is at the head/neck junction with fluoroscopy, and once verified, remove the stylet, attach the syringe, and aspirate (Fig. 26-3, C).
  - In a native hip, bone is felt. Once at the head/neck junction, verify with fluoroscopy and remove the stylet.
  - If aspirating, attach the syringe and attempt to aspirate.
  - If injecting, remove the stylet, fill a 10-mL syringe with air, attach to the needle, and perform an air arthrogram to verify needle is in the joint.
  - If the air stays within the capsule, the needle is intraarticular.

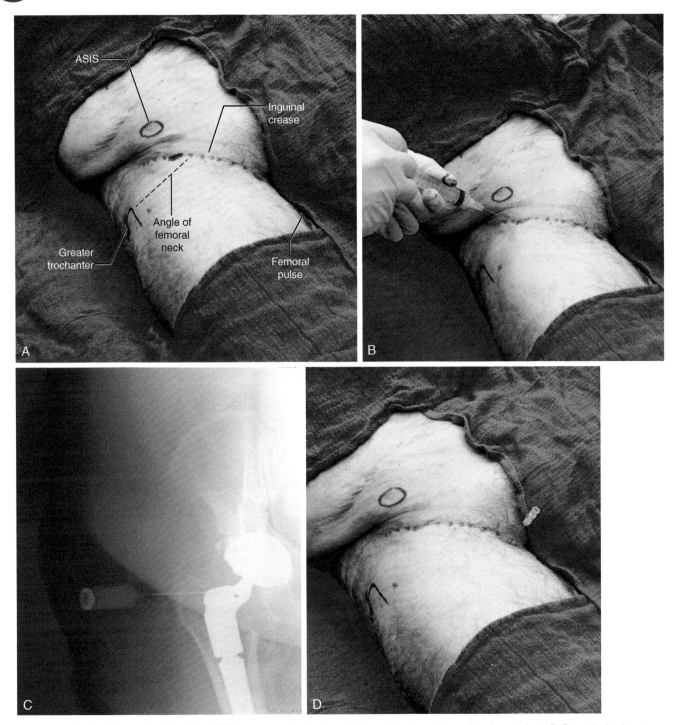

Figure 26-3 **A,** Anterior superior iliac spine *(ASIS),* greater trochanter, femoral artery, trajectory of femoral neck marked out. **B,** Entry site for the antero-lateral hip injection or aspiration. **C,** Fluoroscopic image verifying position of needle in joint. **D,** Entry site for the anterior hip injection or aspiration.

- If the air leaks out, the needle must be repositioned, and the air arthrogram repeated.
- Once verified, remove the empty syringe, attach the new syringe with injection cocktail, and inject.
- The authors recommend saving the air arthrogram for the patient's records.
- Carefully remove the needle and place a bandage at the entry site.
■ Straight anterior (Video 26-8):
- The patient positioning and landmarks that need to be marked are the same as the anterolateral approach.
- This approach is 1 to 2 cm lateral to the femoral artery, so proper marking is imperative. Once the femoral pulse is clearly marked, use a radiopaque object placed on the skin to determine the location of the head/neck junction.
- Mark this area and clean with the standard sterile technique.
- Insert the needle perpendicular to the floor, 1 to 2 cm lateral to the femoral pulse (Fig. 26-3, D).
- Once intraarticular, aspirate or inject in the same manner as in the anterolateral approach.
- Carefully remove the needle and place a bandage at the entry site.

Shoulder Aspiration

■ Posterior (Video 26-9):
- The patient should be sitting up in a chair or bed, with the back supported and the desired shoulder off the side of the chair or bed.
- Having the patient sitting as opposed to standing avoids any issues should the patient become light-headed and faint.
- Once the shoulder and posterior acromion are free, mark out the scapular spine, posterolateral border of the acromion, lateral border of the acromion, and coracoid process.
- Pinch the posterolateral border of the acromion between the thumb and index finger.
- Measure 2 cm distal and 2 cm medial to the posterolateral border of the acromion.
- Mark this spot as the entry site (Fig. 26-4, A). Grasp the humeral head between the thumb and index/middle finger to identify the joint line.
- Once the entry site is marked, clean the skin in the standard sterile technique.
- One hand holds the spinal needle, and one is used put a finger on the coracoid process.
- The authors use an 18-gauge spinal needle for aspirations and a 22-gauge spinal needle for injections.
- Aim the needle toward the coracoid process, roughly parallel to the floor, taking into account the normal retroversion of the glenohumeral joint.
- The stylet is left in the needle until the needle is felt to be intraarticular, and the syringe is only attached once the needle is in the shoulder joint (Fig. 26-4, B).
- The needle is advanced until a pop is felt; this signifies the joint has been entered.
- If the needle hits bone, internally and externally rotate the patient's arm.
- If the needle moves with the bone, the needle is too lateral and is on the humeral head.
- If the needle does not move, it is too medial and on the glenoid.
- Adjust the trajectory of the needle accordingly and feel the pop into the joint.
- Once intraarticular, remove the stylet and attach the syringe for aspiration or injection.
- Carefully remove the needle and place a bandage at the entry site.
■ Anterior (Video 26-10):
- Patient positioning and equipment are the same as previously stated.
- Mark out the coracoid process and acromion as previously stated (see Fig. 26-4, A).

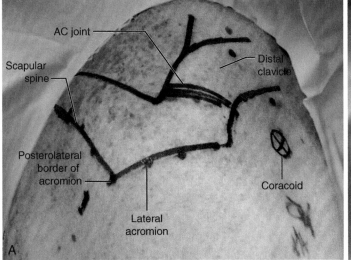

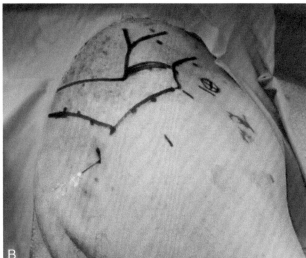

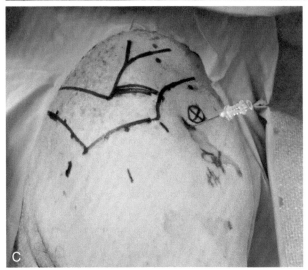

Figure 26-4 A, Posterolateral, lateral, and posterior aspect of acromion, coracoid, acromioclavicular *(AC)* joint, and distal clavicle marked out. **B,** Entry site for the posterior shoulder injection or aspiration. **C,** Entry site for the anterior shoulder injection or aspiration.

- The entry site is just lateral to the coracoid, aiming slightly inferomedial to avoid the musculocutaneous nerve (Fig. 26-4, *C*).
- As with the posterior approach, adjust the needle with the assistance of moving the arm.
- Once intraarticular, inject or aspirate.
- Carefully remove the needle and place a bandage at the entry site.

Elbow Aspiration and Injection (Video 26-11)

- The most common approach to the elbow for injections and aspirations is via the soft spot between a triangle created between the radial head, olecranon, and lateral epicondyle.
- The patient is positioned supine with the elbow slightly flexed.
- Mark out the lateral humeral epicondyle, olecranon, and radial head (Fig. 26-5, *A*).
- Sometimes the radial head can be difficult to feel. Supinate or pronate the wrist to move the radial head and aid in palpation.
- Once marked, feel the soft spot between these bony structures. This is the entry site.
- Clean the skin with the standard sterile technique.
- The authors use an 18-gauge needle for aspirations and a 22-gauge needle for injections.

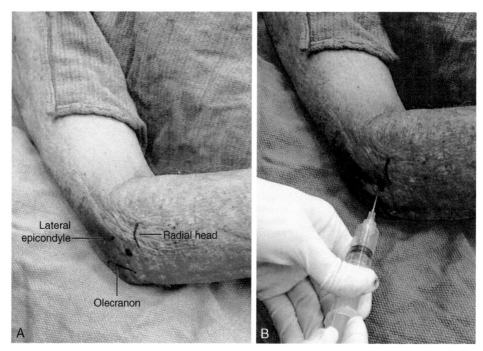

Figure 26-5 **A,** Lateral humeral condyle, olecranon, and radial head marked out. **B,** Entry site for the lateral elbow injection or aspiration.

- The needle is inserted parallel to the distal humerus, aiming anteromedial (Fig. 26-5, *B*).
- The needle is advanced until a pop is felt; this signifies the joint has been entered.
- If the needle hits bone, pronate or supinate the wrist to move the radial head.
- If the needle is felt to move with the bone, the needle is too distal and is on the radial head.
- If the needle does not move, it is too proximal or aimed too posteiror or anterior.
- Adjust the trajectory of the needle accordingly, feel the pop into the joint, and aspirate or inject.
- Carefully remove the needle and place a bandage at the entry site.

Wrist Aspiration and Injection (Video 26-12)

- The wrist is one of the harder joint aspirations and injections to perform because there is little joint space.
- If the surgeon is not comfortable performing this aspiration based on anatomic landmarks, fluoroscopy can be used to aid in and confirm needle placement.
- The patient is supine on the bed with the wrist on a hand table in slight flexion.
- Extend the thumb against resistance to feel the extensor pollicus longus (EPL) and trace it back to Lister's tubercle on the dorsal aspect of the radius (EPL passes ulnar to Lister's tubercle).
- Mark out Lister's tubercle (bump on the distal dorsal radius; Fig. 26-6, *A*).
- Wrist flexion, ulnar deviation, and traction can aid in opening the joint space.
- If aspirating or injecting without an assistant, the hand can be suspended with fingertraps to apply traction and ulnar deviation.
- The entry site is slightly ulnar and 1 cm distal to Lister's tubercle.
- Once the entry site is marked, clean the skin in the standard sterile technique.
- The authors use an 18-gauge needle for aspirations and a 22-gauge needle for injections.
- The needle is inserted aiming slightly proximal (approximately 10 to 15 degrees) to account for the volar tilt of the distal radius (Fig. 26-6, *B*).
- Fluoroscopy can be used to confirm the needle is intraarticular.

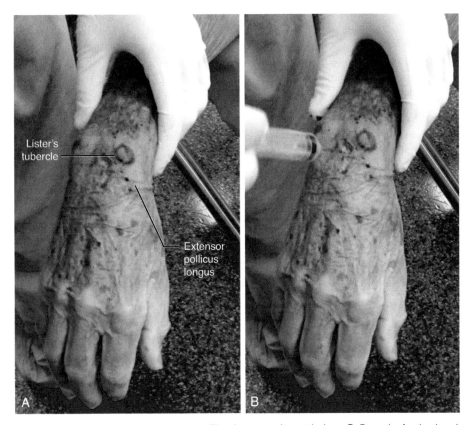

Figure 26-6 A, Lister's tubercle, extensor pollicus longus tendon marked out. **B,** Entry site for the dorsal wrist injection or aspiration.

- If the needle hits bone, flex or extend the wrist and adjust the needle accordingly (if the needle moves while moving the wrist, it is likely in a carpal bone and should be moved proximal, but if it does not move, it is likely in the radius and should be moved distal).
- Once in the joint, inject or aspirate.
  - Carefully remove the needle and place a bandage at the entry site.

BRIEF SUMMARY OF SURGICAL STEPS

- Ensure patient is properly positioned and equipment is gathered
- Obtain a fluoroscopy or mini C-arm if necessary
- Mark the aspiration or injection site
- Clean the site thoroughly with providone-iodine and alcohol or chlordexidine gluconate+isopropyl alcohol
- Insert the needle into the joint
- Ensure proper positioning and aspirate or inject
- If performing aspiration, remove needle and discard; with sterile technique, attach a new sterile needle to the syringe before injecting fluid into tube
- Clean the top of the tubes with chlordexidine gluconate+isopropyl alcohol and alcohol and inject the fluid into the tubes
- Use a new needle for inserting fluid into each tube
- If aspirating, aspirate all fluid possible without causing significant pain because this decreases the patient's pain

REQUIRED EQUIPMENT

18-gauge needle is used for all aspirations (spinal in case of hip and shoulder, or large knee)
22-gauge needle for all injections (spinal in case of hip and shoulder, or large knee)
Alcohol swab or chlordexidine gluconate+isopropyl alcohol
Both red and lavender top tubes
Providone-iodine prep stick, 2
10-mL syringe, 4
Local anesthetic, both short and long acting, as well as a smaller amount of steroid solution (if desired), is needed

TECHNICAL PEARLS

- Avoid hitting cartilage when inserting needle
- Ensure sterile technique to avoid causing a septic arthritis or contaminating a synovial sample
- The authors do not recommend the use of subcutaneous lidocaine for injections because this causes the patient to be stuck twice
- If entering the joint is difficult, moving the joint to see whether the needle moves is a valuable tool to determine in which direction to move the needle

COMMON PITFALLS

(When to call for the attending physician)

- Ensure the needle is in the joint (not in bone or soft tissue) before aspirating
- If no fluid can be obtained from the joint after two attempts, call a senior resident or attending physician
- Use a needle that is long enough to reach the joint; this is especially important in hip and shoulder aspirations and injections and in cases of obese patients for knee injections
- If no fluid is returned, the joint can be flushed with sterile saline solution to obtain a sample and confim appropriate needle placement

POSTOPERATIVE PROTOCOL

After a joint aspiration, the postoperative protocol includes placement of a bandage and instructions to keep the area clean for 24 hours. Ice and over-the-counter nonsteroidal antiinflammatory drugs can be recommended to control pain or swelling associated with the injection. Patients should be instructed that pain may be worse for 1 to 3 days after the injection before improvement is noted. Further definitive management is dependent on the underlying diagnosis.

SUGGESTED READINGS

1. Griffet J, Oborocianu I, Rubio A, Leroux J, Lauron J, Hayek T. Percutaneous aspiration irrigation drainage technique in the management of septic arthritis in children. *J Trauma.* 2011;70(2):377-383.
2. Hansford BG, Stacy GS. Musculoskeletal aspiration procedures. *Semin Intervent Radiol.* 2012;29(4): 270-285.
3. Skeete K, Hess EP, Clark T, Moran S, Kakar S, Rizzo M. Epidemiology of suspected wrist joint infection versus inflammation. *J Hand Surg [Am].* 2011;36(3):469-474.
4. Roberts DW, Roc GJ, Hsu WK. Outcomes of cervical and lumbar disk herniations in Major League Baseball pitchers. *Orthopedics.* 2011;34(8):602-609.

COMPARTMENT SYNDROME
FOUR COMPARTMENT LEG RELEASE TECHNIQUE

John P. Begly | Kenneth A. Egol

Defined as the pathologic elevation of compartment pressure within a closed osteofascial compartment, *acute compartment syndrome* represents a true orthopaedic emergency. Inciting trauma to a given compartment leads to increased tissue pressure, reduced capillary flow, and local cellular anoxia, which in turn further increases edema and elevates compartment pressures. Thus, a vicious cycle of pressure-induced necrosis is created. Irreversible muscle damage may occur in as little as 8 hours after the development of compartment syndrome, and significant nerve damage may occur in only 6 hours. Without efficient and accurate diagnosis and treatment, severe morbidity and long-term disability may result.

A strong clinical understanding of the condition, along with a high degree of awareness, is imperative in the diagnosis and treatment of acute compartment syndrome of the lower extremity. The annual incidence rate of compartment syndrome is 3.1/100,000 persons. The most common cause is tibial fracture (36%), followed by blunt soft tissue injury (23.2%); in their series, McQueen and colleagues found that 7% of patients with acute tibial fractures had development of acute compartment syndrome. Despite the strong association, an acute fracture does not need to be present for compartment syndrome to develop. Any pathophysiologic process that raises compartment pressure, including hemorrhage, burns, and constrictive dressings or casts, places the patient at increased risk.

Acute compartment syndrome is primarily a clinical diagnosis. Classic signs include the five Ps: pain, pallor, paralysis, pulselessness, and paresthesia. Pain on passive stretch and pain out of proportion to examination are the most sensitive examination findings. Examination results, however, may be unreliable, and negative predictive value of the signs and symptoms may be the most valuable aspect of evaluation. In addition, physical examination often can be affected by distracting injuries and is only practical in the responsive patient. Because of these limitations, workup is often supplemented with the direct measurement of compartment pressures. Compartment pressure may be measured with a variety of devices and techniques, including specialized commercial sets, arterial lines, Whitesides' three-way stopcock apparatus, needle manometry, and wick catheters (Figs. 27-1 and 27-2). Compartment syndrome is present when the difference between measured compartment pressures and diastolic blood pressure is less than 30 mm Hg.

Once the clinical diagnosis has been made, with or without confirmatory pressure measurements, the patient should be brought emergently to the operating room. Goals of surgery include decompression of elevated intracompartmental pressure, reestablishment of perfusion, and débridement of necrotic tissue.

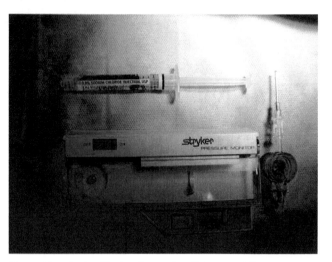

Figure 27-1 Stryker (Stryker Corporation, Kalamazoo, MI) intracompartmental pressure monitor. This kit includes a prefilled syringe, a pressure monitor, a transducer, and a needle. The needle is attached to the transducer, which then is attached to the syringe. The assembled syringe and needle then are placed into the pressure monitor, and the cover is closed and locked.

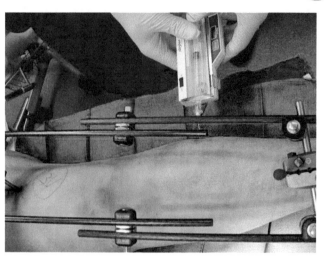

Figure 27-2 Fully assembled pressure monitor in use.

SURGICAL TECHNIQUE

Room Set-up

- A radiolucent table is used in the setting of a planned fracture fixation.
- A large C-arm is positioned on the contralateral side of the affected extremity in the setting of planned fracture fixation.

Patient Positioning

- The patient is positioned supine.
- A small bump may be placed under the ipsilateral hip to faciliate access to the operative extremity. This is particularly useful when the single incision technique is used.
- A tourniquet is applied to the affected extremity but not inflated.

Prepping and Draping

- The affected extremity is prepped and drapped in a sterile manner.
- A wet sterile preparation is used in the setting of open injury.
- The affected extremity is draped free.

Compartment Pressure Measurement

- Use a marking pen to mark relevant anatomic landmarks, including the outline of the fibula, the fibular head, and the lateral malleolus.
  - Lateral compartment: Pressure measurement is taken in line with the fibula or posterior to the fibula (Fig. 27-3).
  - Anterior compartment: Pressure measurement is taken in the muscle belly located between the fibula and the anterior crest of the tibia (Fig. 27-4).
  - Superficial posterior compartment: Pressure measurement is taken over the posteromedial aspect of the gastrocsoleus.
  - Deep posterior compartment: Pressure measurement is taken on the posteromedial border of the tibia in the distal one half of the lower leg.

COMMONLY USED ICD9 CODES

- 958.90—Compartment syndrome, unspecified
- 958.92—Traumatic compartment syndrome of the lower extremity, traumatic compartment syndrome of the hip, buttock, thigh, leg, foot, and toes

COMMONLY USED ICD10 CODES

- T79.A0—Compartment syndrome, unspecified

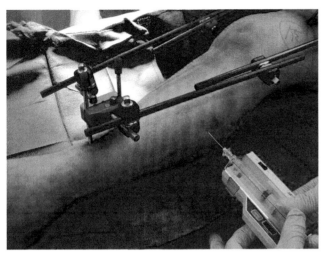

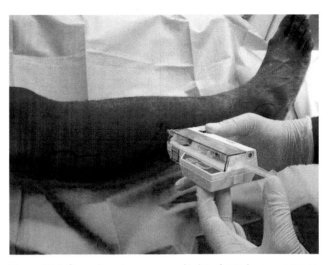

Figure 27-3 Compartment pressure monitoring of lateral compartment.

Figure 27-4 Compartment pressure monitoring of anterior compartment.

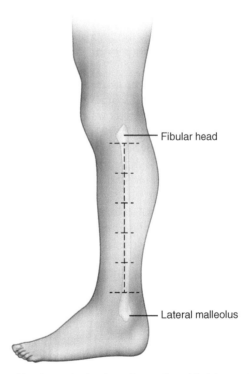

— Fibular head

— Lateral malleolus

Figure 27-5 Lower leg with relevant landmarks and anterolateral incision marked. The anterolateral incision is made between the fibula and the anteiror tibial crest, just anterior to the intermuscular septum between the anterior and lateral fascial compartments.

Double-Incision Technique

- The double-incision technique is the most commonly used technique because of its relative technical ease, predictable compartment release, and safety.
- Anterior and lateral compartments are released with an anterolateral incision (Fig. 27-5).
- A longitudinal incision is placed halfway between the fibula and the anterior tibial crest.
- Incision length is approximately 5 cm distal from the fibular head to 5 cm proximal to the lateral malleolus. Total incision length should be between 15 and 25 cm.

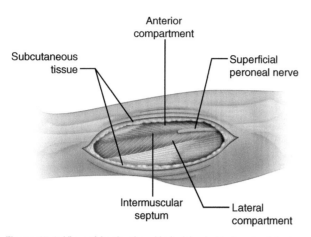

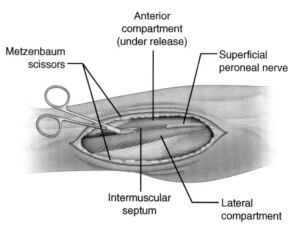

Figure 27-6 View of fascia after skin incision but before fascial release. A small transverse incision should be made in the fascia to allow for direct visualization of the intermuscular septum between the anterior and lateral compartments.

Figure 27-7 Release of the anterior compartment fascia. The tips of the scissors then can be inserted through the previously established rent in the fascia. Note: tips of scissors are kept angled away from the neurovascular structures. Separate longitudinal incisions should be made in both the anterior and the lateral compartments to avoid iatrogenic damage to the intermuscular septum and to the superficial peroneal nerve.

- Dissection of subcutaneous tissue is performed for wide exposure of the fascial compartments (Fig. 27-6).
- Transverse incisions are made over the fascia of the anterior and lateral compartments, below which the intermuscular septum is identified. Care must be taken not to damage the superficial peroneal nerve, which lies just posterior to the septum and may be encountered approximately 10 cm proximal to the lateral malleolus, where it courses from lateral to anterior compartments.
- The skin is retracted anteriorly, and decompression of the entire anterior compartment is performed with Metzenbaum scissors to release the fascia in line with the tibialis anterior (Fig. 27-7).
- The skin is retracted posteriorly, and decompression of the entire lateral compartment is performed by releasing the fascia in line with the fibular shaft (Fig. 27-8).
- The superficial and deep posterior compartments are accessed via a longitudinal incision made on the posteromedial aspect of the lower leg, approximately 2.0 cm posterior to the posterior border of the tibia. Dissection down to the fascia is performed as described previously (Figs. 27-9 and 27-10).
- Identification of the saphenous vein and nerve is performed, crossing the wound from posterior to anterior. Once identified, anterior retraction of the neurovascular structures is performed.
- A transverse incision is made to identify the intramuscular septum.
- Decompression of the entire superficial posterior compartment is performed by releasing the fascia overlying the entire gastrocsoleus complex.
- Decompression of the entire deep posterior compartment is performed by releasing the fascia overlying the flexor digitorum longus. If a soleus bridge is encountered as this release is continued proximally, the soleus should be released from the insertion with electrocautery to access the proximal aspect of the deep posterior compartment and achieve full decompression (Fig. 27-11).

Single-Incision Technique

- A longitudinal lateral incision is made just posterior to and in line with the fibula, beginning 5 cm distal to the fibular head to 5 cm proximal to the lateral malleolus (Figs. 27-12 and 27-13).
- Dissection through subcutaneous tissue is performed, as is identification and incision of the fascia to expose the intermuscular septum.

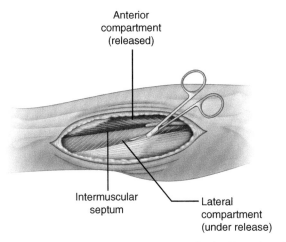

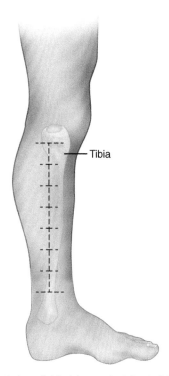

Figure 27-8 Release of the lateral compartment fascia. Note: tips of scissors are kept angled away from the neurovascular structures.

Figure 27-9 Posteriomedial incision marked, located 2 cm posterior to the posterior tibial margin, and used to decompress both the superficial and the deep posterior compartments.

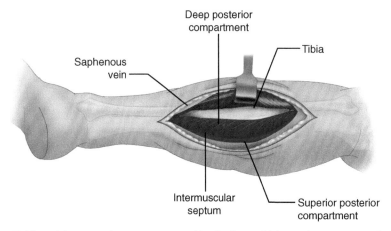

Figure 27-10 View of deep posterior compartment and fascia of superficial posterior compartment before release. Care should be taken to protect the saphenous vein during this approach. Similar to the technique for the anterolateral incision, a small transverse incision should be made in the fascia, which allows for direct visualization of the intermuscular septum between the deep and superficial compartments. After release of the deep compartment fascia, the scissors should be oriented proximally through, and deep, to the soleus bridge to allow for release of the soleus attachment to the tibia.

- Full fascial release of the anterior and lateral compartments is performed as described previously.
- The skin is undermined posteriorly, and the musculature of the lateral compartment is carefully elevated and retracted to allow for identification of the posterior intermuscular septum.
- Complete release of superficial posterior compartment fascia is performed.

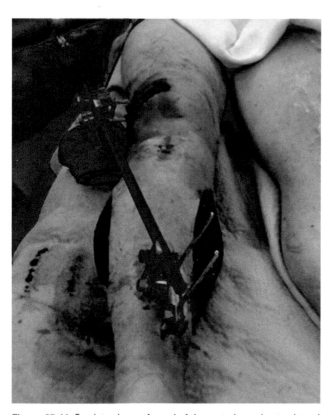

Figure 27-11 Fasciotomies performed of the posterior and anterolateral compartments in conjunction with lower extremity external fixation. (With permission from Cole PA, Lafferty PM, Levy BA, Watson JT. Tibial plateau fractures. In: Browner BD, Jupiter JB, Krettek C, Anderson PA, eds. *Skeletal Trauma: Basic Science, Management, and Reconstruction.* 5th ed. Philadelphia: Elsevier; 2015. Figure 62-2.)

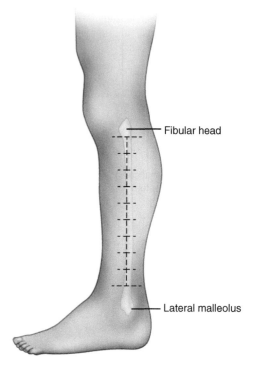

Figure 27-12 Lateral incison for one-incision technique marked.

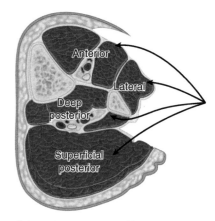

Figure 27-13 Schematic cross section of lower leg compartments, showing access to all four compartments via the single-incision technique.

- The interval between the lateral and the superficial posterior compartments is identified and developed by proximally detaching the soleus from the fibula and subperiosteally dissecting the flexor hallicus longus from the fibula. The fascia is released along this interval.
- Tissue is retracted posteriorly, and the fascial attachment of the tibialis posterior is identified and incised longitudinally.

Débridement and Closure

- Regardless of the release technique used, a dedicated débridement with removal of as much necrotic tissue, if present, as possible is imperitive.
- Many options exist for closure, including delayed primary closure, split thickness skin grafting, dermotraction, and vacuum-assisted wound closure.

BRIEF SUMMARY OF SURGICAL STEPS

- Longitudinal incision is made along full length of the compartment requiring release
- Subcutaneous dissection is performed, with identification of intramuscular septum
- Identification and protection of key neurovascular structures
- Full release of compartment fascia
- Dedicated débridement of necrotic tissue
- Delayed closure of wound to allow for resolution of swelling and avoid unnecessary and harmful closure under tension

REQUIRED EQUIPMENT

Stryker compartment syndrome monitor
Hip bump
Basic orthopaedic set
Electrocautery
Normal saline solution lavage
Closure materials: sutures, elastic bands, or vacuum-assisted closure device
Large C-arm, in event fracture is present and fixation is planned

TECHNICAL PEARLS

- Patients under anesthesia may be at an increased risk for compartment syndrome
  - Blood pressure is a critical factor in the interpretation of compartment pressure measurements
  - Patients under anesthesia are often hypotensive, a state that lowers the absolute pressure at which compartment syndrome develops
- Pressures within a compartment are not uniform
  - Heckman and colleagues found compartment pressures to be highest within 5 cm of injury site
  - Therefore, multiple pressure measurements should be obtained in each compartment, including at the injury site and 5 cm proximal and distal to the injury
- Decompression of all compartments should be performed, regardless of which compartment is most likely affected or in which particular location compartment pressures are measured
- When possible, external fixation or internal fixation of fractures in the setting of compartment syndrome is recommended
  - These modes of fixation allow for stabilization without casts and constrictive dressings, which potentially limit careful monitoring of postoperative neurovascular status and compartment pressures
- The skin incision should be as long as the muscle bulk of the compartment under decompression
  - Cohen and colleagues found that inadequate incisions prevent expansion and may lead to increased compartment pressures despite the completion of full length fasciotomies
- The degree of necrosis and muscle viability may be better assessed with a return to the operating room 2 to 3 days after the index procedure
- The single incision technique may be preferred in certain clinical scenarios, including with severe soft tissue injury, contamination to medial aspect of lower leg, and single vessel distal perfusion and when flap coverage is expected to be necessary
- When performing fasciotomies, keep scissors oriented away from major neurovascular structures
- If possible, preserve perforating vessels to maintain perfusion to the skin flaps
- Small relaxing incisions around the fasciotomy wound can decrease tension and enchance healing

COMMON PITFALLS

(When to call for the attending physician)

- Compartment syndrome is not only an orthopaedic diagnosis; the systemic sequelae, such as myonecrosis, can lead to multiorgan failure and are potentially fatal
  - The surgeon must be aware of any decompensation in patient clinical status and recognize when additional supportive care is necessary
- Inadequate débridement of necrotic tissue
- Failure to completely decompress deep posterior compartment
- Closure of incisions in presence of excess tension on the wounds
- Application of constrictive postoperative immobilization or dressing

POSTOPERATIVE PROTOCOL

After surgery, patients are placed into a nonconstrictive bulky dressing with the ankle and foot in neutral alignment. Elevation of the extremity is emphasized and maintained. Serial neurovascular and compartment checks are performed. Postoperative monitoring for systemic symptoms of compartment syndrome is established, and supportive postoperative care is administered as is clinically indicated. Often, patients are brought back to the operating room 2 to 3 days after the index procedure for repeated débridements or delayed closure. This decision is based on the state of the incisions, the overall condition of the affected extremity, and the postoperative clinical status of the patient.

POSTOPERATIVE CLINIC VISIT PROTOCOL

Patients are instructed to return to the clinic for postoperative assessment approximately 2 weeks after lower limb fasciotomies. After this appointment, patients return to the office for orthopaedic evaluation at 6 weeks, 3 months, 6 months, and 1 year status after index procedure. If postoperative complications occur, this schedule may be adjusted accordingly such that appropriate care is provided.

SUGGESTED READINGS

1. Cohen MS, Garfin SR, Hargens AR, et al. Acute compartment syndrome. Effect of dermotomy on fascial decompression in the leg. *J Bone Joint Surg Br*. 1991;73(2):287-290.
2. Cooper GC. A method of single-incision, four compartment fasciotomy of the leg. *Eur J Vasc Surg*. 1992;6(6):659-661.
3. Heckman MM, Whitesides TE Jr, Grewe SR, Rooks MD. Compartment pressure in association with closed tibial fractures. The relationship between tissue pressure, compartment, and the distance from the site of the fracture. *J Bone Joint Surg Am*. 1994;76(9):1285-1292.
4. Janzing HM, Broos PL. Dermotraction: an effective technique for the closure of fasciotomy wounds: a preliminary report of fifteen patients. *J Orthop Trauma*. 2001;15(6):438-441.
5. Kakagia D, Karadimas EJ, Drosos G, et al. Wound closure of leg fasciotomy: comparison of vacuum-assisted closure vs shoelace technique: a randomised study. *Injury*. 2014;45(5):890-893.
6. McQueen MM, Court-Brown CM. Compartment monitoring in tibial fractures. The pressure threshold for decompression. *J Bone Joint Surg Br*. 1996;78(1):99-104.
7. McQueen MM, Gaston P, Court-Brown CM. Acute compartment syndrome. Who is at risk? *J Bone Joint Surg Br*. 2000;82(2):200-203.
8. Rorabeck CH, Clarke KM. The pathophysiology of the anterior tibial compartment syndrome: an experimental investigation. *J Trauma*. 1978;18(5):299-304.
9. Zannis J, Angobaldo J, Marks M, et al. Comparison of fasciotomy wound closures using traditional dressing changes and the vaccum assisted closure device. *Ann Plast Surg*. 2009;62(4):407-409.

OPEN REDUCTION INTERNAL FIXATION OF TIBIAL PLATEAU FRACTURES

Michael C. Willey | Matthew Karam | J. Lawrence Marsh

COMMONLY USED CPT CODES

- CPT Code: 27530—Closed treatment of tibial fracture, proximal (plateau) without manipulation
- CPT Code: 27532—Closed treatment of tibial fracture, proximal (plateau) with or without manipulation, with skeletal traction
- CPT Code: 27535—Open treatment of tibial fracture, proximal (plateau); unicondylar, includes internal fixation, when performed
- CPT Code: 27536—Open treatment of tibial fracture, proximal (plateau); bicondylar, with or without internal fixation

COMMONLY USED ICD9 CODES

- 823.0—Tibial plateau fracture
- 823.10—Open tibial plateau fracture
- 823.02—Tibial plateau fracture with fibula fracture
- 823.12—Open tibial plateau fracture with fibula fracture

COMMONLY USED ICD10 CODES

- S82.10—Unspecified fracture of upper end of tibia

Dedicated experience with perioperative and operative management of tibial plateau fractures is essential for orthopaedic surgery trainees. Any articular fracture of the proximal tibia is classified as a tibial plateau fracture. This broad classification allows for a wide range of severity of injury to the articular surface, fracture extension to the tibial metaphysis and diaphysis, and soft tissue injury. An orthopaedic surgeon who manages these injuries must have an understanding of how these injury characteristics affect operative management.

High-energy tibial plateau fractures generally occur in young, active individuals with robust bone stock, and low-energy injuries, such as a fall from standing, typically occur in patients with osteoporosis. The magnitude and direction of the force to the extremity affects the injury pattern. Schatzker in 1974 described a classification for articular fractures of the proximal tibia that led to the terms surgeons use to describe these injuries. Learning the language to describe these fractures is important for communication between surgeons. The common terms used to describe this fracture pattern are split, depression, or split-depression, along with the location of the fracture, including medial condyle, lateral condyle, or bicondylar. Figure 28-1 shows the patterns as described by Schatzker. Descriptive terms also are used for common subtypes of fracture patterns, including posteromedial shear fractures (Fig. 28-2), fracture-dislocations (Fig. 28-3), and shaft dissociated patterns (Fig. 28-4). The Association for Osteosynthesis/Orthopaedic Trauma Association (AO/OTA) classification is the alphanumeric classification of these fractures that allows for improved discrimination of injury type and severity. Split depression of the lateral condyle is the most common fracture pattern because of the 5-degree to 7-degree normal alignment of the knee and the propensity of individuals to be struck on the lateral side of the leg. In this pattern, the medial collateral ligament acts as a hinge for the valgus moment at the knee, resulting in failure of the lateral articular surface. Bicondylar patterns generally occur with axial-loading injuries. Medial-sided injuries occur with varus-directed loading.

Severe soft tissue injuries are often associated with bicondylar fractures, fracture-dislocations, and metaphyseal-diaphyseal dissociated patterns. These patients often need spanning external fixation to allow for soft tissue healing before open reduction and internal fixation. Open wounds and fracture blisters are indications for spanning external fixation with delayed internal fixation or definitive external fixation in select cases. Compartment syndrome commonly occurs in patients with high-energy fracture patterns. Stark and colleagues reported compartment syndrome after placement of spanning external fixation in 18% of bicondylar tibial plateau fractures and in 53% of medial plateau fracture-dislocations. This highlights the importance of continued monitoring for compartment syndrome in patients with high-energy patterns, especially fracture-dislocations.

Open reduction and internal fixation of tibial plateau fractures have been reliably performed with modern techniques since the 1980s. Significant advancements have

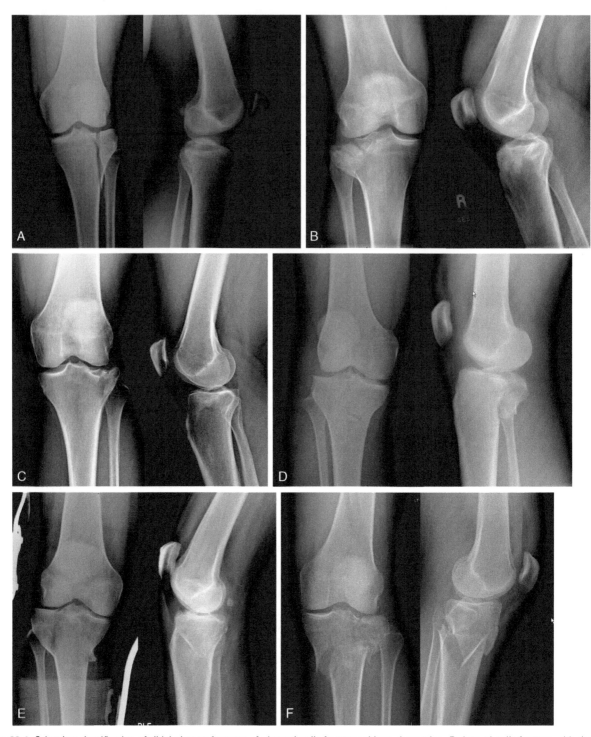

Figure 28-1 Schatzker classification of tibial plateau fractures. **A,** Lateral split fracture without depression. **B,** Lateral split fracture with depression. **C,** Lateral depression fracture without break in the lateral cortex. **D,** Isolated fracture of the medial plateau. **E,** Bicondylar fracture with intact intercondylar eminence. **F,** Bicondylar fracture with proximal tibia fracture dissociating the articular block from the diaphysis.

occurred in approaches, reduction techniques, and methods of fixation. Restoring alignment of the lower extremity has been shown to correlate with improved patient outcomes. In contrast, the articular surface of the proximal tibia has tolerance of modest deformity. The most common approaches used for open reduction and internal fixation of tibial plateau fractures are anterolateral and posteromedial to directly approach the injured side of the joint. These approaches are commonly used in conjunction for select bicondylar fractures. Choosing the correct approach is dependent

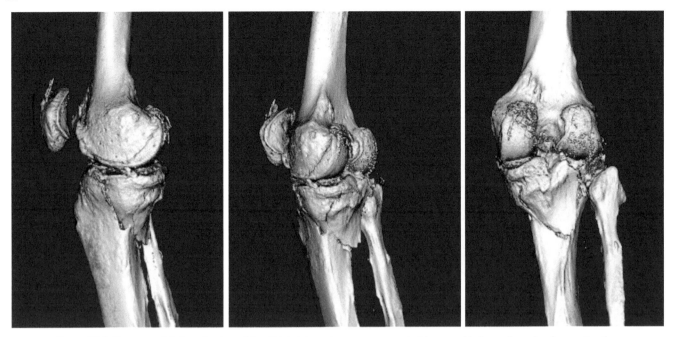

Figure 28-2 Posteromedial shear fracture of the tibial plateau shown on a computed tomographic three-dimensional reconstruction.

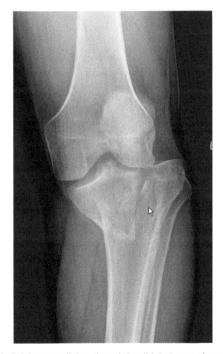

Figure 28-3 Medial fracture-dislocation of the tibial plateau shown on radiograph.

on the fracture pattern and state of the soft tissue envelope. Further sections in this chapter highlight important aspects of approaches, reduction techniques, void filler, and methods of internal fixation important for managing these complex injuries.

SURGICAL TECHNIQUE

Room Set-Up

- A radiolucent operating room table is positioned in the center of the room (Video 28-1) to allow the surgeon, surgical technologist, and anesthesia team appropriate

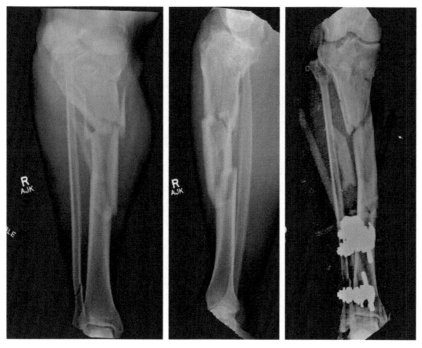

Figure 28-4 Shaft dissociated pattern of tibial plateau fracture.

access to the patient. Large C-arm fluoroscopy is positioned perpendicular to the patient opposite to the operative extremity. Instrument tables and the surgical technologist are positioned behind the surgeon on the operative side.

Patient Positioning

- For fixation of tibial plateau fractures, the patient is most commonly positioned supine. A bump is placed under the hip to neutralize extremity rotation, and the leg is elevated with a nonsterile radiolucent platform or a sterile bump after draping. This allows for easy access to an anterolateral approach or combined anterolateral and posteromedial approaches. In the less common isolated posteromedial shear fracture, a prone position may be more desirable, but this is based on surgeon preference. Access to the posteromedial knee in the supine position requires flexion of the knee and hip with external rotation of the leg (Fig. 28-5).

Prepping and Draping

- The authors' preferred approach is to use an alcohol-based preoperative skin preparation in patients with closed fractures. In patients with severe open fractures, chlorhexidine-only skin preparation is applied. Either a sterile tourniquet is placed after draping or a nonsterile tourniquet prior to draping based on the surgeon preference. The procedure can be performed with or without the tourniquet inflated. Adhesive drapes are used for the procedure, but this is surgeon preference and has not been shown to reduce infection rates (Fig. 28-6).

Anterolateral Approach

- The anterolateral approach is used for isolated lateral condyle fractures and bicondylar fractures. This is the most common approach used for open reduction internal fixation of tibial plateau fractures. Before the surgical approach, anteroposterior and lateral fluoroscopic views of the contralateral and injured knee are taken for later comparison. A longitudinal incision is performed oriented over Gerdy's

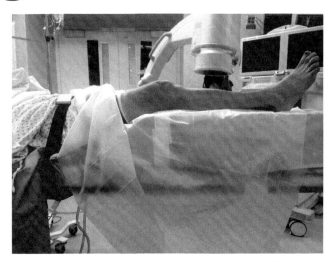

Figure 28-5 Patient positioning for supine approach to tibial plateau fracture.

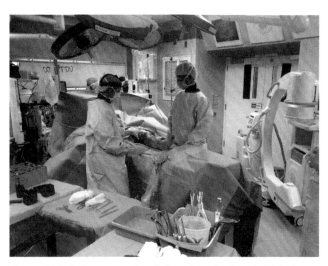

Figure 28-6 Patient prepped and draped for fixation of tibial plateau fracture supine.

tubercle and extending over the anterior compartment muscles (Fig. 28-7). Full-thickness skin flaps are maintained with limited elevation of subcutaneus tissue from anterior compartment fascia. The fascia is incised lateral to the insertion on the tibia to allow a cuff of fascia to close over the plate (Fig. 28-8). Lateral compartment muscles are elevated off the anteriolateral tibia for reduction of split fragments and plate application to bone (Fig. 28-9). Care should be taken over the posterolateral edge of the tibia as the anterior tibial artery passes through the interosseous membrane from posterior. The anterior split fragment is visualized through this exposure. When capsular and iliotibial band insertions are intact on the split fragment, they are left in place to avoid stripping the bone of soft tissue.

- Proximal exposure through an anterolateral approach is variable depending on the surgeon's preferred approach for judging articular reduction. For fluoroscopic or arthroscopic reduction techniques, further dissection proximally into the knee joint is not performed. Depressed articular fragments are accessed through fracture lines. The fragments are elevated with a curette or Cobb, and fluoroscopy or arthroscopy is used to judge reduction (Fig. 28-10). The fragments are held provisionally with K-wires until definitive fixation (Fig. 28-11). Alternatively, in a depressed lateral condyle fracture without a split fragment, the depressed articular fragment is accessed with an anterior cruciate ligament (ACL) tunnel drilling guide to open the lateral cortex. Instruments to elevate the articular cartilage are placed through this opening. Judging reduction and provisional fixation is performed in a similar fashion, but a buttress plate is not required because there is no split fracture in the lateral cortex. Arthroscopic techniques to evaluate reduction have been reported in multiple small series with comparable outcomes.

- Two techniques are used for directly visualizing articular reduction of the proximal tibia. Each technique allows for direct visualization of the articular surface by mobilizing the meniscus. The first technique visualizes the joint from below the meniscus. Skin incision and dissection is carried proximally to the joint capsule. An arthrotomy is made below the lateral meniscus extending posteriorly, and sutures are placed through the periphery of the meniscus to allow for superior retraction. Cross joint distraction can be used to further visualize the proximal tibia articular surface from below the meniscus. The second technique visualizes the articular surface from above the meniscus. A longitudinal anterolateral arthrotomy is performed, with care not to injure the meniscus. The meniscus can be then mobilized by incising the intermeniscal ligament and retracting the anterior horn laterally with the split fragment. Releasing the anterior portion of the coronary

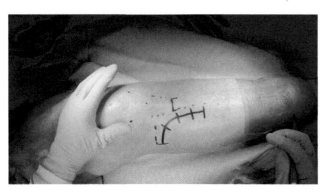

Figure 28-7 Hockey stick incision for anterolateral approach to tibial plateau. Alternatively, a vertical incision can be used rather than the posterior directed proximal arm as shown in this image.

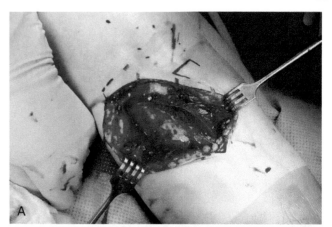

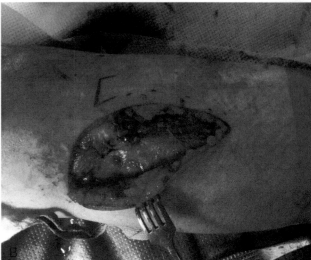

Figure 28-8 A, Incision in the anterior compartment fascia leaving a medial cuff of tissue. **B,** Note the anterior compartment fascia closed completely over the plate at the end of the procedure.

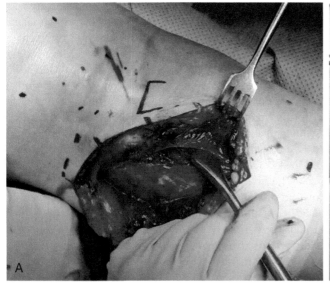

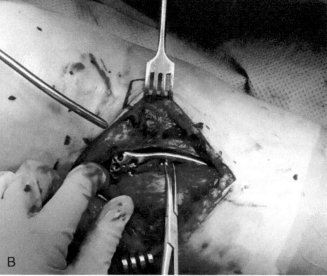

Figure 28-9 A, Elevating the anterior compartment muscles off the lateral tibia. **B,** Sliding the plate along the lateral tibia.

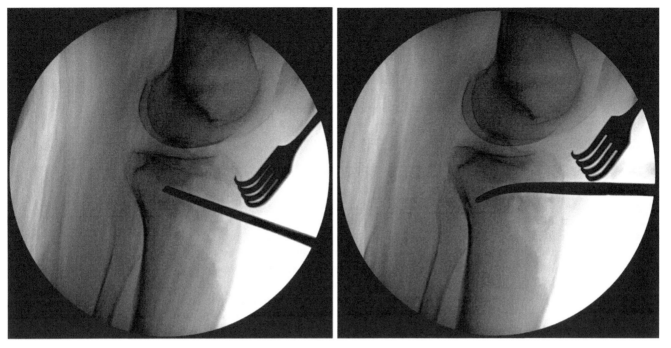

Figure 28-10 Intraoperative fluoroscopy shows technique to elevate depressed articular fragments.

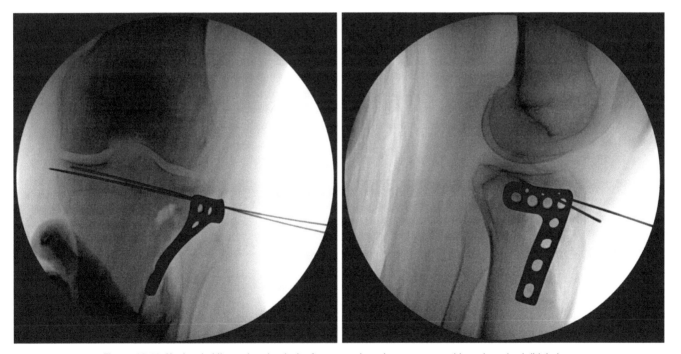

Figure 28-11 K-wires holding reduced articular fragments through a precontoured lateral proximal tibial plate.

ligament can also be performed to increase exposure. After reduction and fixation, the meniscus is repaired through nonabsorbable sutures in the capsule.

Posteromedial Approach

- The posteromedial approach is used for reduction and fixation of medial plateau fractures, including split posteromedial fragments and select bicondylar patterns. Fracture lines in medial patterns can originate in the medial articular surface, in the intercondylar eminences, or to the lateral articular surface. In displaced medial plateau fractures, the lateral femoral condyle can dislocate from the lateral plateau and result in a fracture-dislocation that has a high risk of compartment syndrome. The fracture lines on the posterior medial tibia are generally split and not comminuted, allowing for reliable cortical reduction. For this approach, the patient may be positioned supine or prone based on the surgeon preference. The supine position allows for access to a simultaneous anterolateral approach if required in a bicondylar pattern. Prone position offers the advantage of reduction and fixation with the knee in extension and neutral rotation to avoid varus deforming forces required for exposure in the supine position.

■ An incision is made over the posteromedial border of the tibia. The incision must be posterior enough to allow for posterior to anterior screw paths. Careful dissection is required through subcutaneous tissue to protect the saphenous vein and nerve. The deep interval is between the pes anserinus tendons and the medial head of the gastrocnemius. The neurovascular structures in the popliteal fossa are protected by the medial gastrocnemius; this must be retracted carefully. The popliteus muscle origin is on the posterior aspect of the tibia and must be elevated to expose the fracture. The split medial fracture fragments may be difficult to reduce if widely displaced, and large reduction clamps with elevators with cross joint distraction may be used. Depressed articular fragments can be elevated through the posteromedial fracture lines (Fig. 28-12). Despite reducing extraarticular fracture lines, careful assessment of the articular reduction is important because the fragments can be tilted, resulting in a malaligned limb or articular malreduction.

Bicondylar Tibial Plateau Fracture Patterns

■ Bicondylar fractures patterns of the tibial plateau offer a complex treatment algorithm for the orthopaedic surgeon. Careful consideration of the injury pattern, health of the patient, and state of the soft tissues must be considered. Often these fractures must be treated with 2 to 3 weeks spanning external fixation to allow for soft tissue healing. External fixation pins must avoid the zone of injury when possible and avoid areas of future incisions and internal fixation. The fracture should

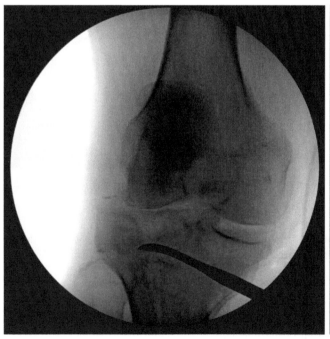
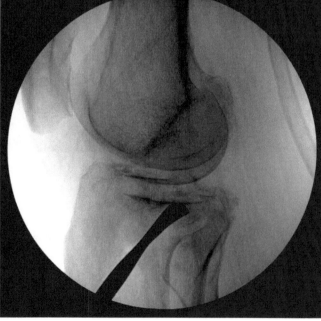

Figure 28-12 Intraoperative fluoroscopy shows reduction of depressed articular fracture through a posteromedial approach.

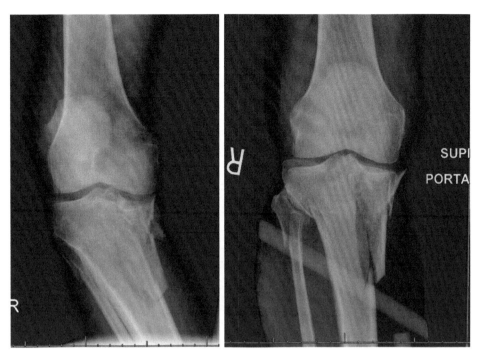

Figure 28-13 Preoperative and postoperative radiographs of a bicondylar tibial plateau fracture treated with temporary spanning external fixation and fasciotomy for compartment syndrome.

be brought out to length and limb aligned properly (Fig. 28-13). Early spanning external fixation is considered in patients with severe open injuries, fracture-dislocations, compartment syndrome, and severe soft tissue injury requiring delayed open reduction internal fixation. Extensile anterior approaches to fix bicondylar fracture patterns of the tibial plateau result in extensive soft tissue stripping and an unacceptable infection rate. Dual anterolateral and posteromedial approaches allow for less soft tissue stripping and direct visualization of important fracture fragments.

■ With treatment of bicondylar fracture patterns, a decision must be made between use of dual plates or lateral locking plate alone. This choice is entirely dependent on characteristics of the medial-sided fracture pattern. Fixation and reduction is improved with a medial antiglide plate when the medial side has a displaced coronal split that results in a posteromedial fragment. If the fragment is not displaced and adequate fixation can be achieved with a lateral locking plate or anterior to posterior screws, a lateral locking plate only can be selected.

■ When performing dual approaches to treat bicondylar tibial plateau fractures, the patient is positioned supine with a bump under the hip and the leg elevated to allow for adequate fluoroscopic imaging. Incisions are 180 degrees from each other to avoid narrow skin bridges. Typically, the posteromedial approach is performed first. Reducing and fixing the medial side first provides a stabilized medial column for the lateral side to be buttressed against (Fig. 28-14). The posteromedial and anterolateral approaches are performed as described previously. Fixation screws in the medial side are directed posterior to anterior to avoid the lateral to medial fixation. Retrospective reviews have shown low but significant complications is these complex injuries, which emphasizes the need for good soft tissue handling techniques.

■ When lateral locking plate only is selected for fixation of a bicondylar pattern, the posteromedial fracture must be carefully evaluated on a computed tomographic (CT) scan. With this technique, the articular block must either be nondisplaced or adequately reduced and stabilized so that it can be aligned with the distal segment (Fig. 28-15). The approach is identical to the anterolateral approach described previously, but less distal dissection is required because the plate can be slid along

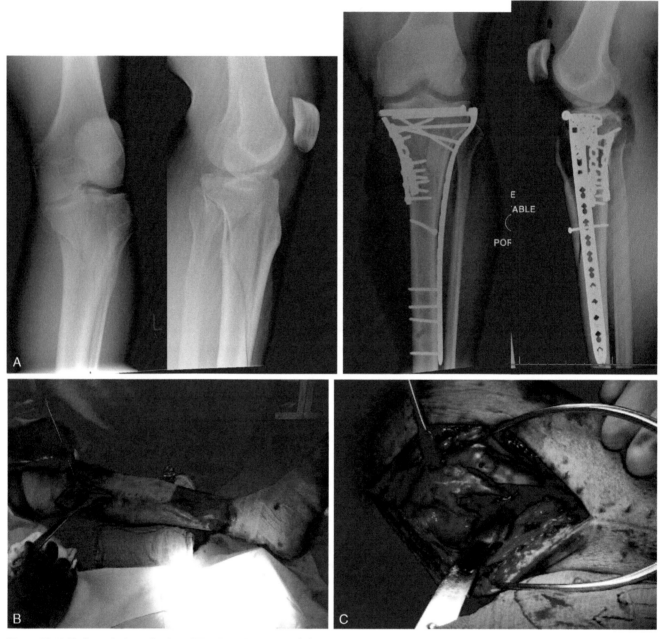

Figure 28-14 Radiograph shows fixation of bicondylar tibial plateau **(A)**, with anterolateral and posteromedial approaches **(B** and **C)**. (Parts B and C with permission from Cole PA, Lafferty PM, Levy BA, et al. Tibial plateau fractures. In: Browner BD, Jupiter JB, Krettek C, Anderson P, eds. *Skeletal Trauma: Basic Science, Management, and Reconstruction.* 5th ed. Philadelphia: Elsevier; 2015. Figures 62-35 and 62-36.)

the lateral tibia and percutaneous guides can be used for distal screw fixation. Areas of metaphyseal comminution can be treated with the "no touch" technique and bypassed with the locking plate. Length and alignment must always be considered when fixing the plate proximally and distally. When placing distal percutaneous screws in longer plates, care must be taken to protect the superficial peroneal nerve and the anterior tibial artery.

Fixation Considerations

- Plates and screws are the most common implants used for fixation of tibial plateau fractures. Generally precontoured periarticular implants are used for anterolateral and posteromedial fixation. Many companies have variations on a similar design

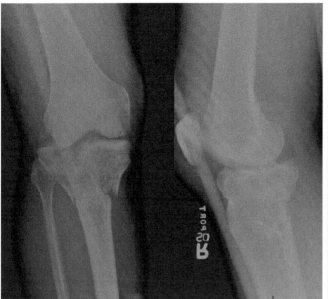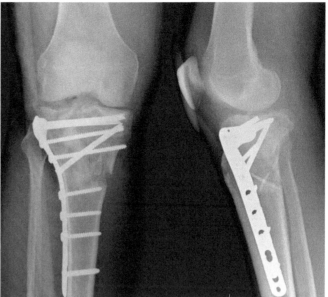

Figure 28-15 Preoperative and postoperative radiographs of a bicondylar tibial plateau fracture treated with lateral locking plate.

for these implants. The function of the plate depends on the fracture pattern and where it is placed on the tibia. On the anterolateral tibia, the plate functions as a buttress that substitutes for the disrupted lateral cortex. There are multiple 3.5-mm holes in the proximal plate to allow for placement of parallel proximal screws. This "rafting screw" technique allows for support under reduced articular fragments to prevent collapse. Posteromedial plates function as an antiglide device to resist shear forces in the posterior tibia. Precontoured plates also allow for minimally invasive, soft tissue–sparing techniques. External guides allow for targeting percutaneous screws distally. Lateral locking plates are used for select bicondylar patterns as described previously because of ability to resist axial, bending, and rotational forces. The plate must be rigid enough to withstand varus deformity in these fracture patterns. Locking plates and screws are commonly used in tibial plateau fracture patterns, and there are reports of maintained reduction and low complication rates in the literature.

■ When reducing depressed articular fragments in the proximal tibia, a void is often created below the fragment. Postoperative settling with loss of reduction is a concern in these patients, and various materials have been used to fill these voids and prevent displacement (Fig. 28-16). Traditionally, autograft bone from the iliac crest was harvested to fill subchondral defects. More recently, allograft bone, bone substitutes, and phase changing cements are preferred by surgeons. A randomized study by Russel and colleagues found that calcium phosphate (Ca-P) cement resulted in less articular subsidence then autograft bone.

■ Definitive external fixation to treat bicondylar tibial plateau fractures is an option for patients with soft tissue injuries too severe for plate fixation even after a period of spanning external fixation. With most external fixation devices, tensioned wires and percutaneous screws are used to fix the articular block (Fig. 28-17). Similar to the technique for lateral locking plate only for fixation of bicondylar tibial plateau fractures, length and alignment must be corrected and maintained.

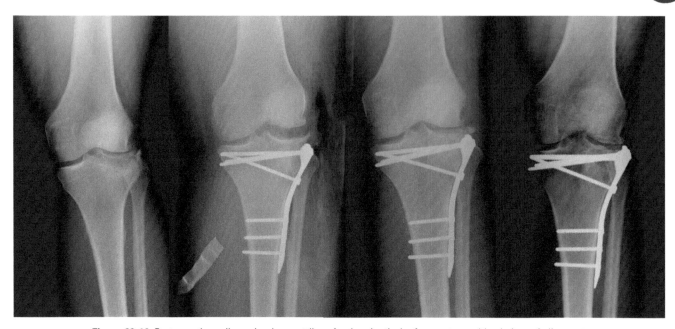

Figure 28-16 Postoperative radiographs show settling of reduced articular fragments resulting in loss of alignment.

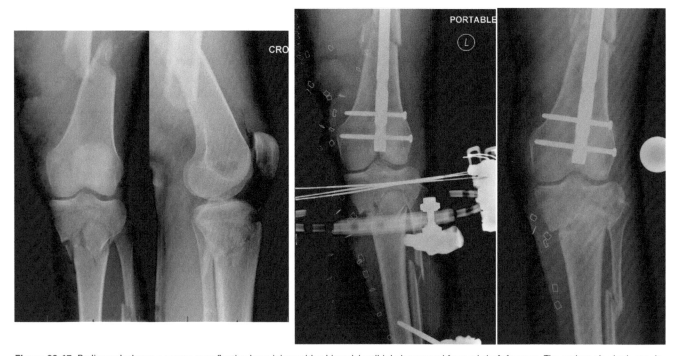

Figure 28-17 Radiograph shows a severe open floating knee injury with a bicondylar tibial plateau and femoral shaft fracture. The patient also had vascular injury. The tibial plateau fracture was treated with definitive external fixation.

BRIEF SUMMARY OF SURGICAL STEPS

- Preoperative planning is essential to determine positioning, appropriate approach, technique to evaluate reduction, and fixation
- Supine positioning with bump under the hip and elevation of the leg or prone positioning can be used for isolated posteromedial approaches
- Perform the appropriate approach
- Execute preoperative plan to perform and evaluate articular reduction
- Provisionally stabilize with K-wires
- Evaluate alignment of the limb with fluoroscopy and clinically
- Place compression screws, buttress plate, or antiglide plate
- Fill defect below the subchondral bone with void filler

REQUIRED EQUIPMENT

Radiolucent operating room table
Positioning devices to bump hip and elevate the leg
Large C-arm fluoroscopy
Tourniquet sterile or nonsterile
Large reduction clamps, Cobb elevator, curette, bone tamp, long K-wires, femoral distractor, anterior cruciate ligament drilling guide
6.5-mm cannulated screws
3.5-mm or 4.5-mm precontoured proximal tibia plates
Bone void filler

TECHNICAL PEARLS

- Properly position the patient so that appropriate approach can be performed without obstruction
- Carefully plan out incisions to minimize soft tissue dissection and prevent narrow skin bridges
- With the anterolateral approach to the tibia, preserve a cuff of anterior compartment fascia on the tibial crest for deep closure over the plate
- Use fracture lines to access depressed articular fragments, and once reduced, provisionally stabilize with K-wires
- Use fluoroscopy to accurately place rafting screws to support reduced articular fragments
- When using an arthrotomy to view the articular reduction, use care not to injure the meniscus and adequately repair during closure
- When using dual approaches for fixation of bicondylar patterns, accurately reduce the medial condyle with minimal fixation to allow for reduction of the lateral condyle and room for lateral to medial fixation
- Always consider overall patient health and soft tissue injury when selecting definitive treatment of tibial plateau fractures

COMMON PITFALLS

(When to call for the attending physician)

- Preoperative evaluation of the computed tomographic scan to identify coronal shear fracture of the medial condyle
- Use good soft tissue handling techniques and avoid stripping bone of soft tissue
- Protect neurovascular structures, including the anterior tibial artery on the posterolateral tibia and saphenous vein and nerve in the subcutaneus tissue, during the posteromedial approach
- Get adequate fluoroscopic images to evaluate reduction and prevent intraarticular placement of screws
- Adequate "rafting screw" fixation and void filling after elevation and reduction of articular fragments
- Ensure that the anterolateral buttress plate is positioned posterior to prevent prominent hardware on the anterior tibia
- Avoid future incisions and implants with external fixation pins
- Always be conscientious of limb alignment before performing definitive fixation

POSTOPERATIVE PROTOCOL

The goal of the postoperative program is to minimize complications, including loss of reduction, while maximizing knee motion and early return to normal function. Modern fixation techniques strive for stable fixation to allow for early motion of the knee either immediately or in the first few weeks after surgery. A hinged knee brace may be used for additional stability with early motion after surgery. Retrospective reviews have indicated that knee stiffness can be an issue in patients immobilized for 2 weeks after surgery. Other studies have shown that knees can gain over 130 degrees of flexion after up to 6 weeks of immobilization in spanning external fixation.

Weight-bearing is generally initiated 6 to 12 weeks after operative fixation depending on the severity of the injury and stability of fixation. Weight-bearing in cast braces or unloader braces is not used commonly but has been described in series with low rates of secondary displacement.

POSTOPERATIVE CLINIC VISIT PROTOCOL

Patients are generally seen in clinical follow-up at 2 to 3 weeks after surgery for suture removal. Knee motion is initiated earlier in the postoperative course in a hinged knee brace. The 2-week to 3-week follow-up visit is flexible based on length of hospital admission for associated injuries in polytrauma cases. The first postoperative radiographs of the knee and tibia are taken at 6 weeks. The patient then is seen again in clinic at 12 weeks when weight-bearing is initiated. Bilateral standing long leg radiographs are taken at that time to assess alignment. Patients then are seen at 6 months and 12 months after surgery with appropriate radiographs.

SUGGESTED READINGS

1. Ali AM, El-Shafie M, Willett KM. Failure of fixation of tibial plateau fractures. *J Orthop Trauma.* 2002;16(5):323-329.
2. Barei DP, Nork SE, Mills WJ, Henley MB, Benirschke SK. Complications associated with internal fixation of high-energy bicondylar tibial plateau fractures utilizing a two-incision technique. *J Orthop Trauma.* 2004;18(10):649-657.
3. Gausewitz S, Hohl M. The significance of early motion in the treatment of tibial plateau fractures. *Clin Orthop Relat Res.* 1986;202:135-138.
4. Haidukewych G, Sems SA, Huebner D, Horwitz D, Levy B. Results of polyaxial locked-plate fixation of periarticular fractures of the knee. *J Bone Joint Surg Am.* 2007;89(3):614-620.
5. Holzach P, Matter P, Minter J. Arthroscopically assisted treatment of lateral tibial plateau fractures in skiers; use of a cannulated reduction system. *J Orthop Trauma.* 1994;8(4):273-281.
6. Marsh JL, Smith ST, Do TT. External fixation and limited internal fixation for complex fractures of the tibial plateau. *J Bone Joint Surg Am.* 1995;77(5):661-673.
7. Russell TA, Leighton RK, Alpha-BSM Tibial Plateau Fracture Study Group. Comparison of autogenous bone graft and endothermic calcium phosphate cement for defect augmentation in tibial plateau fractures. A multicenter, prospective, randomized study. *J Bone Joint Surg Am.* 2008;90(10):2057-2061.
8. Schatzker J. Compression in the surgical treatment of fractures of the tibia. *Clin Orthop Relat Res.* 1974;105:220-239.
9. Stark E, Stucken C, Trainer G, Tornetta P 3rd. Compartment syndrome in Schatzker type VI plateau fractures and medial condylar fracture-dislocations treated with temporary external fixation. *J Orthop Trauma.* 2009;23(7):502-506.
10. Weigel DP, Marsh JL. High-energy fractures of the tibial plateau. Knee function after longer follow-up. *J Bone Joint Surg Am.* 2002;84-A(9):1541-1551.

ANTERIOR SHOULDER STABILIZATION
SURGICAL TECHNIQUE

Rachel M. Frank | Matthew T. Provencher

Anterior shoulder instability remains a growing problem in the young, athletic patient population. For most patients with anterior instability, an anteroinferior labral tear (Bankart lesion) is present and necessitates repair of the soft tissue to the glenoid rim. Arthroscopic stabilization with suture anchors has become the accepted standard of care, with good to excellent clinical outcomes and low recurrence rates in most patients. Arthroscopic anterior shoulder stabilization can be performed in either the beach chair (BC) position or the lateral decubitus (LD) position, depending on surgeon preference, experience level, and the specific intended procedure. The LD position may allow for more inferior suture anchor placement on the glenoid, and because the typical zone of injury in the setting of anterior instability is in the anterior-inferior glenoid quadrant, the surgeon must achieve inferior anchor placement for adequate repair. A variety of arthroscopic techniques can be used for anterior shoulder stabilization, including standard suture anchor repair with a variety of different stitch configurations and knotless suture anchor repair with suture tape. The purpose of this chapter is to provide up-to-date technical pearls for performing a thorough, accurate, and efficient arthrosocpic shoulder stabilization. In this chapter, the technique for stabilization in the LD position is described, although this technique also can be performed successfully in the BC position (Video 29-1).

SURGICAL TECHNIQUE

Room Set-Up

- Ensure that all appropriate equipment is in the room.
- Ensure that all implants and instruments are available and sterile.
- Confirm that the monitors are ergonomically positioned.
- Confirm that the video monitor, pump, and shaver systems are functional.
- The video monitor should be placed opposite the surgeon at head level.

Patient Positioning

- The authors perform arthroscopic shoulder stabilization in the lateral decubitus position.
- Ensure that the bean bag is on the operating table before attempting the transfer. A sheet should be under and on top of the bean bag.
- Transfer the patient to the operating table.
- A team effort is used to roll the patient into the lateral decubitus position on the bean bag, with the operative extremity up.

- Place the axillary roll under the patient, approximately two to three fingerbreadths distal to the axilla against the rib cage, which minimizes pressure on the brachial plexus during the case.
- Position the bean bag as desired to ensure optimal exposure and access to the shoulder and all necessary portals.
- Inflate the bean bag and secure it in place with heavy tape; take care to protect the skin of the patient.
- Ensure that bony prominences are well padded, especially the down arm and down leg at the ulnar nerve and peroneal nerve, respectively. Place a pillow between the legs to minimize pressure on the legs.
- Turn the table 45 to 90 degrees to improve access to the patient for both the anesthesia team and the surgical team (Figs. 29-1 and 29-2).

Prepping and Draping

- The patient is prepped and draped as discussed in the chapter on diagnostic shoulder arthroscopy. For specifics on portal placement for the lateral decubitus position, please see the diagnostic shoulder arthroscopy chapter (Chapter 2).

Landmarks and Portals (Fig. 29-3)

- Draw the following helpful landmarks with an indelible marking pen: acromion ("notch" and posterior and lateral borders), clavicle, coracoid process, acromioclavicular (AC) joint.
- After routine diagnostic glenohumeral arthroscopy is performed with a 30-degree arthroscope (see Chapter 2 on diagnostic glenohumeral arthroscopy), with care taken to note any concomitant pathologies, one can perform the stabilization.

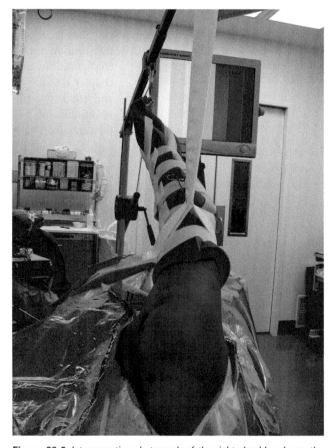

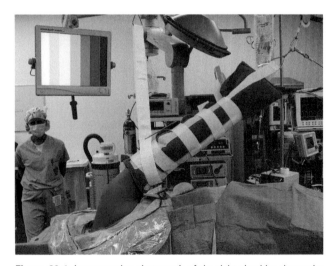

Figure 29-1 Intraoperative photograph of the right shoulder shows the lateral decubitus position with the arm in 30 to 40 degrees of abduction.

Figure 29-2 Intraoperative photograph of the right shoulder shows the lateral decubitus position with the arm in 20 degrees of forward flexion.

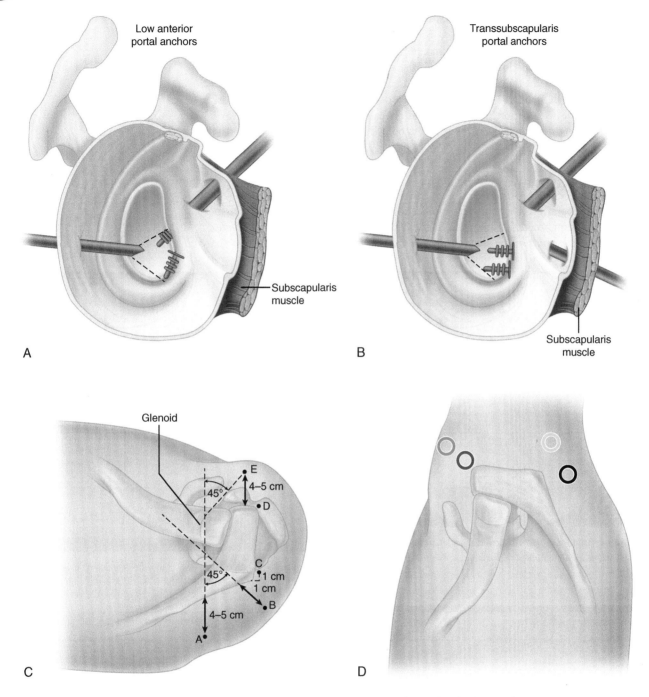

Figure 29-3 A, Sagittal view of the glenoid fossa shows a low anterior portal approach to the inferior glenoid, resulting in inferior anchor angulation. **B,** Sagittal view shows a transsubscapularis portal approach to optimize angulation of the inferior glenoid anchors. **C,** A right shoulder. The positions of the glenohumeral portals are shown: *A,* Posterior portal; *B,* posterolateral portal, which has a 45-degree angle of approach to the posterior glenoid rim; *C,* port of Wilmington, whose location is referenced off the posterolateral acromion; *D,* anterosuperolateral portal; and *E,* anterior portal, which also approaches the glenoid at a 45-degree angle. With the exception of the posterior viewing portal, a spinal needle is used to precisely identify the proper location for each portal. **D,** Superficial markings for shoulder arthroscopy. Reproducible markings based on osseous prominences are excellent guides for portal positions. The standard posterior portal is marked by the *black circle;* the anterosuperior portal by the *red circle;* the midglenoid portal by the *green circle;* and the percutaneous posterolateral portal by the *yellow circle.* With these portals, the entire glenoid labrum can be approached reproducibly. (A and B, Redrawn from Davidson PA, Tibone JE. Anterior-inferior (5 o'clock) portal for shoulder arthroscopy. *Arthroscopy.* 1995;11:519-525. C, Redrawn from Lo IK, Burkhart SS. Triple labral lesions: pathology and surgical repair technique—report of seven cases. *Arthroscopy.* 2005;21(2):186-193.)

■ Identify the anterior-inferior capsulolabral avulsion (Bankart lesion) from a posterior view (Fig. 29-4).

  ● Create an accessory anterior, 5-o'clock portal. This portal is inserted 5 to 12 mm inferior to the superior rolled edge of the subscapularis to allow access to the inferior aspects of the capsule (Fig. 29-3).

  ● Create a posterolateral 7-o'clock portal. This portal is established percutaneously through or just inferior to the teres minor. Because of the proximity of the axillary nerve, one should always use dilators before placing a cannula in this portal (Figs. 29-5 and 29-6).

Arthroscopic Bankart Repair

■ Glenoid preparation is begun with mobilization of the anterior capsulolabral tissue (Bankart lesion) medially along the glenoid neck with an arthroscopic elevator, probe, or dull aspect of the shaver (Figs. 29-7 and 29-8).

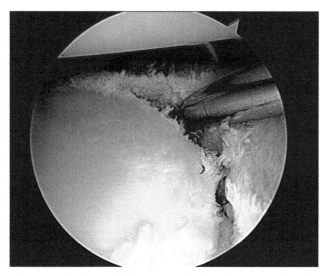

Figure 29-4 Arthroscopic view of the left shoulder in the lateral decubitus position shows an anterior-inferior (Bankart) capsulolabral defect.

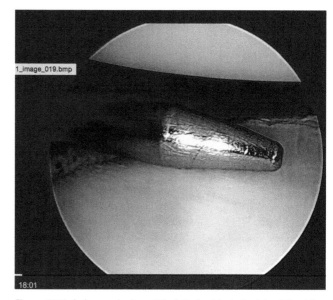

Figure 29-5 Arthroscopic view of the left shoulder in the lateral decubitus position shows establishment of the 7-o'clock portal with a dilator.

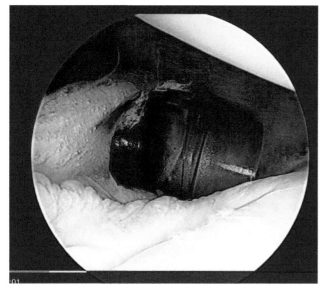

Figure 29-6 Arthroscopic view of the left shoulder in the lateral decubitus position shows establishment of the 7-o'clock portal with a cannula.

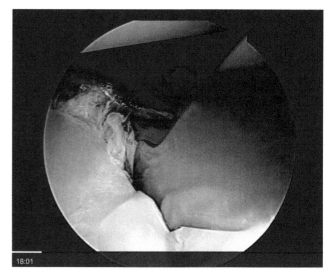

Figure 29-7 Arthroscopic view of the left shoulder in the lateral decubitus position shows elevation of the anterior labrum with an arthroscopic elevator.

- Mobilize and elevate the labrum from 6 o'clock to 3 o'clock, or more, pending the size of the Bankart lesion.
- The soft tissue capsulolabral complex is mobilized until one can visualize the muscle fibers of the subscapularis.
- Adequate mobilization of the labral tissue is critical for ensuring an adequate repair. Test the mobilization by attempting to reduce the labrum back to the anterior glenoid.

- A hooded arthroscopic burr and an arthroscopic rasp then are used to débride the area and create a suitable bed for tissue healing.
  - The glenoid is prepared up to 1 to 2 cm medially to create a bleeding bed of cancellous bone, optimized for soft tissue healing; the inner surface of the labral tissue is also rasped to stimulate soft tissue to bone healing.
- Attention is turned to placing the first anchor in the inferior-most position at approximately 5:30 to 6 o'clock (right shoulder); in some instances, a posterior-inferior suture anchor is also beneficial.
  - The authors aim to place a minimum of three anchors below 3 o'clock (right shoulder) to ensure a stable repair.
- A straight drill guide is inserted through the 7-o'clock portal, placed approximately 2 mm onto the articular rim at a 45-degree angle relative to the glenoid surface (Fig. 29-9).
  - Alternatively, this anchor can be inserted from the accessory anterior 5-o'clock portal or percutaneously through the subscapularis (transsubscapularis).
- After the pilot drill hole is created, the anchor of choice is gently inserted with a mallet with use of direct visualization (Fig. 29-10).
- Once the anchor is implanted, the two-suture limbs (high-strength nonabsorbable no. 2 suture) from the suture anchor are separated.
- A suture retrieval device then is placed through the capsulolabral tissue, and the appropriate suture attached to the anchor then is shuttled through the capsulolabral tissue. In most cases, approximately 1 cm of capsular tissue is plicated to the labrum to eliminate capsular redundancy (Fig. 29-11).
  - The suture retrieval device is placed inferior to the anchor so that when the inferior tissue (anteroinferior glenohumeral ligament) is reduced to the anterior

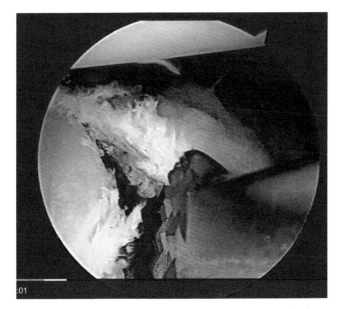

Figure 29-8 Arthroscopic view of the left shoulder in the lateral decubitus position shows preparation of the anterior labrum and glenoid surface with a rasp.

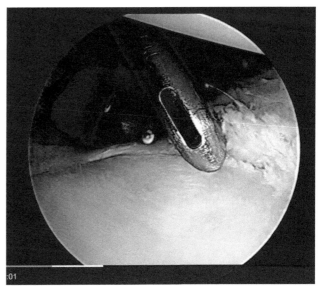

Figure 29-9 Arthroscopic view of the left shoulder in the lateral decubitus position shows a drill guide for the first anchor at approximately 6:30 to 7 o'clock (left shoulder).

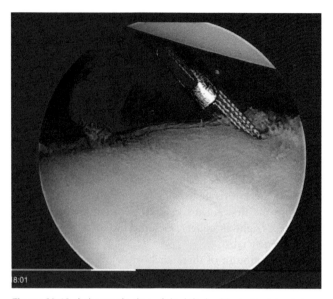

Figure 29-10 Arthroscopic view of the left shoulder in the lateral decubitus position shows suture anchor placement in the drill hole.

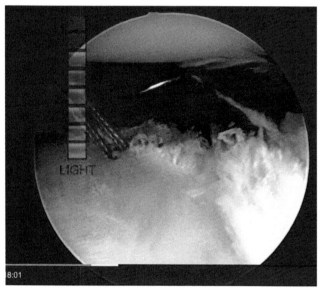

Figure 29-11 Arthroscopic view of the left shoulder in the lateral decubitus position shows the arthroscopic suture passer between the glenoid and caspulolabral tissue.

glenoid rim and the knot is tied down, the capsulolabral tissue is shifted cephalad, forming a "bumper" of capsulolabral tissue onto the labral surface (Fig. 29-12).

- The suture essentially is passed via the suture passer through the capsulolabral tissue at 6 o'clock and is "shifted" from inferior to superior as it is tied down to the anchor at 5:30.
- Knots are tied with the arthroscopic knot-tying technique of choice. The authors prefer a nonsliding knot that consists of reverse posts with alternative half-hitches (RHAP).
  - Other knot-tying techniques are also acceptable.
  - Take care to ensure that the knot sits away from the articular surface to avoid mechanical irritation to the glenoid cartilage.
- All steps are repeated for subsequent anchors, with a goal of at least three anchors below 3 o'clock (Fig. 29-13).
  - Anchors are placed sequentially from inferior to superior, spaced approximately 5 to 7 mm apart, for a secure repair (Fig. 29-14).
- In some cases, with the arm in external rotation, two to three capsular plication sutures can be placed through the capsular tissue in the inferior pouch with the goal of reducing capsular redundancy.
- More recently, knotless fixation constructs with suture tape (i.e., LabralTape, Arthrex, Inc, Naples, FL) have been described, eliminating the need for knots and therefore eliminating the potential for mechanical disruption to the chondral surface from the material of the knot. This technique uses the suture-tape material, anchors (i.e., PushLock, Arthrex Inc, Naples, FL) and polydioxanone suture (PDS) (Ethicon Inc, Somerville, NJ) for passage.

Closure

- Portals are closed with 3-0 nylon sutures with mattress or figure-of-eight sutures.
- Dressings include gauze, abdominal (ABD) pads, and tape, with a sling.

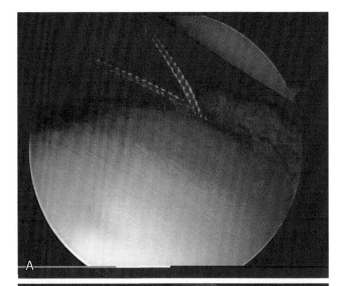

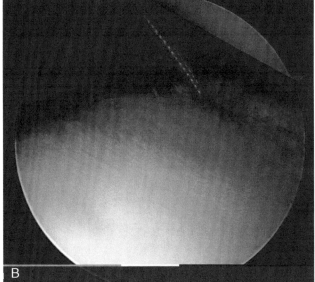

Figure 29-12 A, Arthroscopic view of the left shoulder in the lateral decubitus position shows suture limbs from suture anchor before shuttling with PDS suture from the suture passer. **B,** Arthroscopic view of the left shoulder in the lateral decubitus position shows suture limbs from suture anchor after shuttling with PDS suture from the suture passer (one limb is now deep to the labrum).

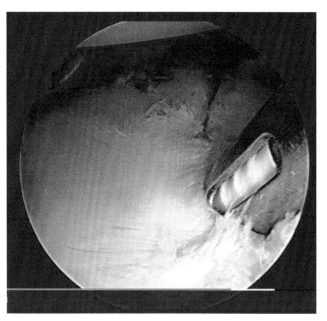

Figure 29-13 Arthroscopic view of the left shoulder in the lateral decubitus position shows the fourth (and final) suture anchor placement at approximately 10 o'clock (left shoulder).

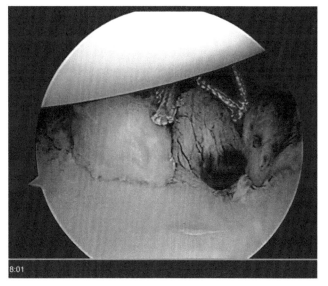

Figure 29-14 Arthroscopic view of the left shoulder in the lateral decubitus position shows the final appearance of the arthroscopic labral stabilization after use of four suture anchors with all knots tied arthroscopically.

BRIEF SUMMARY OF SURGICAL STEPS

- Examination with anesthesia
- Draw landmarks
- Establish portals
- Diagnostic arthroscopy
- Débride rotator interval
- Elevate labrum; prepare surface with elevator, rasp, and shaver; prepare until you can see subscapularis muscle fibers
- Prepare glenoid surface approximately 1 to 2 cm medial to create a bleeding bony surface to improve healing
- Suture passer (i.e., lasso)
- Drill pilot hole for anchor (inferior-most anchor is first; work sequentially from inferior to superior)
- Tap in anchor
- Suture passer penetrates soft tissue around capsulolabral complex (at the glenoid-labrum junction)
- Feed PDS suture through passer
- Shuttle limbs of suture with PDS suture
- Tie suture with reverse posts with alternating half-hitches (or arthroscopic knot of choice)
- Cut suture limbs with arthroscopic scissors
- Repeat all steps for subsequent anchors; goal is at least three anchors below 3 o'clock
- Gently examine shoulder to ensure stability
- First anchor is typically drilled with 7 o'clock portal; subsequent anchors often placed with anterior-superior accessory portal

REQUIRED EQUIPMENT

| 30-Degree arthroscope |
| Traction system with weights and pulleys, bean bag |
| Arthroscopy tower, fluid system, pump, tubing |
| Cannulas |
| Spinal needle |
| Arthroscopic shaver, burr, radiofrequency device |
| Arthroscopic graspers |
| Arthroscopic elevator, probe, wissinger rod, switching sticks, knot pusher, suture passer, PDS suture, suture anchors |

COMMON PITFALLS

(When to call for the attending physician)

- Recognize all concomitant pathology and treat accordingly (symptomatic pathology only)
- Recognize anterior glenoid bone loss and be prepared to convert to a bony augmentation procedure (iliac crest, Latarjet, or allograft) if needed
- Be cautious with suture management and be sure to tie knots sequentially from inferior to superior
- Be cautious with thermal capsulorrhaphy because of the concern for postoperative glenohumeral chondrolysis

TECHNICAL PEARLS

- Establish the 7-o'clock portal with dilators to avoid neurovascular injury
- Aim for a minimum of three anchors below 3 o'clock (right shoulder)
- Place anchors sequentially from inferior to superior
- Add one or more capsular plication stitches in the setting of capsular redundancy

POSTOPERATIVE PROTOCOL

- Weeks 0-4: Passive range of motion (ROM) as tolerated, with goals of 140 degrees forward flexion (FF) and 40 degrees external rotation (ER) at the side; no abduction or 90-90 ER until at least 4 weeks; sling for comfort for weeks 0-2; grip strengthening allowed but no resisted motions.
- Weeks 4-8: Increase passive and active ROM to tolerance without restrictions; begin light isometric exercises with arm at side and advance with therabands as tolerated.
- Weeks 8-12: Increase motion and strengthening as tolerated.

POSTOPERATIVE CLINIC VISIT PROTOCOL

- Days 7-10: First postoperative visit for suture removal and ROM check.
- Weeks 4-6: Second postoperative visit for gait, ROM, and strength check.
- Weeks 8-10: Final postoperative visit.

SUGGESTED READINGS

1. Dickens JF, Owens BD, Cameron KL, et al. Return to play and recurrent instability after in-season anterior shoulder instability: a prospective multicenter study. *Am J Sports Med*. 2014;42(12):2842-2850. doi: 10.1177/0363546514553181.
2. Forsythe B, Frank RM, Ahmed M, et al. Identification and treatment of existing copathology in anterior shoulder instability repair. *Arthroscopy*. 2015;31(1):154-166. doi: 10.1016/j.arthro.2014.06.014.
3. Frank RM, Mall NA, Gupta D, et al. Inferior suture anchor placement during arthroscopic Bankart repair: influence of portal placement and curved drill guide. *Am J Sports Med*. 2014;42(5):1182-1189. doi: 10.1177/0363546514523722.
4. Frank RM, Saccomanno MF, McDonald LS, Moric M, Romeo AA, Provencher MT. Outcomes of arthroscopic anterior shoulder instability in the beach chair versus lateral decubitus position: a systematic review and meta-regression analysis. *Arthroscopy*. 2014;30(10):1349-1365. doi: 10.1016/j.arthro.2014.05.008.
5. Kang RW, Frank RM, Nho SJ, et al. Complications associated with anterior shoulder instability repair. *Arthroscopy*. 2009;25(8):909-920. doi: 10.1016/j.arthro.2009.03.009.
6. Levy DM, Gvozdyev BV, Schulz BM, Boselli KJ, Ahmad CS. Arthroscopic anterior shoulder stabilization with percutaneous assistance and posteroinferior capsular plication. *Am J Orthop*. 2014;43(8):364-369.
7. Mazzocca AD, Brown FM, Carreira DS, Hayden J, Romeo AA. Arthroscopic anterior shoulder stabilization of collision and contact athletes. *Am J Sports Med*. 2005;33(1):52-60.
8. Mologne TS, Provencher MT, Menzel KA, Vachon TA, Dewing CB. Arthroscopic stabilization in patients with an inverted pear glenoid: results in patients with bone loss of the anterior glenoid. *Am J Sports Med*. 2007;35(8):1276-1283. doi: 10.1177/0363546507300262.
9. Nho SJ, Frank RM, Van Thiel GS, et al. A biomechanical analysis of anterior Bankart repair using suture anchors. *Am J Sports Med*. 2010;38(7):1405-1412. doi: 10.1177/0363546509359069.
10. Slabaugh MA, Nho SJ, Grumet RC, et al. Does the literature confirm superior clinical results in radiographically healed rotator cuffs after rotator cuff repair? *Arthroscopy*. 2010;26(3):393-403. doi: 10.1016/j.arthro.2009.07.023.

30

ARTHROSCOPIC ROTATOR CUFF REPAIR

Gregory L. Cvetanovich | Anthony A. Romeo

Rotator cuff pathology includes a disease spectrum that ranges from tendinitis and subacromial impingement, to partial-thickness tears and full-thickness tears, and ultimately to rotator cuff arthropathy. Patients with symptomatic rotator cuff tears typically present with anterolateral shoulder pain that may radiate toward the deltoid insertion. Onset of symptoms is most commonly insidious, although some patients do recall an inciting traumatic event. Pain is dull at rest but worsened with overhead activity and at night while sleeping. Patients, particularly those with large full-thickness rotator cuff tears, also may report weakness and fatigue with overhead activities.

On physical examination, inspection of the shoulder may reveal atrophy of the supraspinatus or infraspinatus, indicative of chronic tears. Impingement signs such as the Neer test and Hawkins-Kennedy test may have positive results. Testing of each rotator cuff muscle then is performed to assess for weakness and positive special tests. Supraspinatus is tested with resisted forward elevation, Jobe test, and drop arm test. Infraspinatus is tested with resisted external rotation with the arm at the side and the external rotation lag sign. Teres minor is tested with resisted external rotation at 90 degrees abduction and 90 degrees external rotation and with the hornblower's sign. Subscapularis is tested with internal rotation weakness, lift-off test, belly press test, and bear hug test. Imaging typically involves plain radiographs to identify degenerative changes, proximal humeral migration, and acromial morphology. Magnetic resonance imaging (MRI) is typically used to determine the muscles involved in the tear, size of the tear, degree of retraction, and fatty infiltration of the rotator cuff musculature. Tears may be classified by size, tendons involved, extent of rotator cuff fatty atrophy (Goutallier classification), partial-thickness (articular, bursal, or intrasubstance) versus full-thickness tear, and tear shape.

Nonoperative treatment with physical therapy, nonsteroidal antiinflammatory drugs (NSAIDs), and subacromial corticosteroid injection is the first line of treatment for most symptomatic rotator cuff tears. Factors to consider when determining whether rotator cuff repair is indicated include severity of the patient's symptoms, response to nonoperative treatment, characteristics of the tear (partial-thickness versus full-thickness, size, retraction, and muscle atrophy), age and activity level of the patient, acute versus chronic tear, preoperative range of motion, and presence of rotator cuff arthropathy. Although open and mini-open rotator cuff repair historically has been quite a successful treatment for rotator cuff tears, arthroscopic techniques have revolutionized rotator cuff repair, including single-row and double-row techniques.

This guide covers the authors' preferred method of arthroscopic rotator cuff repair, with a double-row technique.

CASE MINIMUM REQUIREMENTS

- There are no minimum requirements for rotator cuff repair.
- Residents must log a minimum of 20 shoulder arthroscopy cases, which includes arthroscopic rotator cuff repair.

COMMONLY USED CPT CODES

- CPT Code: 29827—Arthroscopy, shoulder, surgical; with rotator cuff repair
- CPT Code: 29826 [–51 for multiple procedures]—Arthroscopy, shoulder, surgical; decompression of subacromial space with partial acromioplasty, with or without coracoacromial release
- CPT Code: 23430 [–59 for distinct procedural service]—Tenodesis of long tendon of biceps
- CPT Code: 29822—Arthroscopy, shoulder, surgical; débridement, limited
- CPT Code: 29824—Arthroscopy, shoulder, surgical; distal claviculectomy including distal articular surface (Mumford procedure)
- CPT Code: 23412—Repair of ruptured musculotendinous cuff (e.g., rotator cuff) open; chronic
- CPT Code: 23420—Reconstruction of complete shoulder (rotator) cuff avulsion, chronic (includes acromioplasty)

SURGICAL TECHNIQUE

Room Set-Up

- General anesthesia versus regional interscalene block with sedation:
  - The optimal method of anesthesia is determined in conjunction with the anesthesiologist, with the patient's medical comorbidities taken into consideration. General anesthesia can be combined with preoperative interscalene block for improved postoperative pain control.
- Patient positioning: beach chair position versus lateral decubitus:
  - The beach chair position benefits include ease of conversion to an open procedure, ease of arm manipulation during surgery, and more familiar anatomic orientation.
  - The lateral decubitus position benefits include traction on the arm, which allows better access to concomitant glenohumeral pathology. A drawback of this position is traction-related nerve complications.

Patient Positioning

- The authors prefer beach chair positioning for arthroscopic rotator cuff repair procedures (Fig. 30-1).
- The patient is positioned supine, and the head of the bed is elevated 50 to 60 degrees. The knees are flexed with a wedge or pillow under the knees.
- The medial border of the scapula on the operative side is at the edge of the bed, which allows full access to the posterior shoulder for portal placement.
- The head is placed in the head holder with a foam holder to secure it in place.
- A rolled towel is placed just medial to the scapula.
- The patient is well-padded and well-secured.
- A pneumatic articulated arm holder is attached to the bed.
- The bed is rotated to allow adequate surgical access to the operative extremity, and arthroscopy video screens are positioned to allow optimal visualization during the procedure.

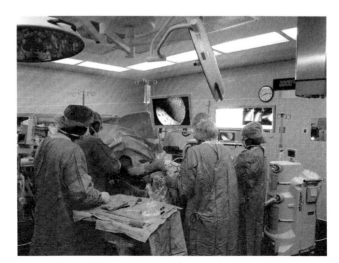

Figure 30-1 Room set-up for arthroscopic rotator cuff repair, with patient in beach chair position, arm in pneumatic arm holder, bed rotated to allow adequate access to all sides of the shoulder, and arthroscopy video screens well-positioned for visualization during the procedure.

Prepping and Draping

- After induction of anesthesia but before prepping and draping, an examination with anesthesia is performed, including range of motion and stability assessment.
- Prepping and draping varies according to surgeon preference.
- Generally, the operative arm is hung, and a clear plastic U-drape is placed. The shoulder and arm then are prepped with the surgical preparation solution of choice.
- A down sheet is placed to cover the legs.
- A sticky blue U-drape is placed from top down, and another is placed from bottom up.
- The arm is taken down from hanging, and an impervious stockinette is placed, followed by Coban wrapping (3M, Minneapolis) to above the elbow.
- Ioban (3M) is used to cover the skin, and an extremity drape then is applied.
- The forearm is placed in a foam wrap for the arm holder, attached to the sterile portion of the arm holder, and overwrapped with Coban wrapping.
- In prepping and draping, care must be taken to leave a field wide enough to allow all potential arthroscopic portals and potential open conversion or mini-open biceps tenodesis.

Portal Placement and Diagnostic Arthroscopy

- Skin markings are placed on standard surgical landmarks: anterior and posterior borders of the clavicle, the edges of the acromion, the scapular spine, the acromio-clavicular (AC) joint, and the coracoid. Typical portals are the standard posterior portal, standard anterior portal, lateral viewing portal, and anterolateral portal (Fig. 30-2).
- Portal sites and sites of any concurrent surgical incisions are marked and anesthetized with 0.25% bupivacaine with epinephrine.
- The posterior portal is located 2 cm medial and 2 cm inferior to the posterolateral corner of the acromion. One can place a thumb in the presumed portal location, long finger on the coracoid, and index finger in the soft spot between the clavicle and scapular spine and then perform a shuck test to verify posterior portal location (Fig. 30-3; Video 30-1).
- An 18-gauge spinal needle is passed through the portal site into the glenohumeral joint, aiming toward the coracoid.

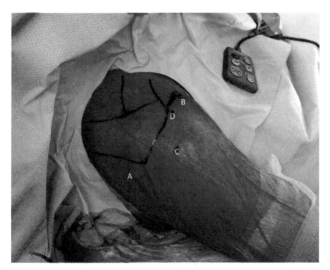

Figure 30-2 Skin markings for arthroscopic rotator cuff repair, with clavicle, acromion, acromioclavicular joint, and coracoid. The authors' preferred portals for arthroscopic rotator cuff repair are shown: *A,* standard posterior portal; *B,* standard anterior portal; *C,* lateral viewing portal; and *D,* anterolateral portal.

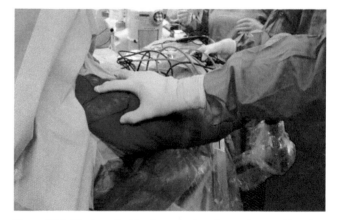

Figure 30-3 Shuck method for determination of posterior portal location. The index finger is placed in the soft spot between the posterior clavicle and scapular spine, the long finger is placed on the coracoid, and the thumb is placed in the presumed portal location.

- The glenohumeral joint is insufflated with 30 mL of normal saline solution.
- A vertical skin incision is made at posterior portal site with a #11 blade.
- A blunt trocar then is aimed toward the coracoid and through the glenohumeral joint.
- The arthroscope is inserted into the posterior portal, typically without a cannula.
- The anterior portal then is established with an outside-in technique with a spinal needle between the supraspinatus and the subscapularis within the rotator interval, entering the skin just lateral to the coracoid (see Fig. 30-2).
- After anterior portal positioning with the spinal needle is confirmed, a vertical skin incision is made and a 5-mm smooth cannula is inserted into the desired location.
- A probe then is inserted from the anterior portal, and a complete diagnostic arthroscopy is performed, including intraarticular débridement and release of the long head biceps tendon from the superior labrum (if indicated for subsequent mini-open subpectoral tenodesis within the bicipital groove).

Subacromial Decompression and Acromioplasty

- A trocar is inserted via the posterior portal, redirected into the subacromial space.
- Slight traction and flexion on the arm with the arm holder can improve visualization of the subacromial space.
- A medial to lateral sweeping motion is performed to confirm subacromial location and to open the subacromial space.
- The arthroscope then is inserted into the anterolateral aspect of the subacromial space from the posterior portal.
- A lateral portal is established with an outside-in technique with an 18-gauge spinal needle. A horizontal incision is used. This is placed at the posterior border of the AC joint and should be placed approximately 2 fingerbreadths below the lateral edge of the acromion to allow unimpeded access to the subacromial space and rotator cuff.
- A shaver is inserted into the lateral portal with the arthroscope viewing through the posterior portal to perform a subacromial bursectomy over the rotator cuff and anterior and lateral subdeltoid space. This allows complete rotator cuff visualization. Care should be taken to not damage the rotator cuff with the shaver by keeping the shaver pointing away from the cuff. One must complete the bursectomy lateral enough, within the gutter, to visualize the location of the lateral row in the double-row rotator cuff repair.
- A radiofrequency device is used through the lateral portal to identify the anterior and lateral acromial edges and release the coracoacromial ligament.
- A distal clavicle excision or acromioplasty can be initiated, if indicated, with a burr through the anterior and lateral portals while viewing from the posterior portal (Fig. 30-4; Video 30-2).
- The arthroscope then is transitioned to view from the lateral portal, and the shaver followed by a burr is used to complete the bursectomy and acromioplasty, with the posterior slope of the acromion as a cutting guide.
- With the view from the lateral portal, an anterolateral portal is established just off the anterolateral edge of the acromion with outside-in 18-gauge spinal needle localization (see Fig. 30-2). A horizontal incision is used, and the spinal needle allows the portal to be centered over the rotator cuff tear. Care is taken not to place this portal too close to the lateral portal to avoid crowding. A threaded 6-mm cannula is twisted in to this portal.

Preparation for Rotator Cuff Repair

- The rotator cuff tear is inspected to determine the pattern and mobility (see Fig. 30-4). The edge of the cuff can be grasped with a tissue grasper to assess cuff mobility to the footprint at the greater tuberosity.

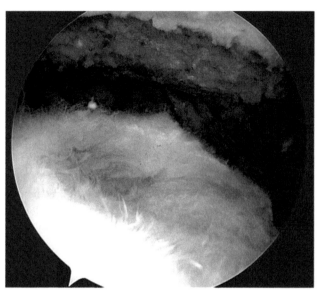

Figure 30-4 The rotator cuff tear is inspected for tear pattern and mobility after adequate subacromial decompression and acromioplasty. The footprint is débrided to punctate bleeding bone before anchor placement to facilitate rotator cuff tendon healing.

- If mobility is inadequate, rotator cuff mobilization is performed with techniques such as releasing the capsule above the superior labrum, removal of superior and posterior rotator cuff adhesions, release of the coracohumeral ligament, rotator interval release, and posterior interval slide.
- Next, the rotator cuff footprint on the greater tuberosity is débrided to bleeding bony surface, with avoidance of complete disruption of the cortex.
- The free edge of the rotator cuff tear is cleaned of devitalized tissue gently with a shaver.
- Margin convergence with free #2 FiberWire (Arthrex, Naples, FL) sutures may be used with U-shaped and L-shaped tears to convert them to crescent-shaped tears before repair with suture anchors.

Anchor Placement and Rotator Cuff Repair: Single-Row

- Depending on surgeon preference and tear configuration, either single-row or double-row rotator cuff repair can be performed.
- In single-row repair, the suture anchors are placed approximately 1 cm lateral to the articular margin on the rotator cuff footprint of the greater tuberosity.
- Anchor placement begins at the posterior edge of the tear, and anchors are approximately 1 cm apart until the anterior aspect of the tear is encountered (commonly at the anterior edge of the supraspinatus).
- Anchor placement occurs via the anterolateral portal, lateral portal, and sometimes additional accessory stab incisions just off the lateral aspect of the acromion.
- After anchor insertion, tug on the sutures to ensure it is well engaged in the bone.
- Sutures are shuttled out of a free portal (commonly anterolateral) until the surgeon is ready to pass them through the rotator cuff.
- Sutures are retrieved through a working portal and passed sequentially through the rotator cuff in a posterior-to-anterior direction.
- Suture passage may be achieved via various devices as per surgeon preference, and suture patterns may include simple sutures versus Mason-Allen stitches.
- After suture passage through the rotator cuff, knots are tied from a posterior-to-anterior direction. A variety of knot configurations has been described, and surgeon preference varies.
- The completed repair is inspected after knots are tied.

Anchor Placement and Rotator Cuff Repair: Double-Row Transosseous Equivalent (Authors' Preferred Technique)

- The authors' preferred double-row transosseous-equivalent technique provides a low-profile transosseous-equivalent repair that maximizes rotator cuff contact with the cuff footprint, which may improve healing and reduce pull-out (Fig. 30-5; Video 30-3).
- Various double-row repair techniques have been described, and the details of technique depend on surgeon preference.
- A medial row of anchors is placed as medial as possible along the articular surface adjacent to the rotator cuff footprint. Typically two to three double-loaded anchors are used based on the size of tear. These are placed from posterior to anterior either via the anterolateral portal or percutaneously via stab incisions just off the lateral edge of the acromion, depending on the necessary trajectory. The lateral portal is used for viewing.
- A punch is malleted down to the laser line (Fig. 30-6). The punch is removed, and the anchor is inserted, with care taken to fully seat the anchor in the bone (Fig. 30-7).
- The authors prefer to use 4.75 Arthrex SwiveLock C (Arthrex, Naples, FL) suture anchor loaded with 2-mm FiberTape (Arthrex, Naples, FL) and #2 FiberWire. The #2 FiberWire then is removed from the anchor and can be used later for a cinch stitch. Sutures are retrieved through the anterolateral portal.
- For the posterior medial row anchor, #1 polydioxanone (PDS) (Ethicon Inc, Somerville, NJ) shuttle suture is passed through the tendon with a Spectrum (ConMed Linvatec, Largo, FL) device through the posterior portal, approximately 1 cm medial to the edge of the tear but remaining lateral to the musculotendinous junction (Fig. 30-8). The PDS is used to shuttle the FiberTape through the tendon and out the posterior portal. Alternatively, a penetrator can be used to pass sutures through the rotator cuff (Fig. 30-9).
- If a posterior dog ear is encountered in the rotator cuff repair, the #2 FiberWire suture previously removed from the anchor can be used as a cinch stitch to avoid the dog ear. A spectrum through the posterior portal is used to pass #1 PDS through the posterior cuff dog ear and out the anterolateral portal. The free FiberWire is folded in half, and the two free ends are pulled together out the posterior portal, with the looped end remaining in the anterolateral portal. The two FiberWire tails then are retrieved to the anterolateral portal from the top of the rotator cuff. The two free ends then are passed through the FiberWire loop, and the tails are pulled tight to cinch the loop down to the tendon. This is pulled tight, and the two free FiberWire ends are transferred to the posterior portal.
- The anterior medial row anchor then is placed in the same fashion as the posterior anchor, either percutaneously or through the anterolateral portal. FiberTape sutures are retrieved from the anterolateral portal, and the FiberWire stutch is removed unless an anterior cinch stitch to avoid an anterior dog ear is desired.
- For the anterior medial anchor, the Spectrum is passed through the anterior portal, with the #1 PDS suture placed through the rotator cuff approximately 1 cm anterior to the posterior suture. The PDS is retrieved from the anterolateral portal. Next, the FiberTape sutures are shuttled through the rotator cuff via the PDS suture and out the anterior portal.
- An anterior cinch stitch can be applied to avoid an anterior dog ear if desired with the free #2 FiberWire, in a manner analogous to the posterior cinch stitch.
- If necessary, a third medial row anchor can be placed, although two medial anchors are typically sufficient.
- Next, the posterior lateral row anchor is placed at the lateral edge of the rotator cuff footprint (Fig. 30-10). The authors prefer a 4.75 Arthrex SwiveLock Anchor, which is unloaded.
- One FiberTape limb from each medial row anchor is retrieved and transferred to the anterolateral portal. The posterior cinch stitch also is retrieved through the anterolateral portal.

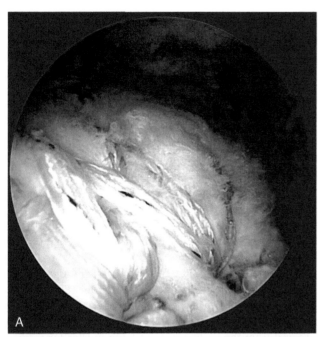

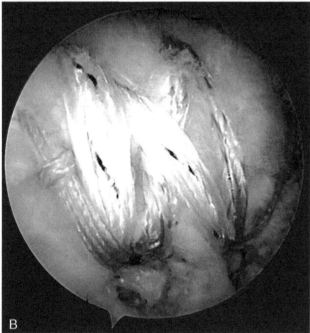

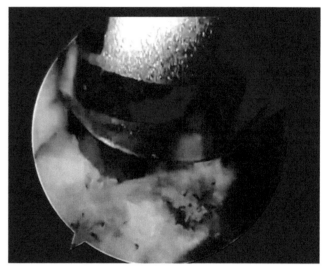

Figure 30-6 A medial row of anchors is placed as medial as possible along the articular surface adjacent to the rotator cuff footprint. Typically two to three double-loaded anchors are used based on the size of tear. A punch is malleted down to the laser line.

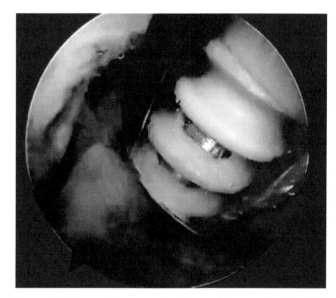

Figure 30-7 The punch is removed, and the medial row anchor is inserted, with care taken to fully seat the anchor in the bone.

Figure 30-5 A, After repair, the repair is inspected to ensure the rotator cuff has maximal contact with the cuff footprint and dog ears are minimized. **B,** The repair in this case was conducted with the authors' preferred technique of double-row transosseous-equivalent repair with anterior and posterior cinch stitches to minimize dog ears, as described in the technique section.

- A punch is inserted via the anterolateral portal and malleted to the laser etch. The SwiveLock Anchor is loaded with the retrieved FiberTape tails and the cinch stitch. Tension the stitches for even rotator cuff reduction and fully seat the posterior lateral anchor.
- The FiberTape and FiberWire sutures can be cut flush with the bone.
- The lateral anterior anchor is placed in an analogous fashion. First, one retrieves the remaining FiberTape limbs from each medial anchor and the anterior cinch stitch into the anterolateral portal.

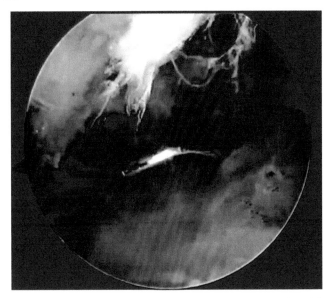

Figure 30-8 A #1 PDS shuttle suture is passed through the tendon with a Spectrum device through the posterior portal, approximately 1 cm medial to the edge of the tear but remaining lateral to the musculotendinous junction. The PDS is used to shuttle the FiberTape through the tendon and out the posterior portal.

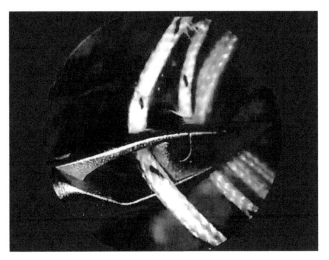

Figure 30-9 A penetrator can be used to pass sutures through the rotator cuff.

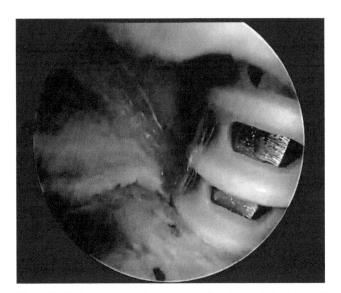

Figure 30-10 Lateral row anchors then are placed at the lateral edge of the rotator cuff footprint. After anchor insertion, sutures are cut flush with the bone.

- A punch is used and malleted to the laser etch. The SwiveLock Anchor is loaded with the two remaining FiberTape limbs and the anterior cinch stitch. These are tensioned for even rotator cuff reduction to the footprint, and the SwiveLock is fully seated.
- The FiberTape and FiberWire sutures can be cut flush with the bone.
- The number of lateral row anchors used is typically the same as the number of medial row anchors. Most commonly, two anchors in each row is sufficient.
- The repair is inspected for integrity (see Video 30-3).
- See Figure 30-11 for an alternative technique tying medial row sutures.

Closure

- The portal sites are closed with interrupted 3-0 Prolene (Ethicon Inc, Somerville, NJ), and a sterile dressing is applied.
- The arm is placed in a sling with a small abduction pillow.

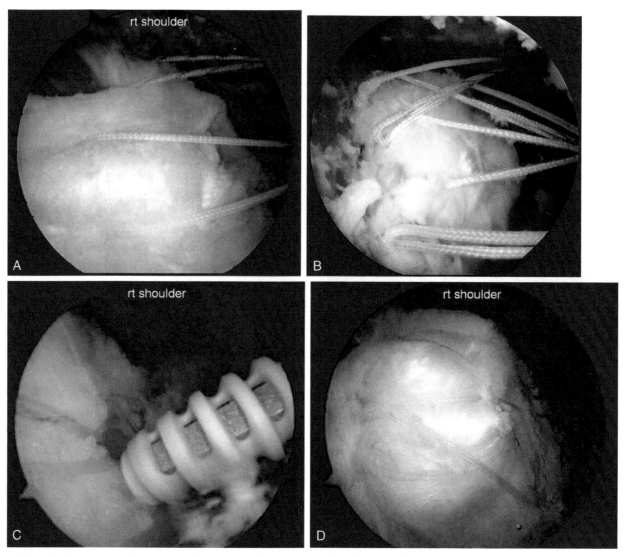

Figure 30-11 **A,** Alternate technique: tying medial row knots. Sutures passed after placement of two medial row anchors. Note four additional suture limbs passed more anteriorly. **B,** Eight sutures from the medial row are tied, resulting in four mattress knots. **C,** Four sutures from the medial row, after knot tying, are incorporated into each of the two lateral row anchors. **D,** Final construct: transosseous-equivalent double-row rotator cuff repair. Four mattress knots tied along the medial row (from two medial row anchors) with sutures incorporated into two lateral row anchors.

BRIEF SUMMARY OF SURGICAL STEPS

- Place posterior and anterior portals and perform diagnostic arthroscopy
- Enter subacromial space and establish lateral portal via inside-out technique
- Complete subacromial decompression and acromioplasty if indicated
- Analyze tear characteristics (pattern, retraction)
- Mobilize rotator cuff and débride degenerative edge of tendon
- Débride cuff footprint on greater tuberosity to punctate bleeding bone
- Establish anterolateral portal and additional stab incisions for anchor placement as needed
- Place medial row of anchors as medial as possible approximately 1 cm apart (two to three anchors)
- Place anchors and pass suture through rotator cuff in posterior to anterior direction
- Arthroscope in lateral portal, use Spectrum through posterior and anterior portals to pass #1 PDS through rotator cuff and out anterolateral portal
- Shuttle FiberTape sutures through rotator cuff and retrieve sutures from posterior and anterior portals
- Apply posterior and anterior cinch stitches with #2 FiberWire to mitigate dog ears (optional)
- Place lateral row of anchors (typically two to three anchors) from posterior to anterior and tension FiberTape to complete second row repair

TECHNICAL PEARLS

- Place lateral portal low so it is parallel to rotator cuff and allows best possible subacromial access, typically 2 fingerbreadths below lateral edge of acromion
- Medial row of anchors in double-row repair should be as medial as possible along articular margin
- Perform suture management and rotator cuff repair in the same reproducible manner every case
- Shuck technique aids in proper posterior portal placement
- Cinch stitches can help avoid posterior and anterior dog ears
- Make additional stab incisions for percutaneous placement of anchors if necessary for proper anchor trajectory
- Bluntly establish the subacromial space by sweeping the trocar in the medial-lateral direction

REQUIRED EQUIPMENT

Standard shoulder arthroscopy set-up in beach chair position with pneumatic articulated arm holder

4.75 SwiveLock suture anchors

Arthroscope, typically 30-degree, 4-mm

Arthroscopic shaver, burr, and radiofrequency (RF) device

#11 blade

18-gauge spinal needles

5-mm smooth cannula

6-mm threaded cannula

COMMON PITFALLS

(When to call for the attending physician)

- Must establish full visualization of rotator cuff and cuff footprint on greater tuberosity via complete subacromial bursectomy, with shaver and RF device, particularly for double-row techniques
- Keep adequate distance between anterolateral and lateral portals to avoid crowding
- Careful fluid management with judicious outflow and limited inflow facilitates visualization and reduces swelling
- Must adequately mobilize rotator cuff to allow repair without undue tension
- If bone is weak, consider larger 5.5 anchor instead of 4.75 to improve anchor pullout strength
- Consider margin convergence to convert U-shaped or L-shaped tears into crescent-shaped tear
- Do not penetrate cortex of greater tuberosity when preparing rotator cuff footprint
- Do not unload anchors inadvertently

POSTOPERATIVE PROTOCOL

After arthroscopic rotator cuff repair, the patient is discharged home on an outpatient basis. The patient remains in a postoperative sling with a small abduction pillow at all times for 6 weeks. Active range of motion of the elbow, wrist, and hand is encouraged. At 6 weeks, the patient is allowed to begin shoulder active-assisted and passive range of motion with outpatient physical therapy. At 12 weeks, active motion and gentle strengthening are begun with outpatient physical therapy. Starting at 16 weeks, strengthening progresses as tolerated.

POSTOPERATIVE CLINIC VISIT PROTOCOL

The incisions are checked and the sutures are removed in the office 7 to 10 days after surgery. Patients are then seen at 6 weeks after surgery to initiate outpatient physical therapy. The next appointment is at 12 weeks to assess range of motion and begin rotator cuff strengthening. Patients then are seen at 6 months, at which point they should be getting close to returning to normal activities.

SUGGESTED READINGS

1. Abrams GD, Gupta AK, Hussey KE, et al. Arthroscopic repair of full-thickness rotator cuff tears with and without acromioplasty: randomized prospective trial with 2-year follow-up. *Am J Sports Med.* 2014;42:1296-1303.
2. Burks RT, Crim J, Brown N, Fink B, Greis PE. A prospective randomized clinical trial comparing arthroscopic single- and double-row rotator cuff repair: magnetic resonance imaging and early clinical evaluation. *Am J Sports Med.* 2009;37:674-682.
3. Cuff DJ, Pupello DR. Prospective randomized study of arthroscopic rotator cuff repair using an early versus delayed postoperative physical therapy protocol. *J Shoulder Elbow Surg.* 2012;21:1450-1455.
4. Franceschi F, Ruzzini L, Longo UG, et al. Equivalent clinical results of arthroscopic single-row and double-row suture anchor repair for rotator cuff tears: a randomized controlled trial. *Am J Sports Med.* 2007;35:1254-1260.
5. Galatz LM, Ball CM, Teefey SA, Middleton WD, Yamaguchi K. The outcome and repair integrity of completely arthroscopically repaired large and massive rotator cuff tears. *J Bone Joint Surg Am.* 2004;86-A:219-224.
6. Gladstone JN, Bishop JY, Lo IK, Flatow EL. Fatty infiltration and atrophy of the rotator cuff do not improve after rotator cuff repair and correlate with poor functional outcome. *Am J Sports Med.* 2007;35:719-728.
7. Hadzic A, Williams BA, Karaca PE, et al. For outpatient rotator cuff surgery, nerve block anesthesia provides superior same-day recovery over general anesthesia. *Anesthesiology.* 2005;102:1001-1007.
8. Lapner PL, Sabri E, Rakhra K, et al. A multicenter randomized controlled trial comparing single-row with double-row fixation in arthroscopic rotator cuff repair. *J Bone Joint Surg Am.* 2012;94:1249-1257.
9. MacDonald P, McRae S, Leiter J, Mascarenhas R, Lapner P. Arthroscopic rotator cuff repair with and without acromioplasty in the treatment of full-thickness rotator cuff tears: a multicenter, randomized controlled trial. *J Bone Joint Surg Am.* 2011;93:1953-1960.
10. van der Zwaal P, Thomassen BJ, Nieuwenhuijse MJ, Lindenburg R, Swen JW, van Arkel ER. Clinical outcome in all-arthroscopic versus mini-open rotator cuff repair in small to medium-sized tears: a randomized controlled trial in 100 patients with 1-year follow-up. *Arthroscopy.* 2013;29:266-273.

HIP ARTHROSCOPY

Marc J. Philippon | Justin T. Newman

CASE MINIMUM REQUIREMENTS

- Persistent pain after a course of nonoperative treatment
- Intraarticular or extraarticular pathology sources of pain based on examination findings and confirmed with magnetic resonance imaging
- Adequate joint space
- Pathology amenable to arthroscopy treatment

COMMONLY USED CPT CODES

- CPT Code: 29916—Labral repair
- CPT Code: 29915—Acetabuloplasty (i.e., treatment of pincer lesion)
- CPT Code: 29914—Femoroplasty (i.e., treatment of cam lesion)
- CPT Code: 29863—Synovectomy/lysis of adhesions; or 29862—Débridement/ having of articular cartilage (chondroplasty), abrasion arthoplasty, or resection labrum

COMMONLY USED ICD9 CODES

- 719.45—Pain in joint
- 843.8—Labral tear
- 726.91—Osteophyte/spur

Arthroscopic surgery of the hip was first described in the 1930s. However, it was not until 1977, when descriptions of the arthroscopic treatment of pediatric congenital hip dislocations appeared, that the technique began to gain popularity. The slow development of hip arthroscopy has been attributed to both difficulties navigating the anatomic constraints surrounding the hip and the delayed recognition of anatomic abnormalities of the hip by surgeons. Refinements in the understanding of hip pathology, diagnostic imaging, and arthroscopic instrumentation have facilitated the rapid expansion of hip arthroscopy to diagnosis and treat disorders of the hip. With the advancements seen in the past decade, there has been a surge in the use of arthroscopy in the treatment of hip disorders.

The differential diagnosis of pain about the hip is extensive and historically has presented a diagnostic dilemma. Consideration must be given to direct, indirect, and sports hernias; retroperitoneal or intraabdominal pathology; gynecologic pain; central or peripheral nervous system contributions; and lumbar, sacral, and pelvic pathology. When the symptoms localize to the hip, it becomes imperative to delineate between intraarticular and extraarticular hip etiology. The patient history is paramount to diagnosis and prognosis. Chronology, inciting event, and exacerbating activities are important.

Physical examination begins with gait and posture. An antalgic or Trendelenburg gait can localize pathology. Postural abnormalities include pelvic obliquity and tilt, leg length discrepancy, scoliosis, and lordosis. Examination of the hip joint includes careful palpation of all associated structures. Tenderness in the adductor or psoas tendons, hip flexor or rectus abdominus musculature, greater trochanteric bursa, or hamstring origin may be an indicator of primary pathology or secondary symptoms from an intraarticular abnormality. Active and passive range of motion in both hips should be evaluated for any asymmetry. Provocative tests can assist with the identification of specific hip abnormalities. An anterior impingement test elicits pain with passive hip flexion, adduction, and internal rotation. This may be indicative of intraarticular pathology that involves the acetabular rim, labrum, or femoral head-neck junction. A posterior impingement test is performed with the hip in a position of extension and external rotation. Pain is caused when the femoral head-neck junction impinges on the posterior acetabulum and labrum. The FABER (Flexion ABduction External Rotation) distance test involves passive flexion, abduction, and external rotation of the hip. This test can help diagnose impingement when compared with the nonsymptomatic hip. A dial test may reveal increased motion in the hip in the presence of hip instability.

Quality radiographs are the first imaging requirement. The presence of either coxa profunda or protrusio acetabuli is an indication of acetabular overcoverage. The presence of acetabular retroversion is determined by identifying a crossover sign or prominent extension of the ischial spine into the pelvis. A posterior wall sign, present when the posterior acetabular wall lies medial to the center of the femoral head, may also be indicative of acetabular retroversion. The presence of dysplasia and risk of instability can be better understood by determining acetabular inclination. This is done with measurement of the Tonnis, the sharp, and the lateral center edge angles. Finally, the anteroposterior (AP) radiograph image also is used to measure joint space narrowing, which has been shown to be a predictor of patient outcome after hip arthroscopy. The cross-table lateral view is assessed for the presence of cam-type impingement, femoral head sphericity, and femoral head neck offset. The alpha angle is typically considered positive for cam impingement with values over 50 degrees. This angle also has been shown to give predictive information for the likelihood of concomitant chondrolabral injury and identification of those with a hip at risk for future symptoms. Magnetic resonance imaging (MRI) has become the modality of choice to supplement the radiographic evaluation and appraise the soft tissue structures around the hip.

SURGICAL TECHNIQUE

Room Set-Up

- The tray should be at the patient's shoulder level (Fig. 31-1).
- The monitor is placed in the direct visual field with the assessory screens positioned for the assistant.
- Pay attention to the location of fluroscopy from the contralateral side, surgical lights, and multiple tables, if required.
- The table is set to a level conducive to surgeon comfort (Fig. 31-2).

Patient Positioning

- The modified supine approach is used.
- The hip is in 15 degrees of flexion to relax the capsule.
- Internal rotation of foot brings the femoral neck parallel to the floor (Fig. 31-3).
- Lateral tilt should be at 15 degrees.
- Abduction of the nonoperative hip is used.
- The operative hip is positioned to neutral, creating a lateralizing force to the femur over the post.
- A large peroneal post is used to avoid excessive peroneal pressure (Fig. 31-4).
- The feet are secured in well-padded traction boots; care is taken to avoid traction neuropraxia (Fig. 31-5).

Prepping and Draping

- Prep is performed consistent with standard of care.
- The skin is prepped, and then four drape towels are used.

COMMONLY USED ICD10 CODES

- M24.151-M24.159—Other articular cartilage disorders, hip [hip impingement syndrome]
- M24.451-M24.459—Recurrent dislocation, hip [hip impingement syndrome]
- M24.551-M24.559—Contracture, hip [hip impingement syndrome]
- M24.851-M24.859—Other specific joint derangements of hip, not elsewhere classified [hip impingement syndrome]
- M25.151-M25.159—Fistula, hip [hip impingement syndrome]
- M25.551-M25.559—Pain in hip [hip impingement syndrome]
- M25.651-M25.659—Stiffness of hip, not elsewhere classified [hip impingement syndrome]
- M25.9—Joint disorder [hip impingement syndrome]
- M25.5—Pain in unspecified joint
- S73.19—Other sprain of hip
- M25.70—Osteophyte, unspecified joint
- M76.20—Iliac crest spur, unspecified hip

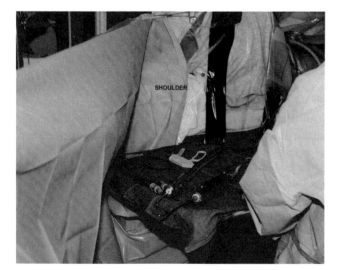

Figure 31-1 The tray for equipment is placed at the patient's shoulder level for easy access.

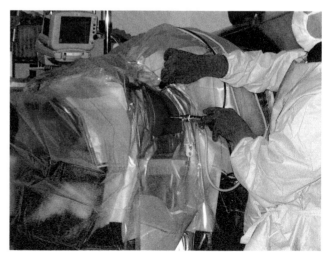

Figure 31-2 The level or height of the table depends on the surgeon. The level should be conducive to the surgeon's comfort.

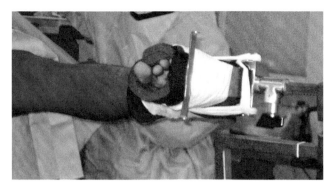

Figure 31-3 The operative leg is placed in internal rotation to bring the femoral neck parallel to the floor.

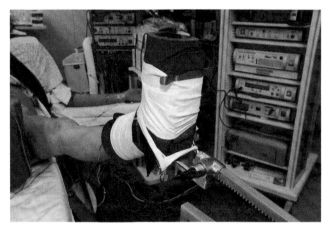

Figure 31-5 The feet are placed in well-padded traction boots. Care should be taken to avoid traction neuropraxia.

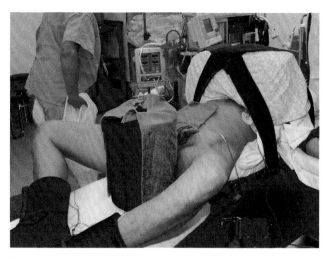

Figure 31-4 A large peroneal post is used to avoid excessive peroneal pressure.

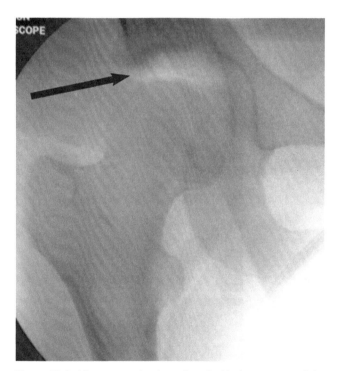

Figure 31-6 Adequate traction is confirmed with the presence of the vacuum sign *(large arrow)* on fluoroscopy.

- Access to the operative site is covered with occlusive dressing to prevent fluid egress and ingress about the surgical field.
- The nonsterile assistant should have access to the lower extremity to manipulate the extremity while allowing the surgeon to assess the location of the extremity.
- A shower curtain or similar draping technique facilitates needs well.

Traction

- Complete muscular paralysis is mandatory, with provider choice of systemic or spinal/epidural combination.
- Meticulous padding of upper extremity pressure points is needed.
- Fluoroscopy can be used to ensure adequate joint distraction as noted by the vacuum sign (Fig. 31-6).

- Both traction time and the amount of traction are critical. The surgeon can alternate between traction for intraarticular work and off of traction with positioning of the leg in space as required for extraarticular work.

Portal Placement

- Accurate portal placement is essential (Figs. 31-7 and 31-8).
- The portal placement provides optimal visualization.
- Anchor placement must be facilitated.
- Avoid neurovascular structures and ligaments.
- Define anatomic landmarks.
- Palpate the tip of the greater trochanter.
- Use fluoroscopic guidance as required.
- The anterolateral portal is placed first and is 1 cm superior and 1 cm anterior to the tip of the greater trochanter (Fig. 31-9).
- The spinal needle is placed first.
- When the intraarticular location of the first wire is confirmed, the stylus is removed and the joint is distended with saline solution to maximal distention (20 to 40 mL

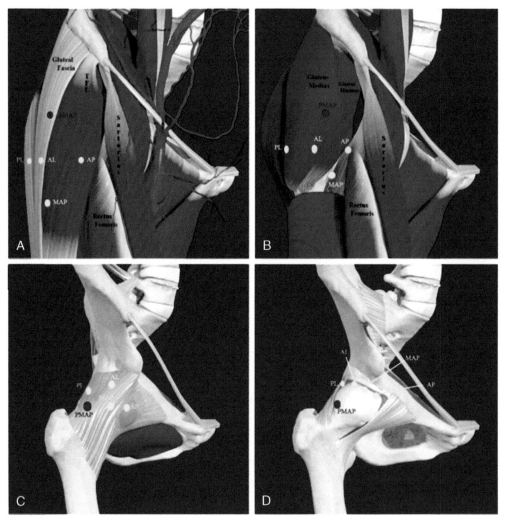

Figure 31-7 Central and peripheral compartment portal locations as they traverse soft tissues surrounding hip from superficial to deep. **A,** The AL portal enters at the junction of the posterior TFL fibers and the anterior gluteal fascial fibers. The AP portal and MAP pierce the TFL. **B,** The AP portal and MAP pass between the gluteus minimus and the rectus femoris via a deep intermuscular plane. The AL portal passes anterior to the hip abductors and should meet little resistance before reaching the hip capsule. **C** and **D,** Portal entry through the capsule to access hip joint and head-neck junction. *AL,* Anterolateral portal; *AP,* anterior portal; *MAP,* mid-anterior portal; *TFL,* tensor fascia lata. (Reprinted with permission. © Primal Pictures Ltd, London.)

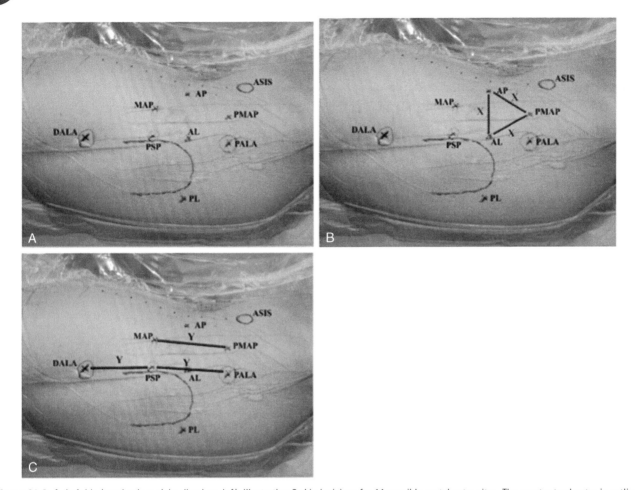

Figure 31-8 **A,** Left hip (proximal on *right,* distal on *left*), illustrating 8 skin incisions for 11 possible portal entry sites. The greater trochanter is outlined. **B,** The AL portal, AP portal, and PMAP form an equilateral triangle with each side equaling X. Likewise, the AL portal, AP portal, and MAP form a second equilateral triangle with all sides equaling X. **C,** The three peritrochanteric portals (DALA, PSP, and PALA) lie in line with the AL portal. The PSP and PALA portals lie posterior to the MAP and PMAP, respectively. The distance between these portals equals Y. The DALA portal lies distal to the PSP at a distance Y. *AL,* Anterolateral portal; *AP,* anterior portal; *DALA,* distal anterolateral accessory portal; *MAP,* mid-anterior portal; *PALA,* proximal anterolateral accessory portal; *PMAP,* proximal mid-anterior portal; *PSP,* peritrochanteric space portal. (With permission from Robertson WJ, Kelly BT. The safe zone for hip arthroscopy: a cadaveric assessment of central, peripheral, and lateral compartment portal placement. *Arthroscopy.* 2008;24(9):1019-1026.)

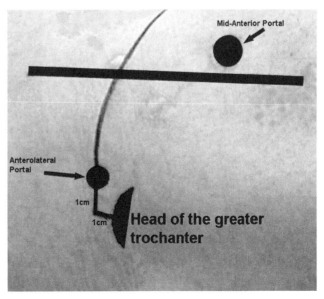

Figure 31-9 The head of the greater trochanter is an anatomic landmark. Anterolateral portal is placed first and is 1 cm superior and 1 cm anterior to the tip of the greater trochanter.

in general). Removal of the syringe with the return of the pressurized saline solution from the needle confirms intraarticular location.

- A flexible guidewire (nitinol) is inserted through the needle, which then is removed over the wire.
- A cannulated system subsequently is introduced through a small skin incision over the guidewire; attention to the cartilage is important, with bevels away from femoral head.
- The cannulated system encounters resistance at the capsule, with controlled entrance to ensure cartilage protection.
- Subsequent portals are established in a similar fashion.
- Additional portals can be added if necessary.
- The midanterior portal is second and localized superficially in the interval between the sartorius and tensor fasciae latae musculature, with direct visualization from the prior portal (Fig. 31-10).
- The transition between portals and for instrument exchange is facilitated by switching sticks and slotted cannulas.
- Intraarticular work is facilitated with capsulotomy.
- After the portals have been established, a beaver blade is introduced and a capsule cut to connect portals, maintaining a minimum of 1 cm of capsule lateral to labrum to facilitate closure at the end of the case (Fig. 31-11).

Labral Repair

- Labral repair is assessed with traction.
- Note presence of an injected, bruised, or torn labrum.
- Measure the width of the labrum to assist with treatment decisions (Fig. 31-12).
- Evaluate for deformities at the chondrolabral junction or a wave sign.
- Detach the labrum if required (Fig. 31-13).
- Prepare the base for repair, and perform pincer resection.
- A motorized angled shaver is used to débride any unstable tissue for the labrum. An arthroscopic osteotome many be used to begin the rim trimming.
- A 5.5-mm round burr is used to completely remove the excess bony overhang (Fig. 31-14).
- During this step, note the preoperative center-edge angle and the measurement of the acetabular surface to avoid resecting too much of the rim, effectively creating a dysplastic acetabulum.

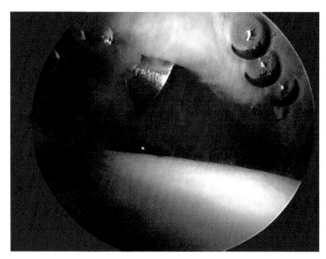

Figure 31-10 The midanterior portal is second and localized superficially in the interval between the sartorius and tensor fasciae latae musculature, with direct visualization from the prior portal.

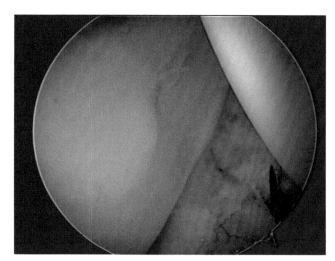

Figure 31-11 After the portals have been established, a beaver blade is introduced and a capsule cut to connect the portals, maintaining a minimum of 1 cm of capsule lateral to labrum to facilitate closure at the end of the case.

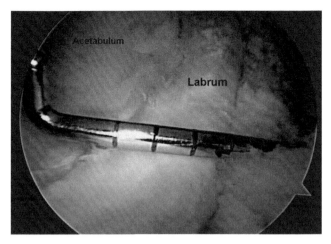

Figure 31-12 The labrum is measured to determine whether adequate tissue is available. The width of the labrum can determine whether a labral repair or labral reconstruction is performed.

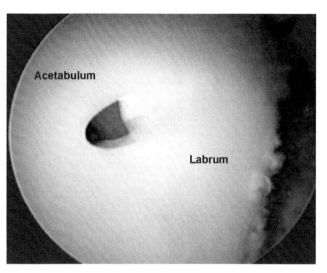

Figure 31-13 The labrum is detached near the tear to prepare the area for repair.

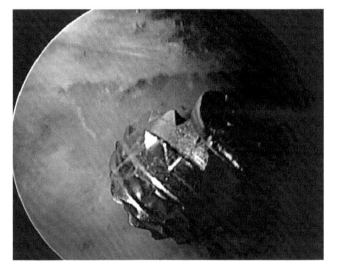

Figure 31-14 A 5.5-mm round burr is used to completely remove the excess bony overhang as a result of pincer impingement.

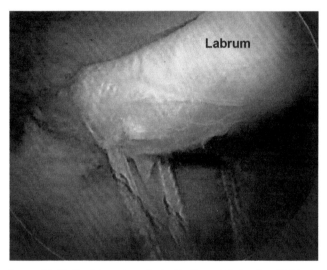

Figure 31-15 The labrum is reattached to the acetabular rim with bioabsorbable suture anchors. The size of anchors and type of suture should be based on anatomic location.

- Create a bleeding bone bed for anchor placement to improve healing.
- The labrum is reattached to the acetabular rim with bioabsorbable suture anchors (Fig. 31-15). While placing the anchor, it is essential to visualize the adjacent articular cartilage to ensure that it is left intact. The location and acetabular rim angle should be considered when placing the anchor (Fig. 31-16).
- Sutures can be looped around the labrum or passed through the labrum. The type of suture is based on the location and amount of labral tissue.
- The knot is recessed and placed towards the capsular side (Fig. 31-17).
- The number of suture anchors is based on the size of the labral tear.

Femoroacetabular Impingement

- The area of resection of a cam lesion is based on the impingement seen on dynamic examination and the associated damage to other tissue (Fig. 31-18).
- Resection is limited by the location of the lateral epiphyseal vessels.

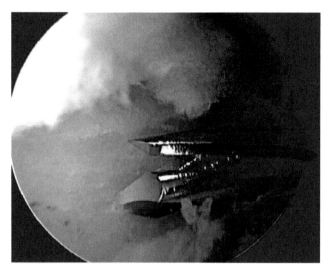

Figure 31-16 The anatomic location should be considered when placing the anchor. The anchor should be close to the cartilage surface and at the appropriate acetabular rim angle.

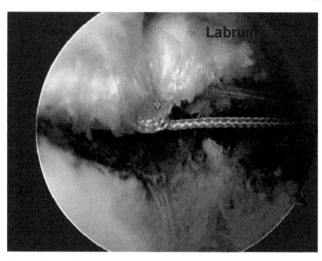

Figure 31-17 After the knot is tied, it is recessed in the hole from the anchor. Always place the suture toward the capsule and away from the cartilage surface.

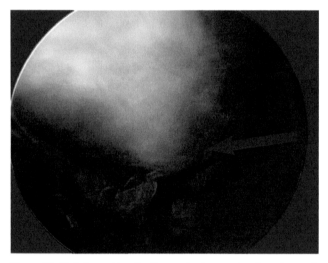

Figure 31-18 Before addressing the cam impingement, a dynamic examination is performed to determine where the abnormal bone on the femoral neck conflicts with other areas.

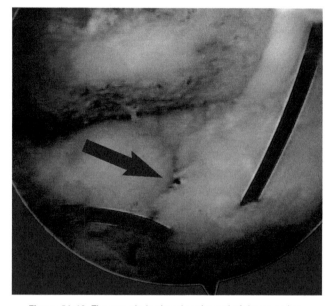

Figure 31-19 The capsule is closed at the end of the procedure.

- The amount of resection should be based on dynamic examination results and decompression of the impingement.
- Overresection should be avoided.
- Pincer impingement is resected at the time of labral repair (see previous).
- Perform dynamic examination to evaluate sufficiency of resection.
- Close the capsule (Fig. 31-19).

BRIEF SUMMARY OF SURGICAL STEPS

- Place feet in boots and provide proper protection
- Apply traction
- When vaccum sign is seen, traction is adequate
- Fluoroscopy should be used if needed for verification of joint space and portal placement
- Accurate portal placement is essential for optimal visualization and anchor placement
- Correct cam and pincer impingement
- Identify labral pathology and treat
- Treat chondral pathology
- Release traction and perform dynamic examination; treat any areas of persistent impingement
- Close capsule

TECHNICAL PEARLS

- Mixed impingement is most common; evaluate the femoral neck and acetabulum for signs of impingement
- Evaluate joint space before arthroscopy
- When damaged labrum is observed, evaluate for etiology
- Measurement of labral width can help with treatment decisions based on algorithm
- Rim trimming can reduce the size of cartilage lesions on the acetabulum
- At the end of the labral treatment, traction should be released and the repaired labrum should be visualized from the peripheral compartment; a dynamic examination of the hip joint should be performed to evaluate the stability of the repair, ensure adequate seal of the labrum around the femoral head, and assess for additional impingement
- Rehabilitation is critical to successful outcomes

REQUIRED EQUIPMENT

Fracture table with adequate adaptations to allow for a controlled and sustained appropriate amount of traction, rotation, and manipulation of the extremity
Well-padded peroneal post
Standard arthroscopy equipment with 70-degree scope
Fluoroscopy
Appropriate patient positioning equipment to allow for stable padding and placement both with and without traction
Long arthroscopic instruments designed for hip arthroscopy
Long cannulae

COMMON PITFALLS

(When to call for the attending physician)

- Unable to create vacuum sign
- Unable to enter joint with first portal
- Visualization of the labrum and articular surfaces is limited
- Increased fluid requirements, pump disturbances, inability to distend the joint, and abdominal swelling are signs of fluid extravasation
- Anchor perforates acetabular surface when placing in acetabular rim during labral repair
- Care must be taken when detaching the labrum to avoid cutting or attenuating the diseased tissue
- Damage to the vessels on the femoral neck

POSTOPERATIVE PROTOCOL

Rehabilitation is initiated immediately. The first stage goals include protecting repairs and soft tissues, diminishing pain and inflammation, maintaining motion within prescribed parameters, and obtaining muscle recruitment. A brace is used for 10 days for protection, to provide proprioceptive feedback, and for motion restriction. Cryotherapy and nonsteroidal antiinflammatory drugs are vital for control of inflammation and pain. The prevention of muscular inhibition is achieved through early strength exercises that limit joint stress while providing the appropriate load through the hip and lower extremity muscles. Aquatic walking with the use of a waterproof dressing in chest-deep water can be initiated on postoperative day 1. Patients progress to the second stage when they have minimal pain, range of motion greater than 75% of the opposite hip, and proper muscle firing patterns. Before beginning the next phase, patients should have progressed to full weight-bearing.

The second phase of rehabilitation includes a progression of range of motion (ROM)/stretching, gait training, and strengthening. Passive range of motion (PROM) and stretching exercises should be continued as needed to achieve full ROM. Gait training should take place both in the pool and on land as the patient is progressed off of crutches. Cardiovascular training is achieved with the use of an elliptical machine or stairclimber during this phase. Impact activities, including treadmills, should be avoided. Advancement to the third phase occurs when the patient has achieved full range of motion, nonantalgic gait, and adequate hip strength.

The third stage of rehabiliation focuses on restoration of muscular strength and endurance, cardiovascular endurance, and neuromuscular control. Advanced strength and neuromuscular control exercises include lunges, water bounding and plyometrics, side-to-side lateral agilities, forward and backward running with a cord, initiation of a running progression, and initial agility drills. Cardiovascular training should continue with progressive biking, elliptic trainer, stairclimber, and swimming. This is followed by sport-specific training. Patients are cleared for return to sports when they have passed the hip sports test.

POSTOPERATIVE CLINIC VISIT PROTOCOL

At postoperative day 1, patients are seen in physical therapy. The surgical dressings are changed and replaced with waterproof dressings. Medications, physical therapy protocol, and operative images are reviewed. Patients are assessed for any focal areas of sensory deficit on the operated lower extremity, including the perineum. Radiographs to assess the cam and pincer resection are obtained in clinic on postoperative day 2 or 3 and include low AP pelvis, frog leg lateral, and cross-table lateral views. The motion is assessed, and the incision sites are evaluated.

At 3 weeks after surgery, patients are followed up via phone or in the office to ensure they are following the physical therapy protocol and continuing to take prescribed medication; they then are instructed on progression off of crutches. Sutures are removed at this time point.

At 6 to 10 weeks after surgery, patients are evaluated in the office. Range of motion, muscle activation, gait, and strength are assessed. Thorough assessment of possible adhesions or scar tissue formation is done with physical examination. Incisions should be well healed. Based on progress, the patient's rehabilitation is updated. Focus is on posterior kinetic chain, core-strengthening program, and gradual progression between the described stages continues.

SUGGESTED READINGS

1. Ayeni OR, Adamich J, Farrokhyar F, et al. Surgical management of labral tears during femoroacetabular impingement surgery: a systematic review. *Knee Surg Sports Traumatol Arthrosc.* 2014;22:756-762.
2. Alradwan H, Philippon MJ, Farrokhyar F, et al. Return to preinjury activity levels after surgical management of femoroacetabular impingement in athletes. *Arthroscopy.* 2012;28:1567-1576.
3. Clohisy JC, Carlisle JC, Beaulé PE, et al. A systematic approach to the plain radiographic evaluation of the young adult hip. *J Bone Joint Surg Am.* 2008;90(suppl 4):47-66.
4. Ganz R, Parvizi J, Beck M, et al. Femoroacetabular impingement: a cause for osteoarthritis of the hip. *Clin Orthop Relat Res.* 2003;417:112-120.
5. Johnston TL, Schenker ML, Briggs KK, Philippon MJ. Relationship between offset angle alpha and hip chondral injury in femoroacetabular impingement. *Arthroscopy.* 2008;24:669-675.
6. McCarthy JC, Noble PC, Schuck MR, et al. The Otto E. Aufranc Award: the role of labral lesions to development of early degenerative hip disease. *Clin Orthop Relat Res.* 2001;393:25-37.
7. Philippon MJ, Maxwell RB, Johnston TL, Schenker M, Briggs KK. Clinical presentation of femoroacetabular impingement. *Knee Surg Sports Traumatol Arthrosc.* 2007;15:1041-1047.
8. Ross JR, Nepple JJ, Philippon MJ, Kelly BT, Larson CM, Bedi A. Effect of changes in pelvic tilt on range of motion to impingement and radiographic parameters of acetabular morphologic characteristics. *Am J Sports Med.* 2014;42:2402-2409.
9. Shearer DW, Kramer J, Bozic KJ, Feeley BT. Is hip arthroscopy cost-effective for femoroacetabular impingement? *Clin Orthop Relat Res.* 2012;470:1079-1089.
10. Skendzel JG, Philippon MJ, Briggs KK, Goljan P. The effect of joint space on midterm outcomes after arthroscopic hip surgery for femoroacetabular impingement. *Am J Sports Med.* 2014;42:1127-1133.
11. Wahoff M, Ryan M. Rehabilitation after hip femoroacetabular impingement arthroscopy. *Clin Sports Med.* 2011;30:463-482.

ELBOW ARTHROSCOPY

Robert Nelson Mead | Felix H. Savoie, III | Michael J. O'Brien

CASE MINIMUM REQUIREMENTS

- Experience with arthoscopy
- 30-Degree arthoscope with interchangeable cannula system
- Arthroscopic equipment including grabbers, punches, and cautery
- Arm holder for lateral position

COMMONLY USED CPT CODES

- CPT Code: 29830—Diagnostic elbow arthroscopy
- CPT Code: 29834—Elbow arthroscopy with removal of loose body
- CPT Code: 29839—Arthroscopy elbow with extensive débridement
- CPT Code: 24343—Repair collateral ligament (lateral) or: 24345 (medial)

COMMONLY USED ICD9 CODES

- 718.12—Loose body in joint, upper arm
- 727.09—Elbow synovitis
- 726.32—Elbow lateral epicondylitis
- 726.31—Elbow medial epicondylitis
- 715.12—Posteromedial elbow impingment (osteoarthritis, localized primary, forearm)
- 732.2—Juvenile osteochondritis dissecans upper extremity, capitellum, humerus
- 841.0—Radial collateral ligament sprain or rupture
- 841.1—Ulnar collateral ligament sprain or rupture

Elbow arthroscopy is one of the most technically demanding arthroscopic procedures. The complexity of the surrounding neurovascular structures and the confined space require a thorough knowledge of the anatomy. In his original study in 1937, Berman actually thought the elbow was not amenable to arthroscopic repair, although he later changed his opinion. With that said, the indications for elbow arthroscopy have expanded significantly since the procedure was first introduced.

Originally, elbow arthroscopy was only indicated for diagnostic purposes and the removal of loose bodies (Video 32-1). Over time, however, the indications have grown to include treatment of pathologies such as synovitis, acute fractures, osteochondral dissecans lesions, instability, lateral epicondylitis, and many others. These indications have expanded in part because more portal sites have been developed to view and work in the entire joint arthroscopically. Although indications have increased, orthopaedic surgeons have to match their skill level with the indicated procedure.

SURGICAL TECHNIQUE

Room Set-Up

- The surgeon is set up on the operative side of the patient with the scrub technician and mayo stand adjacent to the surgeon.
- Place the video monitor and equipment on the opposite side of the operating room table.

Patient Positioning

- Supine:
  - The patient is positioned supine on the operating table with the shoulder abducted to 90 degrees. The hand or forearm is held in traction so that the arm is held in neutral rotation.
- Prone (authors' preferred position):
  - The patient is rolled into the prone position with chest rolls placed to aid in ventilation. Padding is inserted to support the head and face. An armboard or arm positioner is attached and placed parallel to the operating table. The patient's shoulder is abducted to 90 degrees and allowed to hang over the armboard. A rolled blanket is inserted under the upper arm so that the elbow rests at 90 degrees (Fig. 32-1).
- Lateral decubitus:
  - The patient is secured in the lateral decubitus position with a beanbag, and an axillary roll is inserted. The shoulder is flexed to 90 degrees and internally rotated so that the elbow can be flexed over a padded bolster.

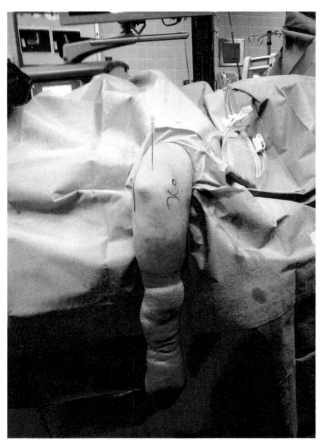

Figure 32-1 The patient is in the prone position. The operative arm is draped over an armboard. This position enables the surgeon to freely move the distal part of the extremity.

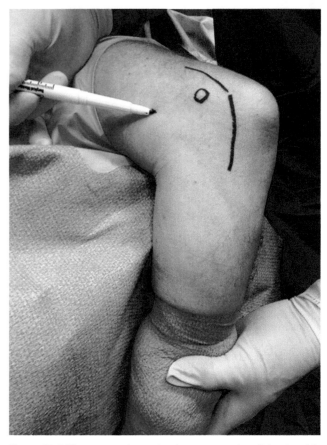

Figure 32-2 The surgeon draws the ulnar nerve and medial epicondyle on the operative arm. The patient is in the prone position with the hand toward the floor.

Prepping and Draping

- Place a nonsterile tourniquet high up on the arm.
- Apply sterile prep to the extremity.
- Drape the patient.
  - Place a sterile down sheet underneath the arm.
  - The hand and distal forearm are inserted into a sterile impervious stockinette.
  - The arm is squared off with sterile blue towels just distal to the tourniquet.
  - A sterile U-drape then is placed around the extremity just distal to the blue towels.
  - Coban wrapping (3M, Minneapolis) is wrapped around the sterile stockinette in a manner that is tight on the forearm to prevent fluid extravasation into the forearm during the surgery.
- Mark anatomic landmarks and anticipated portal sites.
  - Palpate and draw in the course of the ulnar nerve (Fig. 32-2).
  - Include the tip of the olecranon, medial epicondyle, and lateral epicondyle (Fig. 32-3).
- Apply esmarch wrap and inflate the tourniquet to 250 mm Hg.
- Insufflate the joint.
  - Inject 20 to 30 mL of normal saline solution with an 18-gauge needle into the center of the olecranon fossa or into the triad formed by the radial head, capitellum, and ulna, near the location of the soft spot portal, the area formed by the lateral epicondyle, the olecranon, and the radial head.
  - Look for swelling of the joint capsule and slight extension of the elbow joint.

COMMONLY USED ICD10 CODES

- M24.0—Loose body, other site
- M65.80—Other synovitis and tenosynovitis, unspecified site
- M77.10—Lateral epicondylitis, unspecified elbow
- M77.00—Medial epicondylitis, unspecified elbow
- M19.029—Primary osteoarthritis, unspecified elbow
- M93.003—Unspecified slipped upper femoral epiphysis (nontraumatic), unspecified hip
- S53.439—Radial collateral ligament sprain of unspecified elbow
- S53.449—Ulnar collateral ligament sprain of unspecified elbow

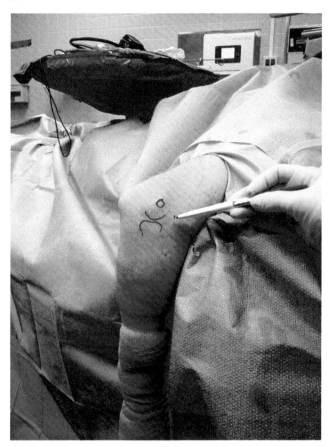

Figure 32-3 The radial head and lateral epicondyle are marked out on the operative arm. Again, the patient is in the prone position with the hand directed toward the floor at the bottom of the image.

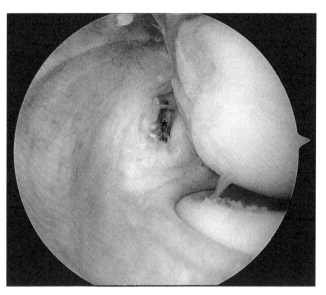

Figure 32-4 The image depicts the initial view from the proximal antero-medial portal. The radiocapitellar joint is on the right of the screen. A tear in the lateral capsule (*) over the extensor carpi radialis brevis origin as seen in lateral epicondylitis is consistent with a Baker grade 3 lesion.

Arthroscopic Surgery Steps

- Arthroscopic surgery begins with entering the joint. The proximal anterior medial portal is established by angling back toward the joint to enter via a soft spot commonly located adjacent to the trochlea (Fig. 32-4). A pop should be felt as the blunt cannula enters the joint. The most common mistakes are traversing anterior to the capsule and missing the joint or entering the joint too far lateral.
- The initial view from the proximal anterior medial portal reveals the radiocapitellar joint, annular ligament, and anterior capsule (Fig. 32-5). Careful retraction of the arthroscope reveals the coronoid process (Fig. 32-6), coronoid fossa (Fig. 32-7), and medial gutter (Fig. 32-8). The lateral portal can be established outside-in with a spinal needle (Fig. 32-9) or by passing a switching stick from medial to lateral (Fig. 32-10).
- The arthroscope then is transferred to the lateral portal, and the medial side of the joint is visualized (Fig. 32-11). This also provides the opportunity to "fix" the medial portal if it entered the joint too far laterally.
- Once the anterior compartment has been evaluated thoroughly, any anterior procedures (e.g., loose body removal [see Fig. 32-11] or extensor carpi radialis brevis débridement [Fig. 32-12]) may be accomplished.
- The inflow then is left anteriorly to flow across the radiocapitellar joint, and a posterior central portal is established (Fig. 32-13). In establishing this portal, one should place the cannula and trocar against the bone in the center of the fossa and then push the cannula down to the bone without withdrawing the trocar to avoid

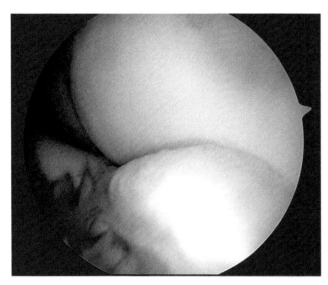

Figure 32-5 The coronoid process viewed from the proximal anterome-dial portal. The radial head and the capitellum are to the far left of the screen and represent the lateral portion of the joint.

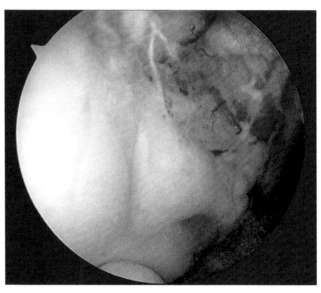

Figure 32-6 The coronoid fossa is visualized in the center of the screen. One can see the tip of the coronoid process in the most inferior part of the screen.

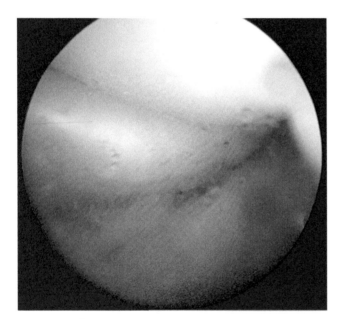

Figure 32-7 The medial gutter is visualized on the inferior and right portion of the screen as viewed from the proximal anteromedial portal.

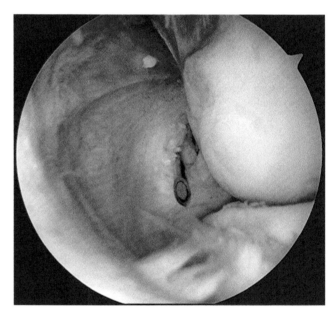

Figure 32-8 A spinal needle represents the starting point of the lateral portal with an outside-in technique. The view is from the proximal antero-medial portal with radiocapitellar joint on the right.

bringing soft tissue into the fossa. Fluid outflow from the cannula should be seen as the trocar is removed.

■ The initial view from the posterior central portal is that of the fossa (Fig. 32-14); one can look superiorly to see the triceps muscle (Fig. 32-15) and then follow the contour of the olecranon tip (Fig. 32-16) toward the lateral gutter. As the arthro-scope progresses toward the lateral gutter, the field of view is rotated until looking medially; and then as the arthroscope progresses down the gutter, the view rotates anteriorly to see the posterior radiocapitellar joint (Fig. 32-17). The arthroscope

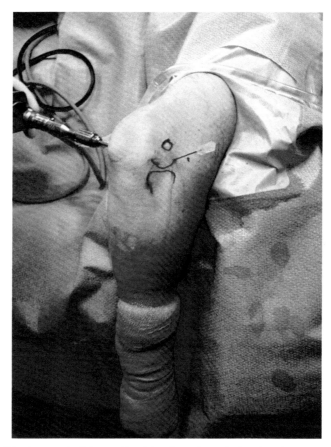

Figure 32-9 This photograph of the outside of the elbow shows the location of the anterolateral portal, located 2 cm proximal and 1 to 2 cm anterior to the lateral epicondyle. The patient is in the prone position with the hand pointed towards the floor.

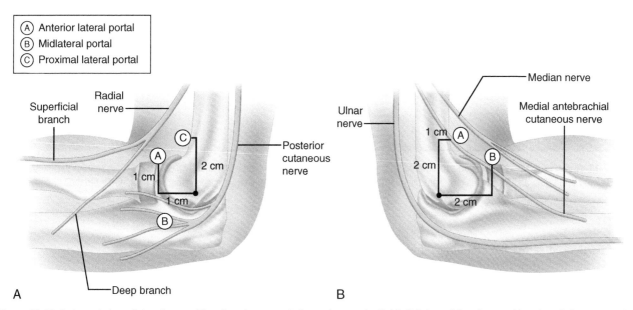

Ⓐ Anterior lateral portal
Ⓑ Midlateral portal
Ⓒ Proximal lateral portal

Superficial branch

Radial nerve

Posterior cutaneous nerve

Deep branch

Ⓒ
Ⓐ
Ⓑ
1 cm
2 cm
1 cm

A

Ulnar nerve

Median nerve

Medial antebrachial cutaneous nerve

Ⓐ
Ⓑ
1 cm
2 cm
2 cm

B

Figure 32-10 **A,** Lateral view of the elbow and location of nerves relative to the portals. **B,** Medial view of the elbow and location of ulnar nerve relative to the portals. Working anterior to the intermuscular septum and proximal to the medial epicondyle, the ulnar nerve stays posterior to the portals. (Redrawn from Raphael BS, Weiland AJ, Altchek DW, et al. Revision arthroscopic contracture release in the elbow resulting in an ulnar nerve transection. *J Bone Joint Surg Am.* 2011;93(Supp1):100-110.)

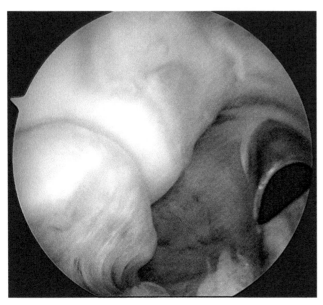

Figure 32-11 The medial side of the joint is on the right side of the image, as viewed from the proximal anterolateral portal. The coronoid process can be seen on the left side of the image.

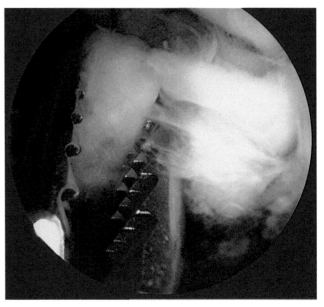

Figure 32-12 Loose bodies are a frequent indication for elbow arthroscopy. This image depicts the removal of a loose body.

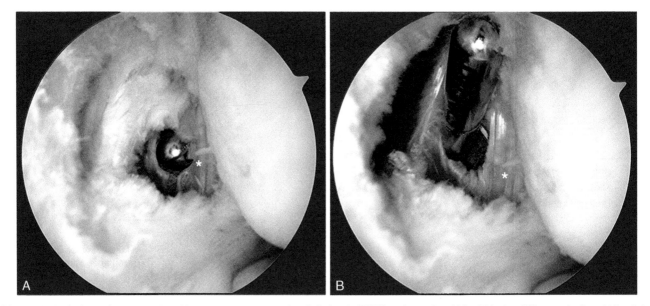

Figure 32-13 A, A tear in the capsule with exposed extensor carpi radialis brevis (ECRB) and associated Nirschl lesion *(*)* is seen in the middle of the screen. **B,** The ECRB origin and Nirschl lesion *(*)* are being arthroscopically débrided in this image, as seen from the proximal anteromedial portal.

may be tracked across the ulnohumeral articulation in the unstable elbow (Fig. 32-18), the drive-thru sign of the elbow.

- The arthroscope is returned to the olecranon fossa and the same steps followed on the medial side to review the medial gutter (Fig. 32-19).
- Procedures are numerous but include loose body removal (Fig. 32-20), débridement, release of the Nirschl lesion in lateral epicondylitis, and microfracture of osteochondritis dissecans (OCD) lesions of the capitellum (Fig. 32-21).

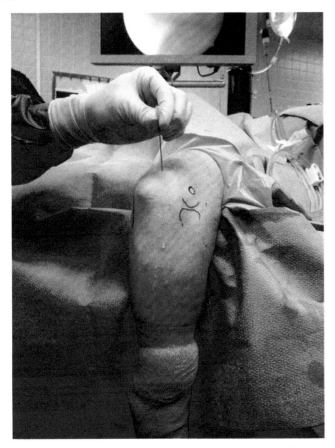

Figure 32-14 The image depicts an outside view of the site of the posterior central portal, located 3 cm proximal to the olecranon process and midline. The patient is in the prone position with the hand directed toward the floor. The surgeon's arm is coming from the patient's feet.

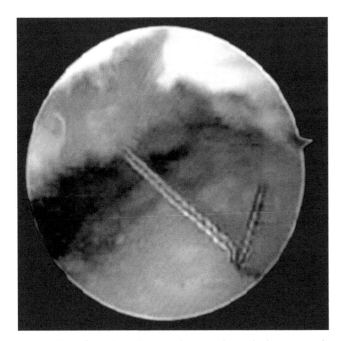

Figure 32-16 Seen from the posterior central portal, the surgeon is viewing a suture anchor in the tip of the olecranon, with a suture passed through a torn triceps tendon and triceps muscle. The tip of the olecranon is located at the bottom right of screen, and the triceps is in the top left of the screen.

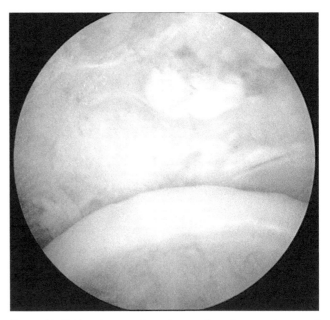

Figure 32-15 The olecranon fossa is seen from the posterior central portal. The olecranon is located in the middle and bottom of the picture.

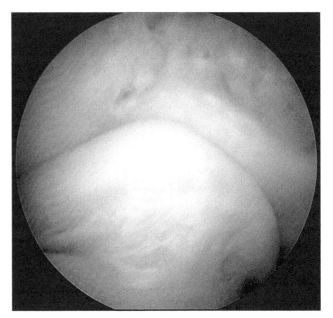

Figure 32-17 The image shows the tip of the olecranon, located in the middle of the screen, as seen from the posterior central portal.

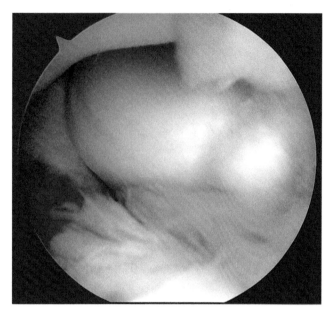

Figure 32-18 The image depicts a view from the posterior central portal of the posterior aspect of the radiocapitellar joint, which is located in the middle and top of the screen. After moving down the lateral gutter, rotate the view anteriorly to see the posterior radiocapitellar joint (plica on the right).

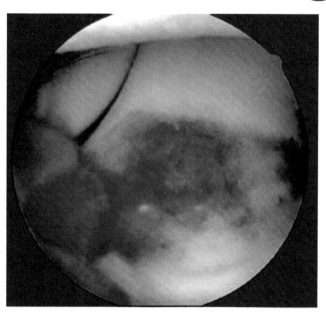

Figure 32-19 The drive-thru sign. If the elbow is unstable, then the arthroscope can be tracked across the ulnohumeral articulation. The arthroscope is in the ulnohumeral articulation, with the humerus at the top of the screen, the ulna on the bottom, and the proximal radioulnar joint in the upper left.

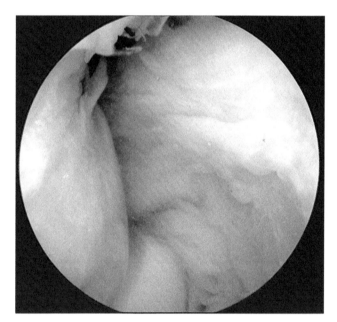

Figure 32-20 The medial gutter, as visualized from the posterior central portal, is seen on the right side of the screen.

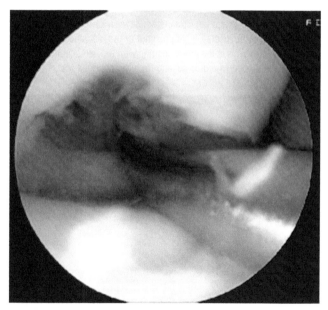

Figure 32-21 The image shows the microfracture of an osteochondritis dissecans lesion in the capitellum. Solid vertical walls have been created around the lesion, and the awl is coming into the middle of the screen to perform the microfracture.

BRIEF SUMMARY OF SURGICAL STEPS

- Begin in the anterior compartment by establishing the proximal anteromedial portal, 2 cm proximal to the medial intermuscular septum and 2 cm proximal to the medial epicondyle
  - Structures to be evaluated: lateral gutter, radial head, coronoid process, trochlea, and the anterior capsule
- Establish the proximal anterolateral portal, 2 cm proximal and 1 to 2 cm anterior to lateral epicondyle; remove loose bodies through this portal
- Evaluate the posterior compartment by starting the posterocentral portal, 3 cm proximal to the olecranon and in the midline posteriorly
- Evaluate the lateral gutter
- Evaluate the medial gutter
- Establish posterolateral portal as the working portal, 3 cm proximal to the olecranon process and lateral to the triceps; remove loose bodies from this portal
- Establish the soft spot portal, located within the space formed by the radial head, lateral epicondyle, and the olecranon; remove loose bodies and evaluate any osteochondral dissecans lesions
- Close the portal sites with Steri-Strips (3M, Minneapolis, MN) or nylon suture
  - Wrap the elbow with a compressive dressing

TECHNICAL PEARLS

- Be sure to draw out anatomic landmarks before establishing portals
  - It helps to orient the surgeon and maintain awareness of key neurovascular structures
- Placing the patient in the prone position causes the neurovascular structures to move away from the joint
- To avoid damage to cutaneous nerves, portals should be made by moving the knife blade across the skin only instead of stabbing the skin
- Retractors may be used to keep important structures out of the way during the procedure

REQUIRED EQUIPMENT

30-Degree arthroscope (with the 70-degree scope available)
3.5-mm and 4.5-mm shavers/burrs
Interchangeable metal cannulas without side ports: large (5.5 mm) and small (4.5 mm)
Switching sticks

COMMON PITFALLS

(When to call for the attending physician)

- Palpate the ulnar nerve as you draw its path instead of where you expect it to be
  - The path of the ulnar nerve may vary in the medial or lateral direction based on the patient; in arthritic or older patients, it tends to "fall" anteriorly in the prone or lateral decubitus position
- Do not use suction on the shaver in the anterior compartment because suction may draw objects into the shaver
- Avoid penetrating the anterolateral inferior capsule to prevent injury to the radial and posterior interosseus nerves when working the anterolateral aspect of the joint
- The ulnar nerve can be damaged during débridement of the medial gutter
  - If you have to work in the medial gutter, it is safer to open explore and retract the ulnar nerve away from the capsule
- Realize that patients with rheumatoid arthritis have attenuated joint capsules and brachialis muscle, so structures like the median and posterior interosseus nerve are at greater risk; never penetrate the brachialis

POSTOPERATIVE PROTOCOL

The postoperative protocol largely depends on the indications for the procedure and the procedure performed. In general, unless a repair or reconstruction was done, the patient is started on range of motion immediately after surgery with a home exercise program consisting of active and active-assisted range of motion. The patients can be given a continuous passive motion device in the recovery room.

Patients who undergo ligamentous repairs often are splinted immediately after surgery in a manner that decreases tension on the repair. The patients are placed in a hinged brace at the first postoperative visit. The patients work on shoulder, periscapular, wrist, and hand exercises. Patients can increase their range of motion as pain and swelling decrease. Physical therapy can become more aggressive once the repair has matured. Once the patient can achieve normal range of motion in the brace, the patient can begin strengthening exercises in the brace. Once the patient can perform strengthening exercises without experiencing pain in the brace, the patient can do the exercises out of the brace.

POSTOPERATIVE CLINIC VISIT PROTOCOL

The patients return to clinic 1 week after the surgery for suture removal. The patients then are brought back to clinic at intervals of 6 weeks, 3 months, and 6 months to monitor their progress. Ajdustments to their occupational therapy or home exercise programs are made accordingly.

SUGGESTED READINGS

1. Abboud JA, Ricchetti ET, Tjoumakaris F, et al. Elbow arthroscopy: basic setup and portal placement. *J Am Acad Orthop Surg.* 2006;14:312-318.
2. Andrews JR, Baumgarten TE. Arthroscopic anatomy of the elbow. *Orthop Clin North Am.* 1995;26: 671-677.
3. Field LD, Altchek DW, Warren RF, et al. Arthroscopic anatomy of the lateral elbow: a comparison of three portals. *Arthroscopy.* 1994;10:602-607.
4. Miller CD, Jobe CM, Wright MH, et al. Neuroanatomy in elbow arthroscopy. *J Shoulder Elbow Surg.* 1995;4:168-174.
5. Kelly EW, Morrey BF, O'Driscoll SW. Complications of elbow arthroscopy. *J Bone Joint Surg Am.* 2001;83-A(1):25-34.
6. Savoie FH. Guidelines to becoming an expert elbow arthroscopist. *Arthroscopy.* 2007;23:1237-1240.
7. Stothers K, Day B, Regan WR, et al. Arthroscopy of the elbow: anatomy, portal sites, and a description of the proximal lateral portal. *Arthroscopy.* 1995;11:449-457.

ANTERIOR CERVICAL DISCECTOMY AND FUSION

Jeffrey A. Rihn

The anterior approach to the cervical spine has been commonly used for more than half a century for treatment of cervical radiculopathy, cervical myelopathy, infection, and traumatic injuries. Anterior cervical discectomy and fusion is the most common surgical treatment performed for cervical disc herniation and spondylosis. Candidates for surgical treatment include those with progressive worsening neurologic deficit, failure of conservative therapy, cervical myelopathy, and intractable pain.

The advantages of the anterior approach include direct access to anteriorly located pathology (i.e., the intervertebral disc) and a minimally invasive approach that does not require much muscle dissection. The approach was first introduced by Smith and Robinson in the mid-1950s, and subsequent modifications have been proposed. The procedure was initially described with use of iliac crest autogenous bone as an interbody graft. Subsequently, however, allograft bone and other bone graft substitutes have been used with great success. Early procedures did not use instrumentation, but over time, screw and plate fixation was reported to increase fusion rate in single-level and multilevel anterior cervical discectomy and fusion (ACDF). Although the use of instrumentation increased fusion rates, it also added the risk of implant-related complications, such as screw and plate breakage and pullout. This procedure has been shown to be effective in treatment of radiculopathy and myelopathy caused by disc herniation and spondylosis (Fig. 33-1, *A* and *B*).

SURGICAL TECHNIQUE

Room Set-Up

- A flat Jackson table or standard operating room table is used (Fig. 33-2).
- The room should have C-arm or intraoperative radiograph capability.
- The instrumentation system depends on surgeon preference.
- Allografts of possible sizes need to be available (if using allograft).
- A high-speed burr, an anterior cervical retraction system, and loupe magnification (preferred) or microscope should be available.

Patient Positioning

- The patient should be positioned supine.
- A small rolled towel or inflatable intravenous bag is positioned behind the scapula.
- The head is in neutral position with no rotation.
- Prep and drape the skin from the neck to the sternum.
- Extend the neck to a desired position to allow access to the anterior neck.
- The arms should be well-padded (Fig. 33-3).
- Gently tape the shoulders and arms at the side, pulling the shoulders down to allow for radiographic visualization (Fig. 33-4).
- Neurophysiologic monitoring leads (if used) are applied.

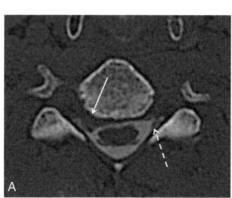
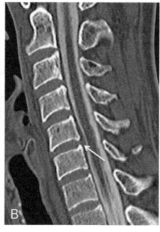

Figure 33-1 **A,** Axial image of a computed tomographic myelogram at the C5-C6 level shows a right-sided disc herniation *(solid white arrow),* with exiting C6 nerve root compression. Note the open foramen on the left side *(broken white arrow).* **B,** Sagittal image of a computed tomographic myelogram shows the C5-C6 disc herniation *(solid white arrow).*

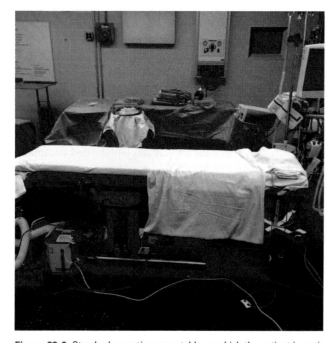

Figure 33-2 Standard operating room table on which the patient is positioned supine. Be sure the draw sheet is long enough to allow the arms to be tucked at the side.

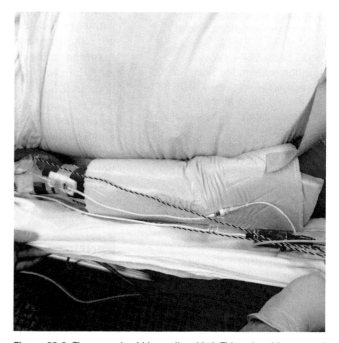

Figure 33-3 The arms should be well-padded. This gel pad is wrapped around the arm to pad the bony prominences, particularly around the elbow and ulnar nerve, before tucking the arm.

Prepping and Draping

- Prep and drape the skin from the chin to the sternum and to the lateral aspect of the neck (Fig. 33-5).
- Prep and drape the anterior iliac crest if using autograft.

Dissection

- Mark out the midline of the chin and the midline of the sternal notch.
- Anatomic landmarks and fluoroscopy can be used to localize the incision site (Fig. 33-6).

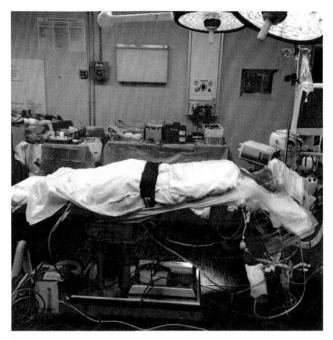

Figure 33-4 Photograph shows patient positioning, supine on an operating room table with the arms taped at the side and the neck in slight extension. Extension is achieved with an inflatable intravenous bag or a rolled towel placed across the upper back, underneath the scapula.

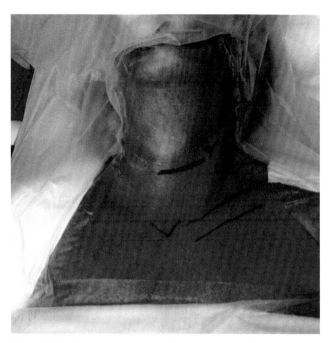

Figure 33-5 Photograph of the area that is to be prepped before anterior cervical surgery. The clavicle and the sternal notch are marked with a marking pen, as is the left-sided transverse incision, in this case, for a C5-C6 approach.

- A left-sided transverse incision is made over the appropriate level.
- Cauterize through subcutaneous tissue to the level of the platysma.
- Lift the platysma with pickups and divide with cautery in line with the skin incision.
- Identify and palpate the anterior border of the sternocleidomastoid muscle (SCM).
- Scissors can be used to develop the plane between the SCM laterally and the strap muscles medially.

Deep Dissection

- The rest of the dissection should be performed bluntly with the index finger down to the anterior cervical spine, medial to the SCM and the carotid sheath (Fig. 33-7).
- Scissors or electrocautery followed by a Kittner dissecting sponge can be used to dissect the prevertebral fascia off of the anterior cervical spine.
- A needle should be placed in the involved disc space, and an intraoperative radiograph or fluoroscopic image should be obtained to confirm the correct level.
- The soft tissues and longus coli muscles can be dissected off of the anterior cervical spine at the involved level.
- After the longus coli muscles are adequately dissected, the soft tissue retractors can be placed (Fig. 33-8).

Discectomy, Fusion, and Instrumentation

- The anterior annulus is incised with a scalpel.
- The intervertebral disc and cartilaginous material is then débrided with a series of curved and straight curettes and pituitary rongeurs back to bleeding endplate bone, working from anterior to posterior and out to the uncovertebral joints bilaterally.
- Caspar pins (Aesculap, Center Valley, PA) can be placed in the vertebrae, and the Caspar distractor (Aesculap, Center Valley, PA) can be used to distract the disc space to allow better access to the posterior aspect of the disc space.

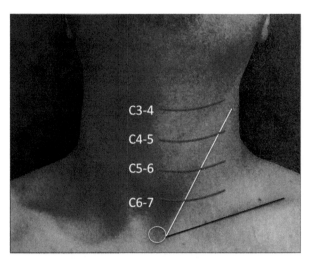

Figure 33-6 Photograph of the anterior neck shows the incision locations for the various cervical levels. The *white line* indicates the location of the sternocleidomastoid muscle, the *black line* indicates the location of the clavicle, and the *white circle* indicates the location of the sternal notch. As a general guideline, the incision for a C6-C7 approach is made 2 fingerbreadths above the clavicle, the incision for a C5-C6 approach is made 3 fingerbreadths above the clavicle, etc. As additional anatomical guides: 1, The cricoid cartilage typically sits directly anterior to the C6 vertebral body; 2, the carotid tubercle that extends off of the C6 vertebral body can oftentimes be palpated, especially in thin patients; 3, the thyroid cartilage typically sits directly anterior to the C4-C5 disc space; and 4, the hyoid typically sits directly anterior to the C3 vertebra.

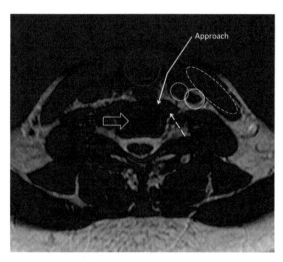

Figure 33-7 The T2-weighted axial magnetic resonance image of the cervical spine at the C6-C7 level shows the left-sided approach *(solid white line/arrow)* to the anterior cervical spine. The approach is performed medial to the sternocleidomastoid muscle *(dashed white circle)* and the carotid sheath containing the internal jugular vein *(dotted white circle)* and the carotid artery *(solid white circle)* and lateral to the trachea *(solid red circle)* and the esophagus *(dashed red circle)*. The longus coli muscles *(dashed white arrow)* need to be dissected off of the anterior aspect of the vertebral bodies *(open white arrow)*.

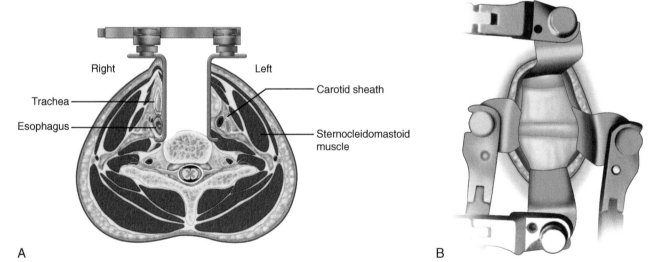

Figure 33-8 Image shows the position of the retractors, with the retractor blades placed underneath the longus coli muscles bilaterally, which have been dissected off of the anterior aspect of the vertebral body and disc space. The trachea and esophagus are retracted medially, and the sternocleidomastoid muscle and contents of the carotid sheath are retracted laterally. This provides access to the anterior aspect of the vertebral bodies and disc. Umbilical tape (30-inch) can be tied around the retractors bilaterally, and with the untied ends thrown off of the sterile field, weights can be tied to the unsterile end and hung from the table to help stabilize the retractors during the procedure. Typically, a 2-lb weight is hung from the umbilical tape that is tied to the medial retractor, and a 1-lb weight is hung from the umbilical tape that is tied to the lateral retractor.

- A high-speed burr is used to remove anterior and posterior vertebral body osteophytes and uncovertebral osteophytes.
- The posterior longitudinal ligament (PLL) is dissected through with a nerve hook or curette and then is resected with a 1-mm or 2-mm Kerrison rongeur.
- The 1-mm and 2-mm Kerrison rongeurs then are used to perform foraminotomies and remove any remaining disc material, PLL, and osteophytes.
- The vertebral endplates are prepared back to bleeding bone with a rasp or a high-speed burr.
- A bone graft (iliac crest autograft or structural allograft) of appropriate size is selected and impacted into the intervertebral space with a tamp and a mallet.
- Caspar pins can be removed after placing the bone graft.
- The plate then is placed over the vertebral bodies, and a drill is used to drill screw holes.
- The screws are placed through the plate and into the vertebral bodies, angled away from the intervertebral space (Fig. 33-9).
- Most plates have a mechanism that prevents screw backout.
- Intraoperative radiographs or fluoroscopy is used to confirm adequate position of the bone graft and instrumentation (Fig. 33-10, *A* and *B*).

Wound Closure

- Hemostasis is obtained, and the wound is irrigated.
- A small drain (e.g., Jackson-Pratt, Cardinal Health, Dublin, OH) is placed so that it sits anterior to the plate and cervical spine and exits either through the incision or through a separate stab incision inferior to the incision.
- Close the platysma with 2-0 absorbable, braided suture.
- Close the subcutaneous layer with 3-0 absorbable, braided suture.
- Close the skin 4-0 absorbable, monofilament suture.

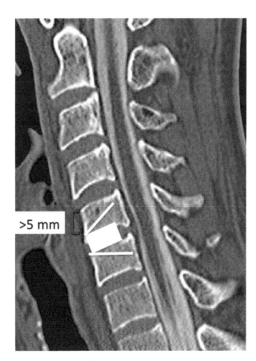

Figure 33-9 Sagittal computed tomographic image of the cervical spine shows, at the C5-C6 level, the ideal placement of the bone graft *(solid white block)* and screws *(white lines)*. The screws in the proximal vertebrae should be at least 5 mm from the adjacent level disc space to minimize the risk of developing adjacent level ossification of the disc.

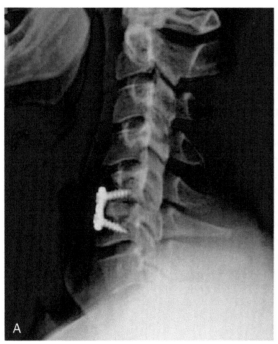
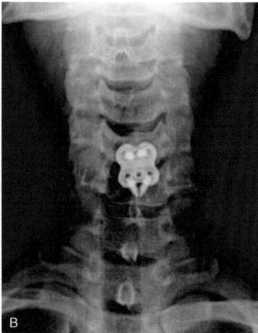

Figures 33-10 A, Postoperative lateral; and **B,** anteroposterior cervical radiograph in a patient who underwent anterior cervical discectomy and fusion at C5-C6 with use of a structural allograft and anterior plate and screws.

BRIEF SUMMARY OF SURGICAL STEPS

- Dissect down to anterior cervical spine
- Confirm level with marker on lateral radiograph
- Annulotomy with scalpel
- Remove disc and cartilagenous material
- Kerrison rongeur used to remove osteophytes and perform foraminotomies
- Endplates are prepared to bleeding bone
- Bone graft is inserted
- The plate and screws are placed and position confirmed on radiograph or fluoroscopy

REQUIRED EQUIPMENT

Standard operating room table

Loupes or microscope

Anterior cervical retractor system

Anterior cervical instrumentation system

High-speed burr

Kerrison and pituitary rongeurs, curettes, nerve hook, scalpel, standard surgical dissecting instruments

Neurophysiologic monitoring equipment (if used)

TECHNICAL PEARLS

- Use retractors during the exposure and surgery to protect the esophagus from injury
- In very spondylotic disc spaces, the high-speed burr may be needed to remove the anterior osteophytes to access the disc space
- Pass a nerve hook out of the foramen and posterior to the vertebral bodies to confirm an adequate decompression
- Floseal (Baxter, Cherry Hill, NJ) is a good hemostatic agent that can be used to control bleeding from epidural veins
- Plate should be at least a 5-mm distance from adjacent level to minimize the risk of ossification of the adjacent disc
- Use a 14-mm drill guide when drilling holes to prevent drilling through the posterior vertebral body into the spinal canal
- Bony bleeding from the anterior vertebral bodies can be controlled with electrocautery or bone wax
- Overzealous or prolonged retraction can increase the risk of nerve injury and postoperative dysphagia; thus, soft tissue retractors should be relaxed every 15 to 20 minutes for a short period of time

COMMON PITFALLS

(When to call for the attending physician)

- Nerve root injury or injury to the spinal cord
- Vascular injury to carotid artey or internal jugular vein
- Recurrent laryngeal nerve injury, most commonly, a traction injury
- Injury to the esophagus
- Injury to the sympathetic chain, which can be encountered with excessive lateral dissection through the longus coli muscles
- Vertebral artery injury
- Spinal fluid leak

POSTOPERATIVE PROTOCOL

Most surgeons place the patient in a cervical collar (soft or hard); however, the use of a postoperative collar, especially for single-level surgery, is controversial. The patient's head-of-bed is elevated to 45 degrees or greater in the early postoperative period to minimize swelling at the surgical site. In addition to the preoperative dose of antibiotics given within 1 hour before skin incision, patients should receive 24 hours of antibiotics after surgery. Sequential compression devices on the bilateral lower extremities and early ambulation are recommended to minimize the risk of postoperative deep venous thrombosis. The drain is typically maintained until postoperative day 1 or until the output is less than 30 mL per 8-hour shift. Patients are typically fairly mobile after this procedure and can expect to go home on postoperative day 1.

Although rare, the devopment of a hematoma in the early postoperatve period can cause airway compromise or neurologic decline. Education of the nursing staff and close observation is important in detecting these issues early to prevent potentially devastating consequences. The most common issues after surgery are related to surgical site pain and swelling, including sore throat, dysphonia, and dysgphagia, all of which typically gradually improve over a period of days to weeks. Intravenous or oral steroids can be helpful in managing these symptoms in the early postoperative period.

POSTOPERATIVE CLINIC VISIT PROTOCOL

After surgery, patients are seen in follow-up for a clinical and radiographic examination at 2 weeks, 3 months, 6 months, 1 year, and then annually. If a collar is used, it is typically discontinued between 2 and 6 weeks after surgery, depending on surgeon preference. Anteroposterior and lateral radiographs are obtained at the 2-week appointment. The addition of lateral flexion and extension radiographs at subsequent follow-up visits can help determine whether the bony fusion is solid. The distance between the spinous processes of the involved level can be measured on the flexion and extension views to determine whether there is still motion at the involved level.

Patients can return to their activities of daily living within a few days of surgery. Nonimpact aerobic (e.g., stationary bicycle, elliptic machine) conditioning and isometric cervical strengthening exercises can start 2 to 3 weeks after surgery. Impact exercise (e.g., jogging) and regular strengthening exercises for the upper and lower extremities can start 6 to 8 weeks after surgery. Patients who play high-impact contact sports (e.g., football or wrestling) should have a computed tomographic scan with documented fusion before returning to play.

SUGGESTED READINGS

1. Bohlman HH, Emery SE, Goodfellow DB, Jones PK. Robinson anterior cervical discectomy and arthrodesis for cervical radiculopathy. Long-term follow-up of one hundred and twenty-two patients. *J Bone Joint Surg Am*. 1993;75(9):1298-1307.
2. Brodke DS, Zdeblick TA. Modified Smith-Robinson procedure for anterior cervical discectomy and fusion. *Spine (Phila Pa 1976)*. 1992;17(10 suppl):S427-S430.
3. Carreon LY, Glassman SD, Campbell MJ, Anderson PA. Neck Disability Index, short form-36 physical component summary, and pain scales for neck and arm pain: the minimum clinically important difference and substantial clinical benefit after cervical spine fusion. *Spine J*. 2010;10(6):469-474.
4. Emery SE, Bohlman HH, Bolesta MJ, Jones PK. Anterior cervical decompression and arthrodesis for the treatment of cervical spondylotic myelopathy. Two to seventeen-year follow-up. *J Bone Joint Surg Am*. 1998;80(7):941-951.
5. Hilibrand AS, Carlson GD, Palumbo MA, Jones PK, Bohlman HH. Radiculopathy and myelopathy at segments adjacent to the site of a previous anterior cervical arthrodesis. *J Bone Joint Surg Am*. 1999; 81(4):519-528.
6. Kepler CK, Rihn JA, Bennett JD, et al. Dysphagia and soft-tissue swelling after anterior cervical surgery: a radiographic analysis. *Spine J*. 2012;12(8):639-644.

7. Riew KD, Buchowski JM, Sasso R, Zdeblick T, Metcalf NH, Anderson PA. Cervical disc arthroplasty compared with arthrodesis for the treatment of myelopathy. *J Bone Joint Surg Am*. 2008;90(11): 2354-2364.

8. Rihn JA, Kane J, Albert TJ, Vaccaro AR, Hilibrand AS. What is the incidence and severity of dysphagia after anterior cervical surgery? *Clin Orthop Relat Res*. 2011;469(3):658-665.

9. Sasso RC, Smucker JD, Hacker RJ, Heller JG. Clinical outcomes of BRYAN cervical disc arthroplasty: a prospective, randomized, controlled, multicenter trial with 24-month follow-up. *J Spinal Disord Tech*. 2007;20(7):481-491.

10. Smith GW, Robinson RA. Anterolateral cervical disc removal and interbody fusion for cervical disc syndrome. *Bull John Hopkins Hosp* 1955;96:223-224.

PROXIMAL HUMERUS FRACTURE FIXATION

OPEN REDUCTION INTERNAL FIXATION AND CLOSED REDUCTION PERCUTANEOUS PINNING

William N. Levine | Jonathan P. Watling

CASE MINIMUM REQUIREMENTS

- Accreditation Council for Graduate Medical Education case minimum requirement: 5 Cases

COMMONLY USED CPT CODES

- 23605—Closed treatment of proximal humeral (surgical or anatomical neck) fracture; with manipulation, with or without skeletal traction
- 23615—Open treatment of proximal humeral (surgical or anatomical neck) fracture, includes internal fixation, when performed, includes repair of tuberosity(s) when performed
- 23616—Open treatment of proximal humeral (surgical or anatomical neck) fracture, includes internal fixation, when performed, includes repair of tuberosity(s) when performed; with proximal humeral prosthetic replacement

Proximal humerus fractures account for up to 5% of all fractures and are the third most common fragility fracture among the elderly population. Although most are considered nondisplaced and may be treated successfully with nonoperative managment, up to 20% require surgical fixation. Proximal humerus fractures follow a bimodal distribution, with the majority occurring in the elderly osteoporotic patient population and a 3:1 predilection toward female patients over males. Patients with proximal humerus fractures present typically with pain and swelling and impaired range of motion in the shoulder after a mechanical fall onto an outstretched arm. A thorough trauma evaluation should be perfomed. Axillary nerve injury is fairly common, observed in up to 45% of cases.

Historically, surgical treatment of proximal humerus fractures has been successful with regard to functional outcome but has also carried a high rate of postoperative complications. Early methods of fixation with nonlocking plate and screw fixation resulted in hardware failure, loss of fixation, and either nonunion or malunion. Advances in implant design, specifically the development of proximal humerus locking plates, have improved outcomes and decreased complication rates, leading to a recent dramatic rise in the rate open reduction internal fixation.

Absolute indications for operative fixation of proximal humerus fractures include open fractures with or without neurovascular injury and unstable displaced intraarticular or periarticular fractures that prevent early range of motion and therefore confer significant functional impairment. When considering surgical intervention, several factors must be taken into consideration, including patient physiologic age, bone quality, fracture pattern, humeral head vascularity, current functional status, patient comorbidities, patient expectations, and surgeon experience. Currently, no true gold standard exists for the surgical treatment of proximal humerus fractures. Goals of surgical fixation include anatomic reduction with stable fixation to allow for early range of motion. Ideally, treatment is geared to minimize posttraumatic arthritis and impingement and to reestablish preoperative strength and range of motion.

SURGICAL TECHNIQUE

Room Set-Up

- The operative table or beach chair should be positioned appropriately under the center of the operating room lights to provide optimal visualization.

- The operative table should be angled in the room to allow for adequate access to the patient by the anesthesiologist and surgeon and proper positioning of the large C-arm fluoroscopy unit.
- The C-arm should be positioned coming in from the head of the patient and parallel to the table to ensure the ability to obtain orthogonal views of the proximal humerus (Fig. 34-1).

Patient Positioning

- The patient may be placed in either the beach chair or the supine position; the authors prefer the beach chair.
- The patient must be positioned as far lateral on the table, toward the operative side, as possible to maximize access to the shoulder.
- Care must be taken in positioning the patient's head to protect the cervical spine while minimizing interference with the surgical field.
- The arm must be free to have unimpeded forward elevation and extension along with internal and external rotation to ensure optimal visualization and fracture reduction (Fig. 34-2).

COMMONLY USED ICD9 CODES

- 812.00—Closed fracture of unspecified part of upper end of humerus
- 812.02—Closed fracture of anatomic neck of humerus
- 812.03—Closed fracture of greater tuberosity of humerus
- 812.09—Other closed fracture of upper end of humerus
- 812.11—Open fracture of surgical neck of humerus
- 812.12—Open fracture of anatomic neck of humerus
- 812.13—Open fracture of greater tuberosity of humerus
- 812.19—Other open fracture of upper end of humerus

COMMONLY USED ICD10 CODES

- S42.20—Unspecified fracture of upper end of humerus
- S42.21—Unspecified fracture of surgical neck of humerus
- S42.22—2-part fracture of surgical neck of humerus
- S42.23—3-part fracture of surgical neck of humerus
- S42.24—4-part fracture of surgical neck of humerus
- S42.25—Fracture of greater tuberosity of humerus
- S42.26—Fracture of lesser tuberosity of humerus
- S42.29—Other fracture of upper end of humerus

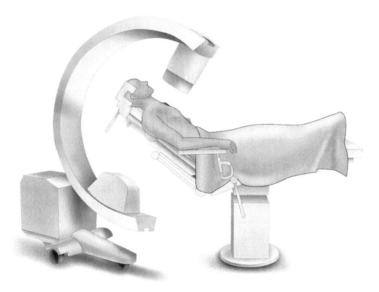

Figure 34-1 C-arm positioning for open reduction internal fixation of a proximal humerus fracture.

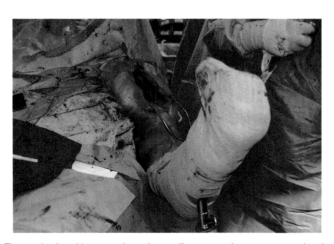

Figure 34-2 The arm is placed in external rotation to allow appropriate anteroposterior visualization and ensure anatomic reduction before provisional fixation. (Figure courtesy of Columbia University Center for Shoulder, Elbow and Sports Medicine, New York.)

Prepping and Draping

- The patient's arm is hung with a rolled gauze bandage or stockinette for preparation.
- The surgical field should be appropriately shaved.
- A plastic drape is placed from medial to lateral, just above the nipple line, traversing under the axilla.
- The shoulder then is scrubbed with chlorhexidine and patted dry with a sterile blue towel.
- The skin is prepared with the cleansing agent of choice (providone-iodine or chlordexidine gluconate+isopropyl alcohol), extending anteromedially to the sternum, inferiorly to the plastic drape, superiorly to just above the crest of the neckline, and as far posterior as the table allows.
- A sterile half sheet is placed under the axilla, covering the lower portion of the patient's body.
- Two blue impervious U-drapes then are placed. The first is placed under the axilla and extends both posteriorly and anteriorly across the chest. The second is placed high along the crest of the neck and extends down the front of the chest and the back to create the surgical field.
- The final drape includes both a cranial and a caudal split sheet. The edges of the surgical field drapes may be reinforced with iodine impregnated incision drapes.
- Stockinette is placed over the hand and forearm of the injured extremity and then wrapped lightly with Coban wrapping (3M, Minneapolis). If a spider arm positioner is used, the arm piece then is placed and secured with additional Coban wrapping.
- The arm then may be placed in the spider arm positioner.

Closed Reduction Percutaneous Pinning (CRPP)

- Closed reduction percutaneous pinning (CRPP) is a minimally invasive method of achieving stable fixation that allows for minimal soft tissue disruption and preserves the biologic environment that facilitates fracture healing.
- CRPP is reserved for patients with good bone quality and relatively simple fracture patterns (two part, three part with large fragments, or four part valgus impacted) to provide maximal oportunity for successful outcome (Fig. 34-3).
- The advantages are less soft tissue dissection, less disruption of vascularity, shorter operating room time, and shorter hospital stay.
- The disadvantages are less stable fixation, pin migration, initial limitation on motion, and stiffness.
- Typical deformity is adduction, anterior displacement, and internal rotation of the humeral shaft from the deforming force of the pectoralis major muscle.
- The reduction maneuver is traction, adduction, and either internal or external rotation to bring both the greater and the lesser tuberosities into alignment. Reduction is attempted before draping.
- Closed reduction is performed, followed by placement of terminally threaded 0.11-inch K-wires or 2.5-mm Schanz pins to achieve fixation. First, reduce the shaft to the head and place the lateral pin; then, place the tuberosity pins or the cannulated screws (Figs. 34-4 and 34-5).
- When placing the pins, the location of relevant anatomic structures must be considered. Lateral pins place the axillary nerve at risk for injury, and slightly more anterolateral pins may damage either the cephalic vein or the long head of the biceps.
- Major complications associated with CRPP include pin migration, which manifests either with loss of fixation or reduction but may also lead to pulmonary or vascular compromise. These patients should be monitored closely for radiographic signs of pin migration, and pins should be removed if there is suspicion for migration. Osteonecrosis and infection also are reported complications, although less common.

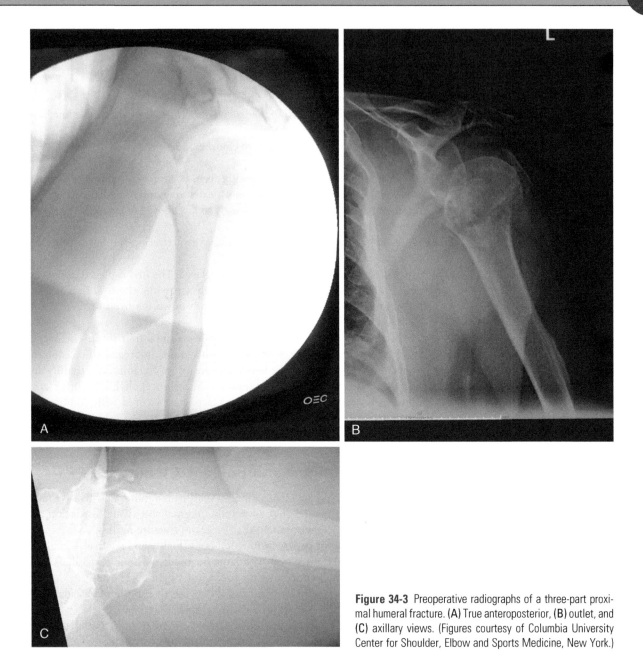

Figure 34-3 Preoperative radiographs of a three-part proximal humeral fracture. **(A)** True anteroposterior, **(B)** outlet, and **(C)** axillary views. (Figures courtesy of Columbia University Center for Shoulder, Elbow and Sports Medicine, New York.)

■ Outcomes for appropriate fracture patterns have shown high union rates with concomitant high American Shoulder and Elbow Surgeons Standardized Shoulder Assessment Form (ASES) scores and low Visual Analog Scale (VAS).

Proximal Humerus Locking Plates

■ The proximal humerus locking plates offer the best and most reliable mode of fixation, especially in patients with osteoporosis and unstable highly comminuted fracture patterns.

■ Its advantages are more stable fixation with regard to angular stability and fatigue resistence, quicker return to range of motion and strengthening, and reduction performed with direct visualization.

■ Its disadvantages are more extensive soft tissue dissection, damage to vascular supply, longer operating time, and longer hospital stay.

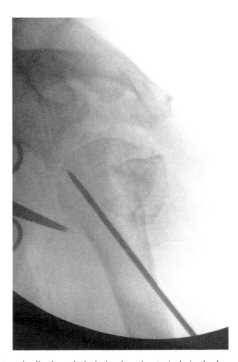

Figure 34-4 A 2.8-mm terminally threaded pin is placed anteriorly in the humeral shaft directed to the humeral articular surface to provisionally fix it. Critically important is that the pin is placed so as to not interfere with anterolateral placement of the proximal humeral locking plate. (Figure courtesy of Columbia University Center for Shoulder, Elbow and Sports Medicine, New York.)

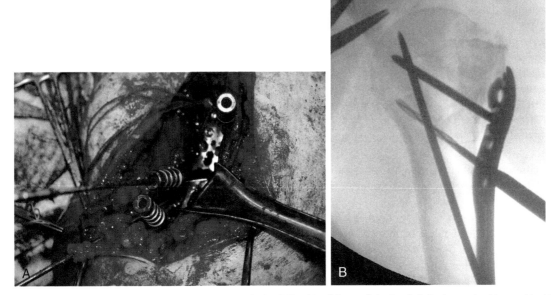

Figure 34-5 **A,** Intraoperative photograph shows the 2.7-mm drill bit in the drill guide of the medial calcar hole in the proximal humeral locking plate; this ensures proper plate height. **B,** The intraoperative fluoroscopic view confirms appropriate plate positioning. (Figure courtesy of Columbia University Center for Shoulder, Elbow and Sports Medicine, New York.)

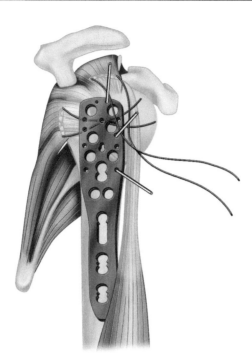

Figure 34-6 Establish preliminary plate fixation and reduction with 0.055-inch K-wires. Note that the bony tuberosities are reduced with #5 suture fixation through the rotator cuff tendon tissue passed through the small plate holes.

- Deltopectoral approach is performed to visualize and mobilize the fracture.
- Provisional fixation with 2.8-mm terminally threaded pin from anterior starting point is critical for maintaining reduction to allow placing the humerus in internal rotation to gain access to the anterolateral humerus where the plate will rest (Fig. 34-6).
- The screw is placed from the neck of the plate to the medial calcar to establish stable fixation.
- After ensuring the distal aspect of the plate is well-aligned along the humeral shaft, locking screws are placed in the humeral head engaging distal subchondral bone for maximal fixation.
- Note that the proximal humerus locking plates are typically positioned 2 to 4 mm posterior to the bicipital groove and 5 to 8 mm inferior to the tip of the greater tuberosity (Fig. 34-7).
- Finally, cortical screws are placed in the distal aspect of the plate to complete the construct.
- The most common complications of open reduction internal fixation (ORIF) with locking plates are intraarticular penetration of screws and osteonecrosis of the humeral head.
- Short-term outcomes with ORIF have been shown to be better with regard to pain, rotator cuff function, and range of motion. Long-term outcomes are equivalent with regard to functional outcomes and pain scores but with higher complication and reoperation rates when compared with CRPP and intramedullary (IM) nailing (Fig. 34-8).

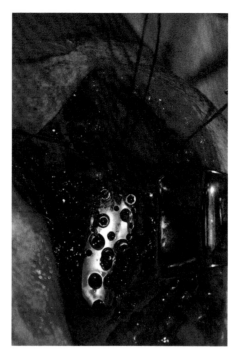

Figure 34-7 Intraoperative photograph shows sutures from the tuberosity/cuff placed into suture holes at the proximal aspect of the locking plate. (Figure courtesy of Columbia University Center for Shoulder, Elbow and Sports Medicine, New York.)

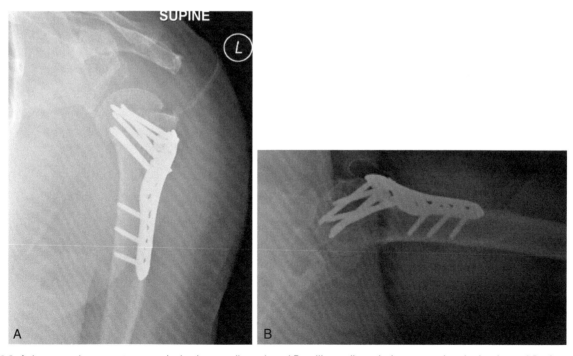

Figure 34-8 **A,** Intraoperative true anteroposterior hard copy radiograph; and **B,** axillary radiograph show anatomic reduction, internal fixation, and appropriate hardware placement. (Figures courtesy of Columbia University Center for Shoulder, Elbow and Sports Medicine, New York.)

BRIEF SUMMARY OF SURGICAL STEPS

- Appropriately position the patient on the operative table; the authors prefer the beach chair position
- Ensure ability to obtain adequate orthogonal radiographic views of the injured shoulder before prep and drape

CLOSED REDUCTION PERCUTANEOUS PINNING:

- Perform reduction maneuver with fluoroscopic guidance before prep and drape
- Place lateral pin first to reduce shaft to humeral head, then place tuberosity pins/cannulated screws to complete fixation; may use accessory incision and skin hook to reduce greater tuberosity

OPEN REDUCTION INTERNAL FIXATION WITH LOCKING PLATES:

- Perform deltopectoral approach
- Identify and mobilize fracture planes and fragments with careful dissection and minimize soft tissue disruption
- Place K-wire from anterior starting point retrograde into humeral head to provide provisional fixation and stable platform for internal/external rotation of humerus
- Place plate on anterolateral surface of humerus while humerus is internally rotated to maximize exposure
- Capture and reduce the greater and lesser tuberosities with #5 suture by passing through the infraspinatus/supraspinatus and subscapularis tendons, respectively; suture may be tied through small holes in the proximal humerus locking plate
- Initial screw should engage the medial calcar to create a stable base for the plate
- After ensuring proper alignment of the plate along the humeral shaft, subsequent locking screws are placed into the humeral head, engaging distal subchondral bone but not penetrating articular surface
- Finally, cortical screws are placed in distal aspect of plate into the humeral shaft to complete the construct
- Shoulder then is taken through full range of motion with live fluoroscopy to ensure that the locking screws have not penetrated the articular surface of the humeral head

TECHNICAL PEARLS

CLOSED REDUCTION PERCUTANEOUS PINNING:

Adequate imaging

Achieving anatomic reduction

- Lateral pin placed first to reduce shaft to humeral head, followed by reduction and pinning of tuberosities
- Do not leave pins protruding out through skin: high risk of infection
- Bend pins underneath skin to prevent pin migration

PROXIMAL HUMERUS LOCKING PLATES:

- Minimal soft tissue dissection during deltopectoral approach
- Tagging sutures in rotator cuff to control tuberosity fragments
- Provisional K-wire fixation: Should be placed anteriorly on the humeral shaft just below the level of the calcar
  - Pin should be directed posterosuperiorly
  - Anterior starting point keeps provisional pin out of the way of the locking plate, maintaining reduction of the fracture while internally rotating the arm
- Full range of motion with flouroscopic guidance to ensure locking screws are not penetrating joint space

REQUIRED EQUIPMENT

Radiolucent table/beach chair
C-arm
Spider arm positioner
Proximal humerus locking plate system
Humeral intramedullary nail
2.8-mm terminally threaded pins

High strength nonabsorbable braided composite sutures (2-0)
Retractors: Richardson, Browne, Link

COMMON PITFALLS

(When to call for the attending physician)

- Inadequate reduction: typically occurs when provisional fixation not performed and arm is placed in internal rotation to apply proximal humeral locking plate
- Inappropriate plate placement: typically occurs with too proximal placement; avoid this pitfall by placing drill into medial calcar hole and confirm with intraoperative fluoroscopy
- Inadequate fixation: typically occurs with osteoporotic fractures and too short plate (three-hole) when there is comminution in the calcar region

POSTOPERATIVE PROTOCOL

After surgery, patients remain in a sling for the first 4 weeks. Full range of motion of the elbow, wrist, and fingers is permitted, regardless of method of fixation. Patients undergoing closed reduction percutaneous pinning (CRPP) are treated more conservatively with regard to range of motion. These patients do not have any shoulder motion after surgery until the pins are removed (typically at 4 weeks).

Terminally threaded pins are typically removed at 4 weeks; this can be done either in the office or in the operating room, dependent on patient-specific and surgeon-specific features. After pin removal, progressive passive, active-assisted, and active range of motion exercises may be started, provided adequate radiographic evidence of healing is evident. Strengthening exercises are often delayed until healing is complete and range of motion exercises are progressing nicely, generally at approximately 12 weeks after surgery.

Patients undergoing open reduction internal fixation with locked plating may be more aggressively rehabilitated after surgery. Pendulum exercises may be started within the first week after surgery and progressed as tolerated. Active-assisted range of motion exercises also may be initiated within the first postoperative month. Strengthening exercises are usually reserved until fracture healing has significantly progressed, again usually at the 12-week mark.

POSTOPERATIVE CLINIC VISIT PROTOCOL

Patients return to the office for their first postoperative visit 7 to 10 days after surgery. At this time, true anteroposterior (Grashey view) and axillary radiographs are taken to ensure maintained fixation and proper positioning of the pins or implants. Careful examination for signs of pin migration is imperative for those patients who underwent CRPP. The incision is inspected, and any sutures may be removed. Gentle passive range of motion is performed. The patient then may be referred for physical therapy to include passive range of motion and active-assisted range of motion of the shoudler. Subsequent office visits should be scheduled for 1 month, 3 months, 6 months, and 1 year after surgery to monitor both fracture healing and progression through rehabilitation.

SUGGESTED READINGS

1. Court-Brown CM, Garg A, McQueen MM. The epidemiology of proximal humeral fractures. *Acta Orthop Scand*. 2001;72:365-371.
2. Gaebler C, McQueen MM, Court-Brown CM. Minimally displaced proximal humeral fractures: epidemiology and outcome in 507 cases. *Acta Orthop Scand*. 2003;74:580-585.
3. Gerber C, Werner CM, Vienne P. Internal fixation of complex fractures of the proximal humerus. *J Bone Joint Surg Br*. 2004;86:848-855.
4. Owsley KC, Gorczyca JT. Fracture displacement and screw cutout after open reduction and locked plate fixation of proximal humeral fractures [corrected]. *J Bone Joint Surg Am*. 2008;90:233-240.
5. Solberg BD, Moon CN, Franco DP, Paiement GD. Surgical treatment of three and four-part proximal humeral fractures. *J Bone Joint Surg Am*. 2009;91:1689-1697.
6. Naranja RJ Jr, Iannotti JP. Displaced three- and four-part proximal humerus fractures: evaluation and management. *J Am Acad Orthop Surg*. 2000;8:373-382.
7. Schlegel TF, Hawkins RJ. Displaced proximal humerus fractures: evaluation and treatment. *J Am Acad Orthop Surg*. 1994;2:54-66.
8. Neer CS II. Displaced proximal humeral fractures: I. Classification and evaluation. *J Bone Joint Surg Am*. 1970;52:1077-1089.
9. Resch H, Povacz P, Frohlich R, Wambacher M. Percutaneous fixation of three- and four-part fractures of the proximal humerus. *J Bone Joint Surg Br*. 1997;79:295-300.
10. Strohm PC, Kostler W, Sudkamp NP. Locking plate fixation of proximal humerus fractures. *Techniques Shoulder Elbow Surg*. 2005;6:8-13.

CHAPTER 35

CLOSED REDUCTION AND PERCUTANEOUS PINNING OF METACARPAL FRACTURES

Joseph Marchese | Jennifer Moriatis Wolf

Metacarpal fractures are common injuries that make up 18% to 44% of all hand fractures. The metacarpals are long tubular bones whose medial and lateral surfaces are enveloped by dorsal and volar interossei and lumbrical muscles. Deep transverse intermetacarpal ligaments are found along the metacarpal neck and limit deformity with low-energy injuries. The extensor apparatus overlies the metacarpophalangeal (MCP) joints, and the collateral ligaments originate from a tubercle on the metacarpal head. Fractures of the metacarpals can disturb this complex mechanism and lead to impairment of hand function. Metacarpal fractures most commonly occur at the metacarpal neck, followed by the shaft and base. The most common injury mechanism involves transmission of an axial load from the MCP joint through the metacarpal, and the resultant fracture pattern depends on the degree of shear, torsion, and energy associated with the applied load. Typically, the fracture at the metacarpal neck or shaft has apex-dorsal malalignment as a result of the pull of the lumbrical and interossei muscles. The optimal treatment for a specific injury is based on the location and extent of bone and soft tissue disruption.

Many metacarpal fractures heal uneventfully and do not require surgical intervention. Often, low-energy transverse or oblique fractures to a single metacarpal heal without any functional deformity, whereas spiral fractures, comminuted fractures, and fractures to several metacarpals are inclined to shorten and rotate, causing tendon imbalance, extensor lag, finger overlap, and loss of finger motion. Surgery is recommended for metacarpal neck fractures when there is any degree of malrotation and greater than 10 degrees of angulation in the index, 20 degrees in the middle, 30 degrees in the ring, and 40 to 50 degrees in the small finger. In the metacarpal shaft, surgery is indicated when there is greater than 10 degrees of angulation in the index or middle fingers or greater than 30 to 40 degrees of angulation in the ring or small fingers. Any rotational malalignment must also be corrected. Clinical assessment of rotation is performed by observing the fingers in flexion for scissoring or overlap. Further indications for surgical reduction and stabilization include open fractures, unstable fractures, shortening of 5 mm, or fractures associated with joint disruption, tendon injury, and neurovascular damage.

Closed reduction and percutaneous pinning is commonly used for low-energy metacarpal shaft and neck fractures (Figs. 35-1 and 35-2). Conversely, this strategy is also well suited for stabilizing simple comminuted fractures and fractures associated with moderate to severe soft tissue injury. With this technique, K-wires are inserted with a power drill for either provisional or definitive fixation. Fracture fixation stability is dependent on the diameter of the K-wire and wire configuration. A commonly used configuration is wire placement in a crossed fashion across the fracture site in either an antegrade or retrograde fashion. The latter is presented here.

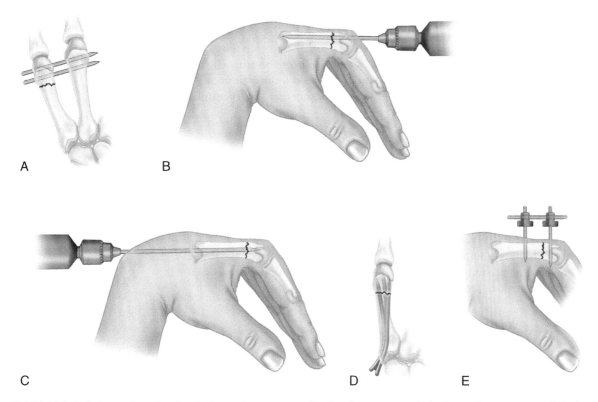

Figure 35-1 Multiple techniques allow closed reduction and percutaneous fixation: **A,** transverse pinning into adjacent metacarpal; **B,** longitudinal, eccentric pin through the metacarpal head; **C,** longitudinal pin through the proximal metacarpal; **D,** several pins passed through the base of the metacarpal; and **E,** external fixator placed percutaneously.

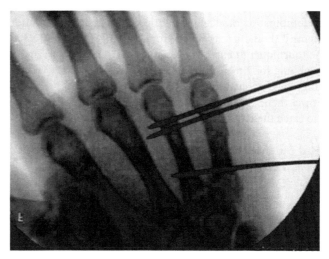

Figure 35-2 A displaced midshaft fracture may be reduced and stabilized by pinning to the adjacent metacarpal.

SURGICAL TECHNIQUE

Room Set-Up

- The operating room table is positioned to provide maximum space for the attached hand table, minifluoroscope, operating surgeons, surgical technicians, instrument table, circulating nurses, and anesthesia personnel.
- Surgical overhead lights are arranged at the head and foot of the hand table to avoid blockage by the surgeon or assistant, above the anticipated position of the patient's

operative extremity. The lighting position then can be adjusted to more suitable positions at various times throughout the operation.

- Once the patient has been positioned, prepped, and draped, the surgeon most commonly sits at the hand table facing the medial or axilla side of the arm. The first assistant sits directly across from the surgeon, and the surgical technician sits at the end of the hand table. The instrument table should be within reach of the surgical technician.

Patient Positioning

- The patient is placed in the supine position on the operating room table with the operative extremity placed on a hand table (Fig. 35-3). The table should be well-padded to prevent pressure sores or injury to the ulnar nerve and is made of a radiolucent material to allow radiography of the hand. The contralateral elbow and wrist should also be well-padded and positioned free from pressure.
- Multiple anesthesia techniques can be used for the surgical treatment of metacarpal fractures. These include local block alone or in conjunction with intravenous sedation, Bier block, regional/brachial plexus blockade, or general anesthesia.

Prepping and Draping

- With the patient properly positioned, a pneumatic tourniquet (generally 18-inch size) is applied on the operative arm as high into the axilla as possible. To prevent injury to the skin beneath the tourniquet, ensure that the tourniquet edges have been well-padded with several layers of cast padding before tourniquet inflation.
- An impervious barrier (such as a 1010™ [St. Paul, MN] drape) is placed just distal to the tourniquet to prevent migration of skin preparation solutions beneath the tourniquet.
- The extremity can be cleansed with a variety of antiseptic solutions. These are generally a combination of alcohol, chlorhexidine, or iodine solutions. The entire upper extremity should be scrubbed from the fingertips to just below the distal edge of the tourniquet to ensure adequate reduction of bacterial skin flora. Continuous scrubbing for 7 to 10 minutes is recommended (Fig. 35-4).
- A sterile three-quarter sheet is placed over the hand table.
- A sterile towel then is clamped over the distal edge of the tourniquet, with care taken not to catch the skin, and a stockinette is applied from fingertip to tourniquet (Fig. 35-5).
- A fenestrated extremity drape with a cuff of plastic is applied over the operative extremity (Fig. 35-6).

COMMONLY USED ICD10 CODES

- S62.30—Fracture of other and unspecified metacarpal bone
- S62.31—Displaced fracture of base of other metacarpal bone
- S62.32—Displaced fracture of shaft of other metacarpal bone
- S62.33—Displaced fracture of neck of other metacarpal bone
- S62.34—Nondisplaced fracture of base of unspecified metacarpal bone
- S62.35—Nondisplaced fracture of shaft of other metacarpal bone
- S62.36—Nondisplaced fracture of neck of other metacarpal bone
- S62.39—Other fracture of other metacarpal bone

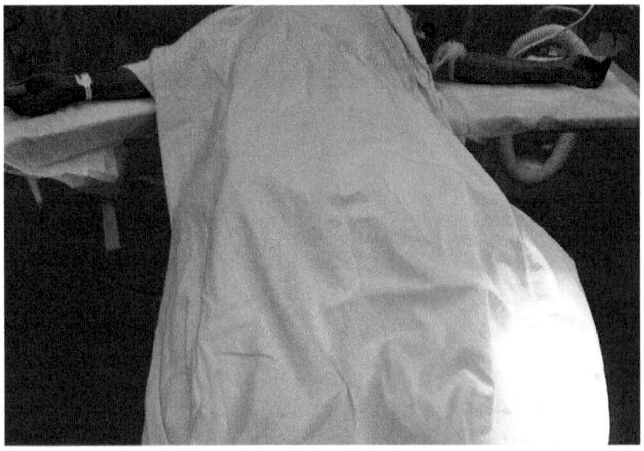

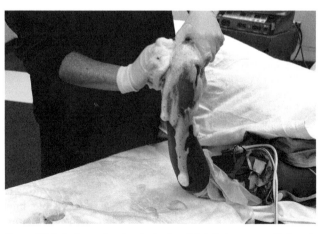

Figure 35-3 The patient is placed in a supine position on the operative table with the operative extremity placed on an adjoined hand table.

Figure 35-4 An impervious barrier is placed distally to a pneumatic tourniquet, and the operative extremity is cleansed with an antiseptic solution.

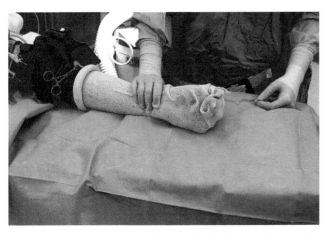

Figure 35-5 A sterile towel is clamped distal to the tourniquet, and a stockinette is applied from fingertip to tourniquet.

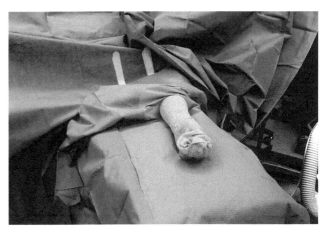

Figure 35-6 A fenestrated extremity drape is applied over the operative extremity as the final draping step.

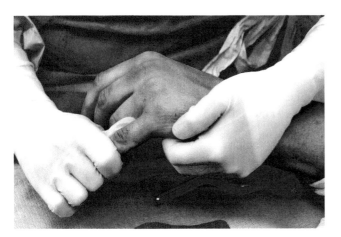

Figure 35-7 The Jahss maneuver.

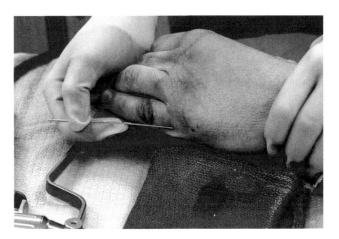

Figure 35-8 A K-wire is introduced by hand in a retrograde manner at the metacarpophalangeal joint.

Reduction Maneuver

- Traction is applied to the affected finger.
- The MCP joint is flexed, and the proximal phalanx and metacarpal head is pushed dorsally to realign the neck and shaft, a technique commonly known as the Jahss maneuver (Fig. 35-7; Video 35-1).

Procedure

- To better control the distal fragment and subsequent pin placement, flex the MCP joint of the indicated digit.
- Gently insert a 0.045-inch smooth K-wire by hand from the MCP joint in a direction oblique to the fracture plane (Fig. 35-8). Flexing the MCP joint to 90 degrees allows retrograde pins to enter near the origin of the collateral ligaments and avoids injury to the articular surface.
- Confirm placement in the coronal plane by assessing a posteroanterior view and the sagittal plane by assessing an oblique or lateral view (Fig. 35-9).
- Using power, advance the wire into the metacarpal shoulder and through the bone to the fracture site (Fig. 35-10).
- Reduce the fracture and advance the wire across the fracture site to seat it in the bone of the metacarpal shaft or base.

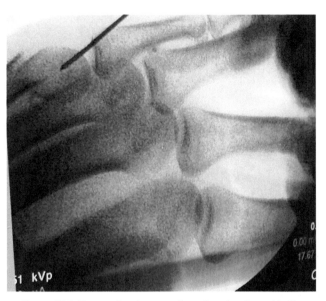

Figure 35-9 Proper wire placement is confirmed radiographically.

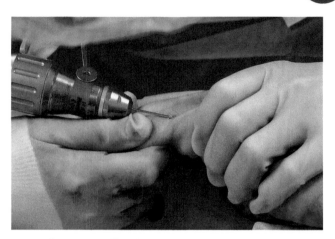

Figure 35-10 The wire is advanced to the fracture site.

- Pass a second wire to complete fracture stabilization, with care taken to derotate the finger as needed to avoid malrotation, typically by internally rotating the digit (Video 35-2). Optimal reduction and fixation is obtained when the wires cross the fracture site.
- The wires should cross proximal to the fracture site for maximal stability (Fig. 35-11).
- After satisfactory wire placement, use a large needle driver to stabilize and bend each wire and cut its tip with a wire cutter (Fig. 35-12).

BRIEF SUMMARY OF SURGICAL STEPS

- Obtain alignment in a closed fashion with traction and Jahss maneuver (Video 35-1)
- Flex the metacarpophalangeal joint to 90 degrees and pass K-wire oblique to fracture plane (see Fig. 35-8)
- Confirm placement on anteroposterior, lateral, oblique views (see Fig. 35-9)
- Advance K-wire into metacarpal shoulder, to the fracture site (see Fig. 35-10)
- Reduce, advance K-wire across fracture site to metacarpal shaft or base
- Pass second wire to complete stabilization; derotate the finger with internal rotation as needed (see Fig. 35-11; Video 35-2)
- Bend wire ends with needle driver and cut (see Fig. 35-12)

REQUIRED EQUIPMENT

Mini fluoroscope

0.035-inch to 0.045-inch diameter K-wires

Powered wire driver (wired or wireless/battery)

Wire cutter

Large needle driver or bulldog clamp

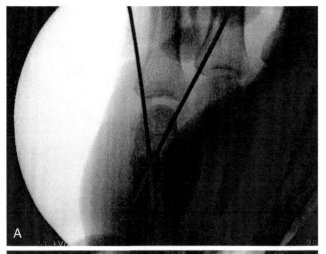

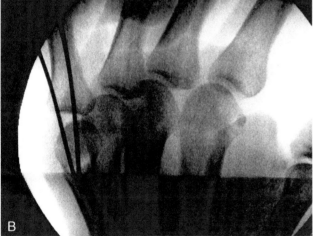

Figure 35-11 **A,** Posteroanterior radiograph confirming satisfactory reduction of metacarpal neck fracture. **B,** Pronated lateral view in fluoroscopy which rotates the small finger into view for evaluation of reduction.

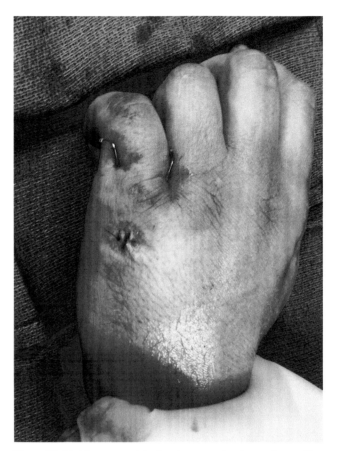

Figure 35-12 After successful wire placement, the tips are bent with a needle driver and cut with a wire cutter.

TECHNICAL PEARLS

- Most metacarpal fractures respond to nonoperative treatment with good functional outcomes
- There is usually some element of disturbance to the extensor mechanism, metacarpophalangeal joint capsule, or intrinsic muscles with surgery
- Rotational malalignment is poorly tolerated and must be corrected
- When advancing the wire through the intramedullary canal, consider using a mallet rather than power to remain intramedullary
- More stable internal fixation is recommended when early motion is desired (i.e., associated extensor tendon injury)
- Pin tract infections are common in areas with increased skin mobility, such as the metacarpophalangeal joint
  - Keep pins covered and clean with peroxide during splint or cast changes
  - For cellulitis or locally irritated skin, oral antibiotics are required
- If addressing the fracture at 10 days or more from injury, early callus may not allow closed reduction
  - Be prepared to make a 5-mm longitudinal incision at the level of the fracture and use a freer elevator to disimpact the fracture (Fig. 35-13)

COMMON PITFALLS

(When to call for the attending physician)

- When misplaced pins cause metacarpal head comminution
- When closed reduction techniques fail; this is when a small open incision may be needed and a freer is used to gain acceptable reduction

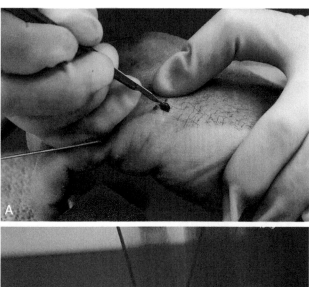

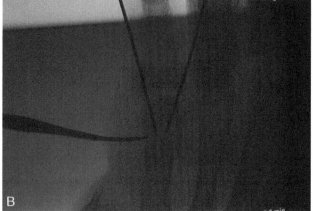

Figures 35-13 A, When closed reduction is not possible, an incision is made and a freer elevator is introduced to aid fracture disimpaction and reduction. **B,** Posteroanterior radiograph showing the freer elevator used to add stability to fracture while driving wires across the fracture site.

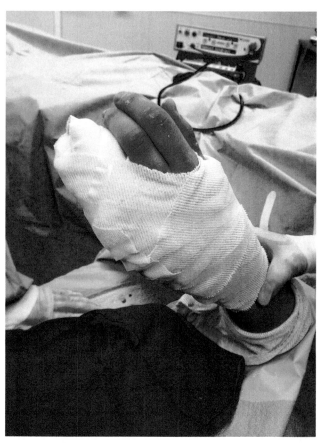

Figure 35-14 An intrinsic-plus, bulky ulnar gutter splint is applied after surgery for fourth and fifth metacarpal fractures.

POSTOPERATIVE PROTOCOL

A postoperative bulky intrinsic-plus ulnar gutter splint is typically placed for 7 to 10 days to allow for postoperative swelling to resolve (Fig. 35-14). An ulnar gutter cast then is placed after pin site cleaning. The rehabilitation plan is individualized and dependent on the stability of fixation, the soft-tissue envelope, the treatment of associated injuries, and patient compliance. To promote tendon gliding and prevent capsular contraction, immediate active and active-assisted motion of the interphalangeal joints is encouraged in compliant patients. K-wires are removed at 4 weeks after surgery. Radiographic evaluation for callus growth should be obtained at each postoperative visit, noting that callus formation may be visualized in a delayed fashion. Active and passive MCP joint motion is begun 4 weeks after surgery when there are clinical signs of union because this allows maximal extensor excursion over the fracture site. Strengthening exercises are typically added at 8 weeks.

POSTOPERATIVE CLINIC VISIT PROTOCOL

The patient is seen at 7 to 10 days after surgery, and the ulnar gutter splint is removed and the pin sites cleaned with peroxide. The patient then is placed into a short arm ulnar gutter cast, which is maintained until the patient is seen at 4 weeks after surgery. Pins typically are removed at this visit, and the patient is placed into a metacarpal fracture brace that leaves the MCP and carpometacarpal joints free.

SUGGESTED READINGS

1. Facca S, Ramdhian R, Pelissier A, Diaconu M, Liverneaux P. Fifth metacarpal neck fracture fixation: locking plate versus K-wire? *Ortho Traumatol Surg Res*. 2010;96(5):506-512.
2. Faraj AA, Davis TR. Percutaneous intramedullary fixation of metacarpal shaft fractures. *J Hand Surg [Br]*. 1999;24(1):76-79.
3. Jahss SA. Fractures of the metacarpals: a new method of reduction and immobilization. *J Bone Joint Surg Am*. 1938;20A:178-186.
4. Kelsch G, Ulrich C. Intramedullary k-wire fixation of metacarpal fractures. *Arch Orthop Trauma Surg*. 2004;124:523-526.
5. Wong TC, Ip FK, Yeung SH. Comparison between percutaneous transverse fixation and intramedullary K-wires in treating closed fractures of the metacarpal neck of the little finger. *J Hand Surg [Br]*. 2006;31(1):61-65.

CHAPTER 36

OPEN REDUCTION AND INTERNAL FIXATION OF DISTAL RADIUS FRACTURES

Laith M. Al-Shihabi | Mark S. Cohen

ractures of the distal radius are the most common closed and third most common open fracture encountered by orthopaedic surgeons, comprising up to 25% of pediatric and 18% of adult fractures annually. Amongst children, peak incidence occurs from ages 8 to 11 in boys and 11 to 14 in girls; elderly women are the most commonly affected subgroup overall. Most fractures share a common mechanism of injury, a fall or impact onto an outstretched hand. However, the wide range of fracture energy and patient bone density lead to a broad spectrum of injury complexity. Although many fractures are amenable to closed reduction and immobilization, especially in elderly and low-demand cases, surgeons should recognize the clinical and radiographic characteristics of fractures best treated operatively. Intraarticular incongruity at the radiocarpal or radioulnar joints may not correct with closed manipulation, and those fractures with significant initial displacement, shortening, angulation, or severe metaphyseal comminution are unlikely to retain acceptable alignment (Fig. 36-1), even if an excellent initial reduction can be achieved. With moderate evidence, the 2011 American Academy of Orthopaedic Surgeons Clinical Practice Guidelines recommend open reduction and internal fixation (ORIF) for fractures with radial shortening more than 3 mm, dorsal tilt more than 10 degrees, or intraarticular displacement/step-off greater than 2 mm after closed reduction. In addition, inherently unstable fracture types, such as shear (Barton's) injuries, should also be treated operatively because they are predisposed to further displacement over time. If the nature of the fracture cannot be fully understood from plain radiographs, a computed tomographic scan of the distal radius (preferably with coronal, sagittal, and three-dimensional reconstructions) can be obtained.

Many different surgical techniques and implants have been developed for the management of distal radius fractures, and understanding the advantages and disadvantages of each is necessary to properly apply them. The simplest surgical technique, percutaneous pinning with immobilization, remains a valuable means of maintaining fracture reduction in simple extraarticular fractures when cast treatment alone is insufficient. Children and adolescents are often ideal candidates because bone quality is excellent, permanent implants are avoided, and any slight residual displacement corrects with bony remodeling. External fixation relies on the principle of ligamentotaxis to maintain displaced fracture fragments in acceptable alignment and historically was popular for unstable fractures that would lose reduction with plaster alone. Although it remains a viable option if extensive soft-tissue injury precludes immediate ORIF, as a means of definitive fixation, it has been largely replaced. Temporary bridge plating across the wrist for extensively comminuted, unreconstructable fractures achieves a similar reduction while avoiding the need for an external frame, and for reconstructable fractures, internal plating has become an alternative option. Compared with other forms of treatment, ORIF more consistently restores fracture alignment and offers improved early function. Broadly, modern plates draw on one of two philosophies to maintain fracture reduction: fixed-angle volar locking plates or fragment-specific locking plates. Volar locking plates are the most common form of

COMMONLY USED CPT CODES

- CPT Code: 25607—Open treatment of extraarticular distal radial fracture or epiphyseal separation, with or without fracture of ulnar styloid, with or without internal or external fixation
- CPT Code: 25608—Open treatment of intraarticular distal radial fracture or epiphyseal separation, with internal fixation of two fragments
- CPT Code: 25609—Open treatment of intraarticular distal radial fracture or epiphyseal separation with internal fixation of three or more fragments
- CPT Code: 25651—Percutaneous fixation ulnar styloid fracture
- CPT Code: 25652—Open treatment ulnar styloid fracture

COMMONLY USED ICD9 CODES

- 813.4—Fracture of lower end of radius or ulna closed
- 813.5—Fracture of lower end of radius or ulna open

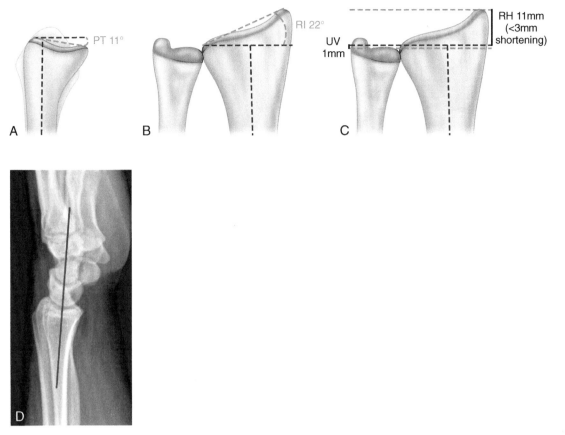

Figures 36-1 **A,** Normal values for palmar tilt *(PT);* **B,** radial inclination *(RI);* **C,** radial height *(RH)* and ulnar variance *(UV),* along with acceptable values for closed reduction in parentheses. In addition, on the lateral radiograph **D,** it should be possible to subtend a line near the center of the radial shaft, radiocarpal joint, lunate, and capitate.

fixation, and the technique for their use is the focus of this chapter. They effectively treat most fracture types, are well-tolerated, and allow for direct visualization of the extraarticular fracture reduction. Fragment-specific fixation uses separate plates to support the individual facets of the distal radius. These are indicated for specific fractures that would be poorly supported by routine volar plating, such as shear fractures of the radial styloid or volar or dorsal lunate facet injuries. In all cases, the surgical technique chosen is only a means to obtain and maintain fracture reduction; careful preoperative evaluation of the fracture is necessary to determine how best to do so.

SURGICAL TECHNIQUE

Room Set-Up

- A hand table, pneumatic tourniquet, and a minifluoroscopy unit are all necessary. Instruments and implants should be available and in the room before starting the case.
- Display preoperative imaging on view boxes or monitors that can be easily seen during the case.
- Adjust hand table and seat height before prepping.
- If using a traction table or weights, verify the presence of required finger traps, rope, or other equipment.

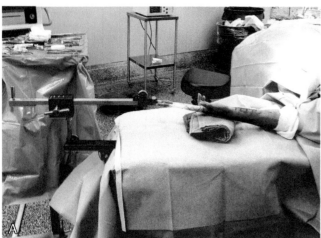
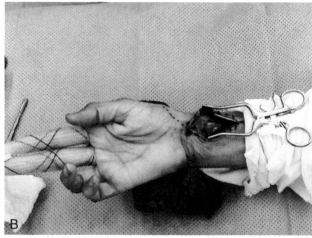

Figure 36-2 A, A table-mounted traction apparatus (Wrist Fracture System, Allen Medical, Acton, MA) can be used to assist in reduction of the fracture by bringing it out to length. Sustained traction also allows for stress-relaxation of the forearm musculature, which may allow the reduction to be performed more easily. **B,** Exposure of the fracture with the assistance of external traction. (Images courtesy of Brian Bear, MD, and Brian Foster, MD.)

Patient Positioning

- The patient is positioned supine on the operating room bed, with the operative extremity placed in the center of the hand table.
- A pneumatic tourniquet is placed on the upper arm before prepping.
- A unipolar cautery grounding pad is placed on the thigh or abdomen.
- Focus the operating room lights on the wrist such that they will not need to be moved again during the case.

Prepping and Draping

- The skin of the arm is prepared.
- Drape the arm with an extremity sheet covering the hand table, and a halfsheet or fullsheet to cover the remainder of the operating room bed.
- Drape the minifluoroscope with a sterile cover.
- If using intraoperative traction, apply liquid adhesive to the index and longer fingers followed by finger traps. Attach the traction apparatus or weights and apply traction through the wrist and forearm sufficient to bring the fracture out to length (Fig. 36-2).
- Pass instrument cords, such as for cautery or power tools, across the patient's body and secure them at the base of the hand table.
- Exsanguinate the arm and inflate the tourniquet.

Approach and Exposure

- Palpate the flexor carpi radialis (FCR) volarly, and mark its course from the distal volar wrist crease proximally.
- Mark a 6-cm to 8-cm incision directly over the FCR extending proximal from the distal volar wrist crease. The authors' preference is to create an ulnar-based flap at the distal extent of the incision to assist with distal exposure (Figs. 36-3 and 36-4), although a straight incision can also be used.
- Incise the skin to the level of the subcutaneous veins with the tip of a #15 blade scalpel.
- Cauterize small bridging skin veins crossing the field.
- Elevate the distal skin flap and tie down the apex to the ulnar side using a 4-0 nylon stitch.

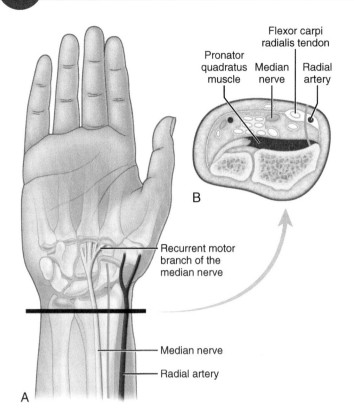

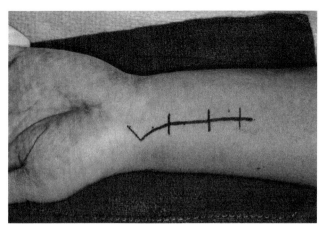

Figure 36-4 The planned surgical incision. Proximally, the incision follows the flexor carpi radialis (FCR) tendon. As it approaches the proximal volar wrist flexion crease, a slight curve radially is made, followed by a 90-degree angulation ulnarly to the distal volar flexion crease overlying the FCR tendon. This creates a skin flap that aids in distal exposure. (Copyright Mark S. Cohen.)

Figure 36-3 A, Approach through the flexor carpi radialis (FCR) tendon sheath floor. **B,** The approach is between the FCR tendon and the radial artery. Avoid excessive traction on the median nerve: 1, radial artery; 2, flexor carpi radialis tendon; 3, median nerve; 4, recurrent motor branch of the median nerve; and 5, pronator quadratus muscle.

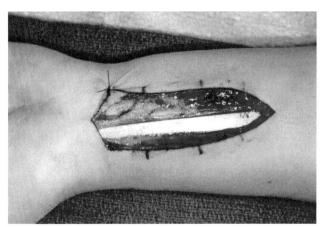

Figure 36-5 Dissection is carried down through the skin and subcutaneous fat to the level of the flexor carpi radialis tendon. The roof of the tendon sheath is incised to expose and mobilize the underlying tendon. (Copyright Mark S. Cohen.)

- With the scalpel, dissect down to and through the FCR tendon sheath (Fig. 36-5). Reflect the FCR ulnarly and place self-retaining (Gelpi) retractors. The palmar cutaneous branch of the median nerve lies along the ulnar aspect of the FCR floor and should be protected. Take care that the Gelpi retractors are placed superficially on the radial side so as not to injure the radial artery (Fig. 36-6).
- With a Ragnell retractor to retract proximally then distally, continue with the scalpel through the thin floor of the FCR tendon sheath, with care taken not to cut the underlying muscle. Distally, this fascial layer is confluent with the transverse carpal ligament and can be released. If a full carpal tunnel release is required, however, this should be done through a separate palmar incision.
- At the distal end of the incision, identify and either protect or cauterize the superficial crossing branch of the radial artery.
- Use a gauze pad to sweep the flexor pollicis longus (FPL) muscle belly ulnarly, exposing the radial shaft and pronator quadratus. Readjust the ulnar arms of the Gelpi retractors to hold the FPL ulnarly and out of the field (Fig. 36-7).

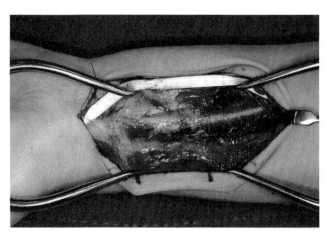

Figure 36-6 The flexor carpi radialis (FCR) tendon is retracted ulnarly, protecting the palmar cutaneous branch of the median nerve. This exposes the floor of the FCR tendon sheath, which is incised to reveal the muscle belly of the flexor pollicis longus. (Copyright Mark S. Cohen.)

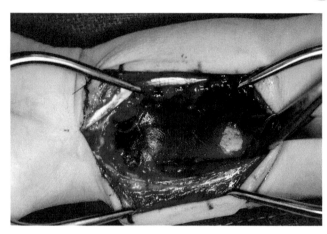

Figure 36-7 The flexor pollicis longus (FPL) is swept ulnarly with the digital flexor tendons, exposing the pronator quadratus (PQ), which is incised longitudinally in the center of the radius to the level of the red-white junction. Radial and ulnar flaps of the PQ are reflected off of the bone, exposing the fracture and radial shaft. Note the claw clamp on the radial shaft proximally. This helps control the shaft during the reduction maneuver. (Copyright Mark S. Cohen.)

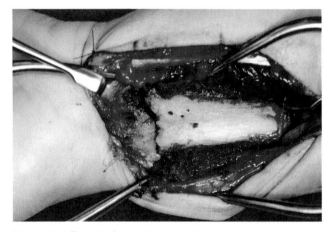

Figure 36-8 The volar fracture lines are fully exposed and cleared of any entrapped muscle, periosteum, or fracture callus that may block reduction. (Copyright Mark S. Cohen)

- A lobster claw is placed on the radial shaft proximally at this time to provide proximal fragment control.
- With unipolar cautery, the pronator quadratus (PQ) is divided longitudinally. Care is taken not to extend distally because this can damage the volar radiocarpal ligaments and destabilize the wrist.
- Dissect the PQ off of the radius radially and ulnarly; the ulnar corner is key to confirming reduction at the distal radioulnar joint and must be well-exposed (Fig. 36-8).
- The brachioradialis tendon is released from the radial styloid to prevent it from acting as a deforming force. This is accomplished by dissecting out and protecting the first dorsal compartment tendons as they cross the radial styloid; the brachioradialis tendon is readily identified just proximal to this at its attachment to the radius. With a scalpel or small rongeur, clean the fracture edges and any muscle or callus from the fracture site that may impede reduction.

Reduction and Fixation

- Once the fracture has been cleared of any obstructive debris, it can be reduced. Most dorsally displaced fractures are reduced with a combination of downward (dorsal-directed) force on the radial shaft along with volar and ulnar translation of the distal fragment (Fig. 36-9).
- A traction table can assist in pulling the fracture out to length (see Fig. 36-2, *B*), but this is rarely necessary. Manual manipulation is most important in correcting translation and angulation before fixation.
- If the fracture remains "short" or dorsally translated, a freer elevator can be placed into the fracture site to lever it up and into position on the proximal shaft. Care should be taken not to break any of the fracture spikes, which aid in reduction.
- If necessary, a 0.062-inch K-wire can be placed from the styloid across the fracture to help maintain the reduction. Smaller K-wires can also be used to help keep smaller, partial articular fractures in place.
- Confirm reduction with anteroposterior and lateral fluoroscopy. Carefully assess the restoration of gross length and alignment and the quality of the articular reduction at the radiocarpal and distal radioulnar joints.
- Reduction is maintained with the assistant using downward pressure on the radial shaft while the operative hand is placed over a rolled towel, maintaining volar flexion and translation at the fracture site.
- Place the selected distal radial plate on the volar cortex. Generally, the plate should be centered on the distal radius, but specific fracture patterns may benefit from slight radial or ulnar plate translation.
- Place a nonlocking cortical screw into the oblong shaft hole of the plate and fine-tune the plate's position with fluoroscopy. The distal locking screws should run distal enough to capture and protect any intraarticular comminution while safely staying out of the joint. Care is taken to subtract 1 to 2 mm from all distal screw measurements to decrease the potential for extensor tendon embarrassment.
- Place the distal, fixed-angle locking screws in to the distal fracture fragment, followed by the remaining proximal locking screws (Figs. 36-10 and 36-11).
- Use fluoroscopy to confirm the reduction and appropriate placement of fixation.

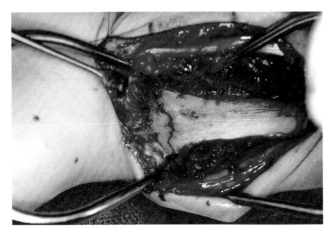

Figure 36-9 The fracture is reduced anatomically. For most dorsally angulated fractures, this is performed with volar translation of the distal fragment while applying a dorsally directed force to the radial shaft. The radial shaft may have to be translated ulnarly as well to achieve the reduction. A rolled towel underneath the wrist and distal fracture fragment can assist in maintaining reduction and volar tilt. (Copyright Mark S. Cohen.)

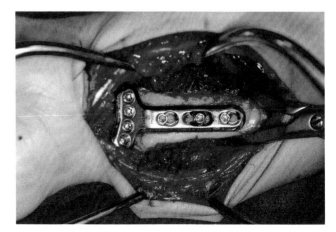

Figure 36-10 A volar locking plate is applied. A cortical screw is placed in the oblong hole of the plate first, which allows for fine-tuning of the distal-proximal placement and rotation of the plate. The distal locking screws are placed next, from ulnar to radial, followed by the remaining cortical shaft screws. (Copyright Mark S. Cohen)

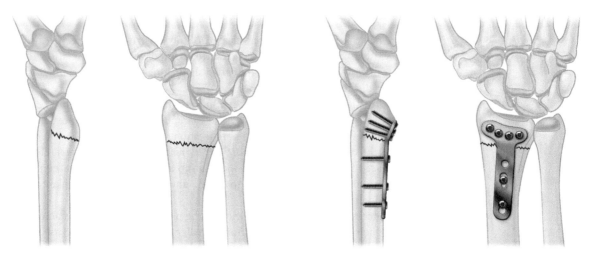

Figure 36-11 Anteroposterior and lateral views of distal radius fracture before and after open reduction internal fixation with volar plate.

Closure and Dressing

- The authors do not routinely close the PQ over the plate because it does not appear to affect outcomes.
- The dermal layer of the skin is closed with 4-0 absorbable suture, followed by horizontal mattress sutures of 4-0 nylon to close the skin.
- The incision is dressed with petroleum gauze, dry cotton gauze, and cast padding followed by a short-arm volar splint for comfort. Dressings should not obstruct motion of the thumb or finger metacarpophalangeal joints.

BRIEF SUMMARY OF SURGICAL STEPS

- The distal radius is approached volarly with an incision overlying the flexor carpi radialis (FCR) tendon
- Dissection is carried through the floor of the FCR tendon, retracting the carpal tunnel contents ulnarly and the radial artery laterally
- The fracture is exposed by dividing and reflecting the pronator quadratus, then cleaning it of callus and entrapped periosteum and muscle
- Reduce the fracture; for most dorsally displaced and angulated fractures, this requires a combination of traction, volar and ulnar translation of the distal fragment, and dorsally applied force to the proximal radial shaft
- Apply a volar locking plate to the proximal shaft with a single nonlocking screw in the oblong hole
- Confirm the plate position and reduction, and insert the distal locking screws; all screws should be 1 to 2 mm shorter than measured length
- Insert the remaining shaft screws
- Close the skin and dress the wound with a volar splint and compressive bandage

REQUIRED EQUIPMENT

Hand table, with a traction setup if desired
Pneumatic tourniquet
Minifluoroscopy unit
Basic hand instrument tray
A pneumatic, electric, or battery-powered drill and K-wire driver
Distal radius fracture implant and tool trays
Suture and dressings for closure

TECHNICAL PEARLS

- Critically assess preoperative radiographs or computed tomographic scan to determine the optimal approach, reduction technique, and fixation; although most fractures can be treated with volar locking plates, this may not be the best technique
- For fractures with extensive comminution or bone loss, obtain preoperative radiographs of the uninjured wrist
- The volar approach allows direct visualization of extraarticular fracture lines, but to fully assess the articular surface, either an open dorsal or arthroscopic approach is also required
- With the traditional volar approach, the flexor carpi radialis tendon and flexor pollicis longus musculature are swept ulnarly to help protect the median nerve and its branches
- Exposure of the fracture must be carried over to the volar, ulnar corner of the distal radius because this fracture key corresponds to the reduction of the distal radioulnar joint
- Reduce the fracture correctly once and keep it reduced; repeated reduction attempts disrupt fracture keys stability
- Radial-ulnar translation of the plate must be correct before placing a screw in the oblong hole; distal-proximal translation and rotation of the plate can be corrected after the oblong screw hole is filled, while radial-ulnar translation is fixed
- Once all hardware is in place, move the wrist through flexion, extension, pronation, and supination to confirm a smooth arc of motion; if instability of the distal radioulnar joint (DRUJ) is present along with an ulnar styloid fracture, it should be fixed

COMMON PITFALLS

(When to call for the attending physician)

- Improper incision placement:
  - The incision should extend proximally from the distal wrist flexion crease over the flexor carpi radialis (FCR) tendon
  - Common errors are to place the incision too distal or proximal, or mistake the palmaris longus tendon for the FCR
  - The FCR can always be felt along a line from the distal pole of the scaphoid to the medial epicondyle of the elbow
- Damage to the palmar cutaneous nerve:
  - Although it is generally ulnar to the FCR tendon (running between the FCR and flexor pollicis longus), in rare instances or revision cases, it may be more radial and injured by careless dissection
- Injury to the radial artery with overly radial dissection or puncture with sharp self-retaining retractors
- Reflecting the pronator quadratus from the radius distal to the red-white junction, which may detach the volar radiocarpal ligaments and destabilize the wrist
- Incomplete visualization of the fracture and consequent malreduction
- Failure to appreciate and correct articular depression, which may also lead to intraarticular hardware placement, even if gross alignment and angulation is restored
- Intraarticular or prominent dorsal hardware. Fluoroscopic images parallel to the lunate facet on the anteroposterior and radial styloid on the lateral best assess for articular penetration; oblique views can help with dorsal screw prominence
- Failing to have a backup plan for complex fractures
  - A combination of approaches or techniques may be required for atypical or highly comminuted fractures

POSTOPERATIVE PROTOCOL

Most patients are discharged home on the day of surgery and are instructed to keep their surgical dressings in place until their first postoperative clinic visit. For high-energy injuries or with concerns for postoperative swelling, an overnight stay with elevation and regular neurologic checks is warranted. Active and passive finger motion exercises are encouraged to help decrease swelling and maximize digital motion. At 7 to 10 days, the operative dressings and stitches typically are removed. The patient is fitted for a removable short-arm splint, which is worn full-time, apart from formal therapy and motion exercises. At 6 to 8 weeks, the splint is weaned and isometric strengthening initiated, followed by lightweight dynamic strengthening at 10 weeks. If patients are doing well by 12 weeks, they are allowed to slowly return to activity as tolerated.

POSTOPERATIVE CLINIC VISIT PROTOCOL

7-10 days: Remove operative dressings and sutures. Apply custom or prefabricated removable splint and start rehabilitation program under the supervision of an occupational therapist.

6-8 weeks: Wean from the splint and start isometric strengthening. Continue with non–weight-bearing activity. Dynamic strengthening can begin 2 weeks later.

12 weeks: Transition to a home therapy program and slowly return to activity as tolerated.

Patients who are doing well can opt to follow-up on an as-needed basis. Patients with complicated or slower recovery should be seen for additional scheduled follow-up visits as indicated.

SUGGESTED READINGS

1. Arora R, Lutz M, Deml C, Krappinger D, Haug L, Gabl M. A prospective randomized trial comparing nonoperative treatment with volar locking plate fixation for displaced and unstable distal radial fractures in patients sixty-five years of age and older. *J Bone Joint Surg Am*. 2011;93(23):2146-2153.
2. Court-Brown CM, Caesar B. Epidemiology of adult fractures: a review. *Injury*. 2006;37(8):691-697.
3. Court-Brown CM, Bugler KE, Clement ND, Duckworth AD, McQueen MM. The epidemiology of open fractures in adults. A 15-year review. *Injury*. 2012;43(6):891-897.
4. Egol KA, Walsh M, Romo-Cardoso S, Dorsky S, Paksima N. Distal radial fractures in the elderly: operative compared with nonoperative treatment. *J Bone Joint Surg Am*. 2010;92(9):1851-1857.
5. Hershman SH, Immerman I, Bechtel C, Lekic N, Paksima N, Egol KA. The effects of pronator quadratus repair on outcomes after volar plating of distal radius fractures. *J Orthop Trauma*. 2013;27(3):130-133.
6. Koval K, Haidukewych GJ, Service B. Zirgibel BJ. Controversies in the management of distal radius fractures. *J Am Acad Orthop Surg*. 2014;22(9):566-575.
7. Lafontaine M, Hardy D, Delince PH. Stability assessment of distal radius fractures. *Injury*. 1989;20(4):208-210.
8. Lichtman DM, Bindra RR, Boyer MI, et al. American academy of orthopaedic surgeons clinical practice guideline on: the treatment of distal radius fractures. *J Bone Joint Surg Am*. 2011;93(8):775-778.
9. Nellans KW, Kowalski E, Chung KC. The epidemiology of distal radius fractures. *Hand Clin*. 2012;28(2):113-125.
10. Ruch DS, Ginn TA, Yang CC, Smith BP, Rushing J, Hanel DP. Use of a distraction plate for distal radial fractures with metaphyseal and diaphyseal comminution. *J Bone Joint Surg Am*. 2005;87(5):945-954.

TOTAL SHOULDER ARTHROPLASTY

Peter N. Chalmers | Alexander W. Aleem | Leesa M. Galatz

CASE MINIMUM REQUIREMENTS

- N = 0

COMMONLY USED CPT CODES

- CPT Code: 23472—Total shoulder arthroplasty or reverse total shoulder arthroplasty
- CPT Code: 23470—Hemiarthroplasty
- CPT Code: 23332—To be used in association with 23472 for revision total shoulder arthroplasty
- CPT Code: 23331—To be used in association with 23470 for revision hemiarthroplasty

COMMONLY USED ICD9 CODES

- 715.91—Degenerative joint disease or osteoarthritis of the shoulder
- 716.11—Traumatic arthropathy of the shoulder
- 714.00—Rheumatoid arthritis
- 733.41—Avascular necrosis of the head of the humerus
- 812.00—Proximal humerus fracture
- 718.01—Shoulder articular cartilage disorder

COMMONLY USED ICD10 CODES

- M19.01—Primary osteoarthritis, shoulder
- M12.51—Traumatic arthropathy, shoulder
- M05—Rheumatoid arthritis with rheumatoid factor
- M87.02—Idiopathic aseptic necrosis of humerus
- S42.2—Fracture of upper end of humerus
- M24.11—Other articular cartilage disorders, shoulder

Since the popularization of shoulder hemiarthroplasty by Neer in the 1950s, shoulder arthroplasty has been performed with increasing frequency, with more than 27,000 total shoulder arthroplasties (TSAs) and 20,000 hemiarthroplasties (HAs) performed in the United States in 2008 alone. TSA is indicated for primary osteoarthritis, rheumatoid arthritis, posttraumatic arthritis, and instability arthropathy (as long as the rotator cuff is intact and functional), which makes it a crucial portion of the shoulder surgeon's armamentarium. TSA has been shown to have excellent long-term outcomes with sustained pain relief, function, and range of motion.

The main contraindications include active infection, axillary nerve palsy, rotator cuff insufficiency, and severe glenoid bone loss that would preclude adequate fixation of the glenoid component. Rotator cuff dysfunction can lead to eccentric loading of the glenoid component with the "rocking horse glenoid phenomenon" and accelerated glenoid loosening. After surgery, the most common early complications include infection, hematoma, neurologic injury, periprosthetic fracture, and instability. The most common late complication is proximal humeral migration from rotator cuff dysfunction with resultant glenoid loosening.

SURGICAL TECHNIQUE (VIDEO 37-1)

Room Set-Up

- Shoulder surgery is generally performed with the table at a 45-degree angle with respect to the room, with the surgeon positioned at the anterior aspect of the shoulder, the operative assistants at the lateral and posterior aspects of the shoulder, the scrub nurse on the contralateral or ipsilateral side of the patient, and the anesthesia team at the head of the bed toward the contralateral side.
- The surgeon can use an adjustable, articulated, pneumatic arm holder (McConnell, Inc., Greenville, TX), a padded mayo stand, or a short armboard for intraoperative positioning of the operative arm. Generally, a second mayo stand is positioned over the patient's abdomen.

Patient Positioning

- TSA is usually performed with the patient in the beach chair position. First, the patient must be positioned in the bed so that the "break" within the bed falls at the patient's hips.
- The patient's anterior superior iliac spine is positioned 1 handbreadth above the break in the bed. The head is positioned with a commercial head holder with a foam facemask to ensure cervical spine stability and patient safety. A foam wedge or pillow is placed under the knees to take pressure off the sciatic and peroneal nerves during surgery.

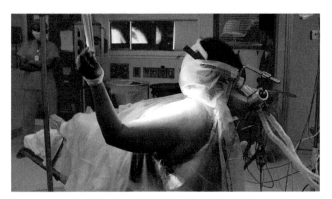

Figure 37-1 Room set-up and patient positioning before skin preparation and draping.

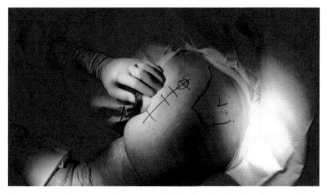

Figure 37-2 Set-up of the surgical field after draping but before placement of adherent, occlusive iodinated dressing.

- Pneumatic sleeves are routinely used on lower extremities for deep venous thrombosis prophylaxis. The back of the bed is then raised to 60 to 70 degrees, with close observation of the patient's blood pressure for orthostasis. The head then must be readjusted to maintain neutral cervical alignment.
- Kidney rests are placed to keep the patient's torso from shifting. An armrest can be placed for the contralateral side.
- Specialized shoulder tables are available to give access to the posterior aspect of the shoulder. If such a table is not available, the patient must be shifted as far toward the operative side as possible before positioning the head and raising the back of the bed. The "leg" portion of the table then can be flexed to provide additional knee flexion.

Prepping and Draping

- The operative field should be shaved and then sealed from the remainder of the body with adhesive plastic drapes, ensuring that the scapula, clavicle, and neck are prepped into the field (Fig. 37-1).
- After sterile skin preparation, the authors drape the body with a half sheet and seal the operative field with adhesive U-drapes from the neck down and the torso up. The arm then is draped to just below the axilla with an impervious stockinette fixated with self-adherent wrap (Coban, 3M, Inc, St. Paul, MN).
- If the surgeon chooses to use an arm holder, it can be placed at this time (Fig. 37-2). The authors also prefer to seal the skin of the operative field with an occlusive iodinated adherent drape (Ioban, 3M Inc, St. Paul, MN).
- The surgeon should perform an appropriate surgical time-out to confirm the patient, the procedure, and the surgical site and that preoperative antibiotics have been administered.

Approach

- A standard deltopectoral approach is used with an 8-cm to 12-cm incision from the coracoid process toward the insertion of the deltoid (Figs. 37-3 and 37-4). Electrocautery is used to dissect through the fat, with self-retaining retractors proximally and distally.
- While dissecting superficially, the surgeon should err medially because the deltoid tends to "drape" over the coracoid. The coracoid is consistently palpable and can serve as a guide to locating the deltopectoral interval. In addition, a conserved triangle of fat can aid the surgeon in identifying the proximal aspect of the interval (Fig. 37-5).

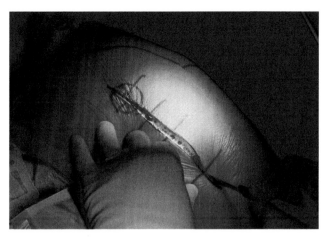

Figure 37-3 Incision extends from the coracoid process to the deltoid insertion.

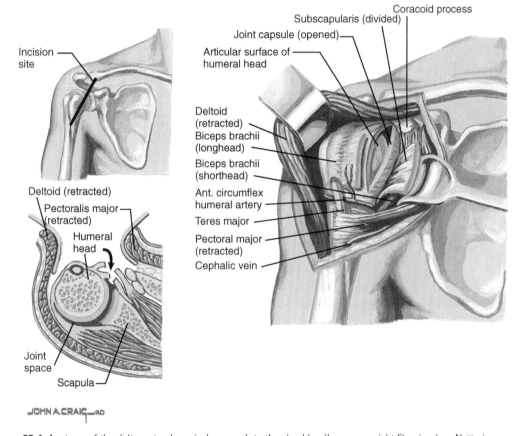

Figure 37-4 Anatomy of the deltopectoral surgical approach to the shoulder. (Image copyright Elsevier, Inc., Netterimages.com.)

- The surgeon then can use scissor dissection technique to open the interval and to free the medial aspect of the cephalic vein so that it can be mobilized laterally with the deltoid.
- Place a Richardson retractor under the deltoid and the vein and bluntly release any subdeltoid bursal scarring, working from distal to proximal and using a Cobb elevator and curved mayo scissors as necessary.
- The rotator cuff should be protected during this mobilization. The clavipectoral fascia overlying the lateral aspect of the conjoint tendon is released. The proximal 2 cm of the pectoralis major humeral insertion is released with electrocautery if

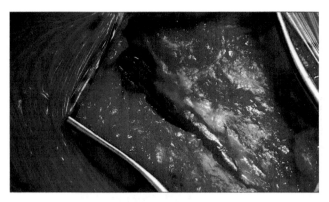

Figure 37-5 This image shows the deltopectoral interval and the cephalic vein. Proximally, the vein can be seen to extend into the deeper tissues with an overlying, conserved triangle of adipose tissue.

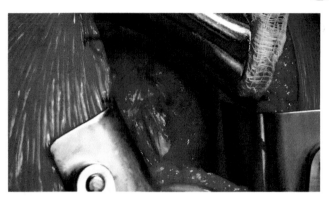

Figure 37-6 Wound appearance after placement of the Buxton. A slit has been made in the bicipital sheath with the electrocautery.

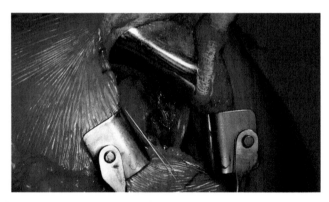

Figure 37-7 The rotator interval has been released, and a traction stitch has been placed in the subscapularis.

additional exposure is needed, with care taken not to violate the bicipital sheath deep to the pectoralis major insertion.

- The surgeon should palpate and identify the axillary nerve as it courses inferiorly and laterally superficial to the anterior aspect of the subscapularis, turning posterior at the inferior border to travel beneath the inferior glenoid neck toward the quadrilateral space. The surgeon must be aware of the location of the axillary nerve at all times because an axillary nerve injury is a devastating and debilitating complication.

- A self-retaining retractor, such as a Buxton, a Kolbel, or a "baby" Balfour, can be placed under the deltoid and the conjoint tendon, with care taken not to place traction on the axillary or musculocutaneous nerve (Fig. 37-6).

- Identify and tag with stout nonabsorbable sutures the lateral aspect of the subscapularis tendon. The anterior humeral circumflex artery and its two accompanying veins, the "three sisters," course along the inferior one third of the subscapularis and can be cauterized (or suture ligated) to control bleeding. Just lateral to the lesser tuberosity is the intertubercular groove. The groove is unroofed, and biceps tenotomy or tenodesis is performed. Release the rotator interval along the superior rolled border of the subscapularis as it travels toward the coracoid (Fig. 37-7). Electrocautery then can be used to release the soft tissue from the medial aspect of the intertubercular groove, traveling distal to the insertion of the subscapularis to release the latissimus.

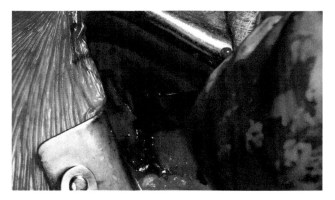

Figure 37-8 Lesser tuberosity osteotomy.

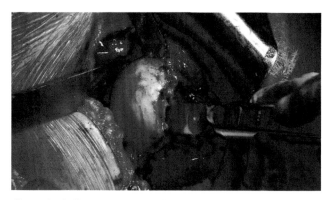

Figure 37-9 Humeral neck cut with placement of protecting retractors.

Subscapularis Takedown

■ Several options exist for management of the subscapularis, including tenotomy, release of the tendon directly from the bone, a peel, or osteotomy of the lesser tuberosity.

■ One technique has not emerged definitively as superior to another technique; however, subscapularis insufficiency is debilitating. Therefore, a careful takedown and repair is critical. The authors prefer to make an osteotomy of the lesser tuberosity with a curved half-inch osteotome, starting from the base of the groove. The bone is scored with the osteotome and then an osteotomy of the tuberosity is performed (Fig. 37-8). The subscapularis then can be released in a full-thickness sleeve with the capsule off the inferior calcar and humeral neck while adducting, externally rotating, and flexing the arm to progressively dislocate the humeral head.

■ During this process, the surgeon must be careful because the axillary nerve is at risk. Use short bursts of electrocautery to avoid excess heat build-up and remove the self-retaining retractor to take the nerve off tension.

Humeral Preparation

■ Expose the humeral neck with two Darrach retractors, one under the neck to protect the pectoralis and the axillary nerve and one intraarticularly. Excise marginal osteophytes as needed with a curved osteotome, with care taken not to compromise the teres minor insertion posteriorly.

■ A large Bankart elevator then can be placed at the insertion of the rotator cuff with a sponge to protect the deltoid. Before making the humeral head cut, the surgeon must have adequate visualization of the anatomic neck, the insertion of the rotator cuff, and the bare area.

■ To match the patient's anatomic version, the plane of the osteotomy shoulder intersects the chondral border, passing through the middle of the bare area and exiting just medial to the insertion of the rotator cuff (Fig. 37-9). A cut parallel to the forearm is neutral version by definition. Little to no bone should remain adjacent to the superior-most aspect of the cuff; however, the bare area should remain more posterior, or the osteotomy will be too retroverted.

■ The steps for humeral preparation differ slightly depending on the implant system selected. Generally, the canal is opened with progressive reamers and broaches. A trial stem then is implanted, with care taken to ensure that anatomic version is recreated and that the stem seats evenly (Fig. 37-10). The osteotomy can then be coplaned. The surgeon should err on the small side to avoid overstuffing the joint.

■ An oversized head results in increased cuff tension and joint reactive forces that lead to cuff failure and glenoid wear. The eccentric trial head is rotated until the optimal coverage is selected, and this position is marked with electrocautery and

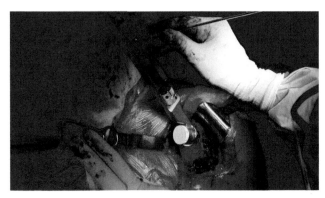

Figure 37-10 Placement of the humeral trial, positioned to avoid varus and anteversion.

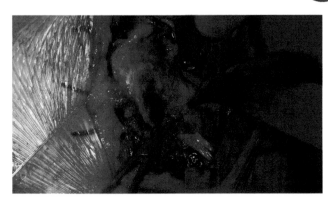

Figure 37-11 Subscapularis mobilization. The cancellous surface of the lesser tuberosity osteotomy fragment can be seen in the center of the wound.

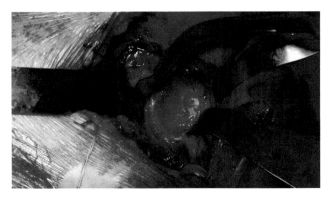

Figure 37-12 Optimal placement of retractors for glenoid visualization.

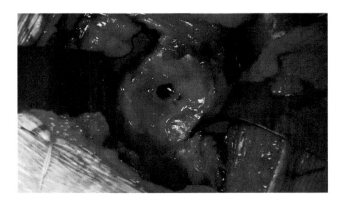

Figure 37-13 Placement of the glenoid center hole and appearance of the glenoid after reaming.

communicated to the scrub nurse. The head trial then can be removed to improve the glenoid exposure.

Glenoid Preparation

- Abduct and externally rotate the arm and place two Bankart retractors at the posterior and posterosuperior aspects of the glenoid. With the retention sutures placed previously for traction on the subscapularis, perform a circumferential release of the rotator interval and anterior and inferior capsule around the subscapularis with mayo scissors (Fig. 37-11), with care taken to protect the axillary nerve along the anterior and inferior aspects of the subscapularis. During this process, the superior glenohumeral ligament and middle glenohumeral ligament are resected. A Bankart retractor can then be placed anterior to the glenoid, completing the glenoid exposure (Fig. 37-12).
- Any residual labrum, biceps anchor, and cartilage then can be sharply removed from the glenoid. Mark the center of the glenoid and place a guide pin for reaming. Generally, reaming must continue until the glenoid has a smooth surface, but the surgeon must be diligent not to ream into subchondral bone because this weakens the bone (Fig. 37-13). The glenoid is prepared according to protocol for the chosen prosthesis. The authors prefer a pegged glenoid.

Cementation of Implants

- While the scrub nurse is mixing the cement on the back table, use pulsatile irrigation to clean the glenoid. Pack cement into the glenoid with syringe and sponge pressurization, twisting the syringe while extracting it to avoid pulling cement out

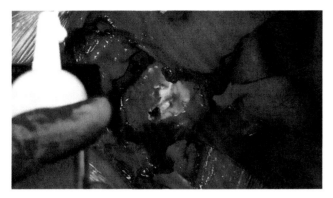

Figure 37-14 Pressurization of cement for the glenoid component. The syringe used for pressurization can be seen to the left of the image.

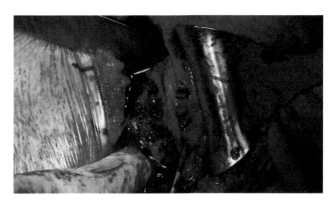

Figure 37-15 Placement of drill holes for passage of transhumeral, stout, reinforced, nonabsorbable sutures for later repair of the lesser tuberosity osteotomy.

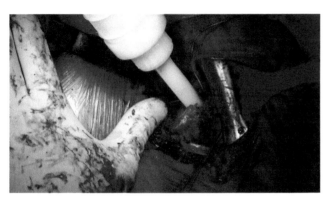

Figure 37-16 Cementation of the humeral component.

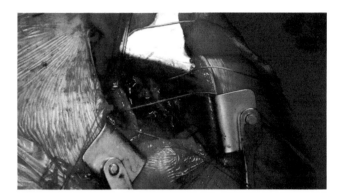

Figure 37-17 Passage of the lesser tuberosity osteotomy sutures through the subscapularis before suture tying.

(Fig. 37-14). Insert and impact the glenoid component and then maintain thumb pressure against the component while clearing excess cement with a freer elevator. Once the cement has hardened, carefully remove the retractors, with care not to scratch or damage the glenoid component.

- Expose the proximal humerus with Darrach retractors and a deltoid retractor. Remove the humeral trial and assemble the humeral component on the back table. While the scrub nurse is mixing cement, clean the humerus with pulsatile irrigation. Place three drill holes just lateral to the intertubercular groove and pass three stout, reinforced, nonabsorbable sutures through these holes for repair of the lesser tuberosity osteotomy (Fig. 37-15). The bottom two canal limbs of the suture pass around the stem of the prosthesis and are positioned appropriately in anticipation of stem insertion. The authors typically use proximal cement technique, placing a moderate amount of cement into the proximal canal (Fig. 37-16). Monitor the component during insertion to avoid varus or anteversion. Once the component is seated, hold pressure until the cement hardens. Alternatively, a cementless prosthesis can be used according to surgeon preference.

Closure

- Reduce the humeral head and place the arm into neutral rotation. Stability is assessed, and the prosthesis should slide posteriorly but spontaneously reduce with release of translation forces.
- Place a retractor under the deltoid. Pass the stitches previously placed through the humerus through the musculotendinous junction of the subscapularis just medial to the lesser tuberosity and use these to reduce the lesser tuberosity fragment (Fig. 37-17).

- Tie the sutures, starting with the middle, proceeding to the inferior, and finishing with the superior, ensuring that tension is maintained while tying.
- After closure of the subscapularis, assess the posterior translation of the humerus head, which should be roughly 50% of the width of the glenoid with spontaneous reduction.
- Also check the axillary nerve by placing one finger under the nerve as it passes around the anterior subscapularis and another finger under the nerve as it travels on the undersurface of the deltoid, with a tug on one finger transmitted into the other finger.
- Irrigate the wound. The authors routinely place a subdeltoid drain, although this step also depends on surgeon preference. Close and dress the wound in the usual fashion. Place a sling before changing the patient's position.

BRIEF SUMMARY OF SURGICAL STEPS

- Position the patient in the beach chair position
- Incise along the deltopectoral interval
- Open the deltopectoral interval, retracting the cephalic vein laterally
- Release subdeltoid adhesions, open the clavipectoral fascia, and release the proximal aspect of the pectoralis major insertion
- Open the intertubercular groove, follow biceps into the rotator interval, and perform tenotomy
- Open the rotator interval
- Perform a lesser tuberosity osteotomy and release the humeral inferior capsule
- Perform the humeral neck cut and prepare the metaphysis and diaphysis of the humerus
- Place trial humeral components
- Mobilize the subscapularis circumferentially, releasing anterior and inferior capsule
- Expose the glenoid and remove the labrum
- Ream the glenoid and machine for a peg or keeled component
- Cement the glenoid component
- Place three stout, reinforced, nonabsorbable sutures through the anterior humeral cortex for later repair of the subscapularis
- Cement the humeral component
- Reduce the shoulder and repair the subscapularis
- Irrigate and close

REQUIRED EQUIPMENT

Adjustable operating room table to allow beach chair positioning

Full set of shoulder retractors, including Bankart, Buxton, Darrach, and deltoid retractors

Stout, reinforced, nonabsorbable sutures for subscapularis repair

At least two bags of cement; the authors prefer to include 1.2 g of tobramycin per 40 g of cement

A total shoulder arthroplasty system, with the appropriate reamers, broaches, instruments for machining the glenoid, trial components, etc.

Power with a set of drills and a saw blade

TECHNICAL PEARLS

- Proper patient positioning and draping is a critical portion of the procedure; ensure that the head is stabilized and that the entirety of the shoulder girdle is included in the sterile field
- Develop a consistent and reproducible mechanism to position the arm during surgery; the authors prefer a pneumatic, adjustable, articulated arm holder
- During exposure, the coracoid and the proximal triangle of fat can be guides to assist in locating the deltopectoral interval
- Retract the cephalic vein laterally with the deltoid because there are fewer medial than lateral tributaries
- Release the superior aspect of the pectoralis major insertion to improve exposure
- Identify the long head of the biceps tendon to identify the rotator interval and subscapularis insertion
- Replicate the patient's anatomy with the humeral neck osteotomy
- Circumferentially mobilize the subscapularis to fully expose the glenoid
- A lesser tuberosity osteotomy can improve glenoid exposure, as can a complete inferior capsular release, resection of osteophytes, resection of excess calcar bone, and reaming of the anterior glenoid in cases of retroversion
- Do not oversize the humeral head
- Pressurize the cement in the glenoid
- After closure, ensure that the patient has maintained 50% posterior translation of the humeral head with spontaneous reduction

COMMON PITFALLS

(When to call for the attending physician)

- Improper positioning can make intraoperative visualization near impossible
- Ensure that the deltopectoral interval is identified before splitting muscle fibers to avoid possibly denervating a portion of the anterior deltoid
- Use scissors dissection around the cephalic vein; maintenance of the vein improves physiologic venous return from the arm and aids in identification of the deltopectoral interval in future revision surgery
- Identify the axillary nerve before subscapularis takedown and studiously protect it through the procedure
- Avoid injuring the superior or posterior cuff insertion in the humeral neck osteotomy
- Avoid overstuffing the joint during selection of a humeral head size
- Avoid violating the subchondral surface of the glenoid or leaving any irregularities in the glenoid
- When cementing the glenoid, twist the syringe while extracting it to avoid pulling cement out
- Inadequate release of anterior capsule, inferior capsule, and rotator interval can make glenoid exposure difficult
- Monitor the humeral component during preparation, trialing, and implantation to avoid varus position or anteversion of the component
- Ensure that tension is maintained on the suture during repair of the subscapularis and that square knots are tied

POSTOPERATIVE PROTOCOL

Initial postoperative management depends on subscapularis technique. If an osteotomy is performed, the patient wears a sling for 7 to 10 days. If tenotomy is performed, a longer period of immobilization is used, up to 6 weeks. This protocol is for patients with an osteotomy. The sling is removed the first postoperative day for waist-level activity and elbow, wrist, and hand range of motion. Active-assisted flexion and continuous passive motion machine is started on postoperative day 1. Patients progress from active-assisted range of motion to active range of motion as tolerated but are restricted from actively internally rotating or extending the shoulder for 6 weeks to protect the subscapularis repair. Range of motion goals are 90 degrees of forward elevation, 20 degrees of external rotation, and 75 degrees of abduction at 1 week and 120 degrees of forward elevation, 40 degrees of external rotation, and 75 degrees of abduction at 2 weeks. The most important aspect of therapy in the first several weeks after surgery is recovering range of motion. When motion returns, strength follows. Most patients are on a home program and only go to supervised physical therapy if range of motion goals are not attained.

POSTOPERATIVE CLINICAL VISIT PROTOCOL

Patients generally follow-up at 2 weeks after surgery to ensure that the wound is healing and that no hematoma has formed. Subsequent visits occur at 3 months, 6 months, and 1 year. The authors see patients every other year thereafter for surveillance radiographs to monitor for osteolysis, subsidence, and wear.

SUGGESTED READINGS

1. Defranco MJ, Higgins LD, Warner JJP. Subscapularis management in open shoulder surgery. *J Am Acad Orthop Surg.* 2010;18(12):707-717.
2. Flatow EL, Bigliani LU. Tips of the trade. Locating and protecting the axillary nerve in shoulder surgery: the tug test. *Orthop Rev.* 1992;21(4):503-505.
3. Franklin JL, Barrett WP, Jackins SE, Matsen FA. Glenoid loosening in total shoulder arthroplasty. Association with rotator cuff deficiency. *J Arthroplasty.* 1988;3(1):39-46.
4. Gerber C, Pennington SD, Yian EH, Pfirrmann CAW, Werner CML, Zumstein MA. Lesser tuberosity osteotomy for total shoulder arthroplasty. Surgical technique. *J Bone Joint Surg Am.* 2006;88(suppl 1 Pt 2):170-177. doi:10.2106/JBJS.F.00407.
5. Groh GI, Simoni M, Rolla P, Rockwood CA. Loss of the deltoid after shoulder operations: an operative disaster. *J Shoulder Elbow Surg.* 1994;3(4):243-253. doi:10.1016/S1058-2746(09)80042-6.
6. Harryman DT. Common surgical approaches to the shoulder. *Instr Course Lect.* 1992;41:3-11.
7. Kim SH, Wise BL, Zhang Y, Szabo RM. Increasing incidence of shoulder arthroplasty in the United States. *J Bone Joint Surg Am.* 2011;93(24):2249-2254. doi:10.2106/JBJS.J.01994.
8. Raiss P, Bruckner T, Rickert M, Walch G. Longitudinal observational study of total shoulder replacements with cement: fifteen to twenty-year follow-up. *J Bone Joint Surg Am.* 2014;96(3):198-205. doi:10.2106/JBJS.M.00079.
9. Raiss P, Schmitt M, Bruckner T, et al. Results of cemented total shoulder replacement with a minimum follow-up of ten years. *J Bone Joint Surg Am.* 2012;94:e171(1-10).
10. Young A, Walch G, Boileau P, et al. A multicentre study of the long-term results of using a flat-back polyethylene glenoid component in shoulder replacement for primary osteoarthritis. *J Bone Joint Surg Br.* 2011;93(2):210-216. doi:10.1302/0301-620X.93B2.25086.

MIDSHAFT CLAVICLE FRACTURE OPEN REDUCTION AND INTERNAL FIXATION

Sanjeev Bhatia | Joshua A. Greenspoon | Maximilian Petri | Peter J. Millett

CASE MINIMUM REQUIREMENTS

- There are no ACGME case minimum requirements for clavicle fracture fixation.

COMMONLY USED CPT CODES

- CPT Code: 23515—Clavicle fracture open reduction and internal fixation

COMMONLY USED ICD9 CODES

- 810.0—Clavicle fracture

COMMONLY USED ICD10 CODES

- S42.021A—Displaced fracture of shaft of right clavicle
- S42.022A—Displaced fracture of shaft of left clavicle, initial encounter for closed fracture
- S42.023A—Displaced fracture of shaft of unspecified clavicle, initial encounter for closed fracture
- S42.024A—Nondisplaced fracture of shaft of right clavicle, initial encounter for closed fracture
- S42.025A—Nondisplaced fracture of shaft of left clavicle, initial encounter for closed fracture
- S42.026A—Nondisplaced fracture of shaft of unspecified clavicle, initial encounter for closed fracture

Clavicle fractures are extremely common and comprise 2.6% to 5% of all fractures in adults, with midshaft injuries accounting for almost 75% of all fracture types. Clavicle fractures typically occur when an axial load is applied to the bone, usually in the form of a sudden point load to the apex of the shoulder. When these fractures displace, the proximal fragment generally is pulled superiorly by the sternocleidomastoid muscle while the distal fragment is pulled laterally by the weight of the arm.

Most nondisplaced or minimally displaced clavicular fractures can be managed nonsurgically simply by placing the arm in a sling. In these instances, the nonunion and malunion rates are extremely low. However, when midshaft clavicular fractures present with complete displacement or significant shortening, the risk of nonunion is significantly higher with conservative management. The surgical decision making remains a matter of debate. At present, the only absolute indications for surgical treatment of clavicular fractures include open injuries and fractures associated with evolving skin compromise. Relative indications for open reduction and internal fixation of midshaft clavicular fractures include injuries with 15 to 20 mm of shortening, completely displaced fractures, fractures with significant comminution, floating shoulder injuries that involve a concomitant glenoid neck fracture, painful nonunions, and midshaft clavicular fractures in certain multisystem trauma cases.

Depending on fracture morphology, either closed or open reduction and intramedullary pin fixation or open reduction and plate fixation can be performed. Biomechanically, both methods provide similar repair strength for middle-third clavicle fractures. After hardware removal, clavicles previously treated with intramedullary fixation were shown to be stronger than those treated with plate fixation. Clinically, open reduction and internal fixation of clavicular fractures has shown marked success for union in a relatively predictable time frame with low complications. Intramedullary fixation offers the advantage of smaller scars and lower refracture potential but also bears the potential risk of hardware prominence and a slightly higher incidence of nonunion. General principles for a successful surgical outcome involve minimizing soft tissue disruption and periosteal stripping as much as possible during exposure, achieving an anatomic reduction, and preventing hardware irritation and wound complications as much as possible with appropriate soft tissue hardware coverage. Either dynamic compression plates or locked plating constructs can be used, depending on bone quality and fracture type. In general, the plate is placed on the anterosuperior, or tension side, of the clavicle to result in the most biomechanically sound construct.

SURGICAL TECHNIQUE

Room Set-Up

- The operating room table likely is rotated from the initial position to allow ease in accessing the shoulder.
- Fluoroscopy should be positioned over the top and from the cephalad portion of the operating room bed. Be sure to confirm that an anteroposterior view and 45 degree cephalic/caudad tilt views are possible before draping.

Patient Positioning

- The patient is placed in the modified beach chair position (Fig. 38-1).
- The ipsilateral arm can be positioned in a specialized arm holder or can simply be secured over the belly.
- A bump underneath the medial border of the ipsilateral scapula is helpful for achieving better length at the fracture site.

Prepping and Draping

- The clavicle is prepped and draped in a sterile fashion.
- Wide draping is used so distal and proximal clavicular ends are free and accessible (Fig. 38-2).

Incision Placement

- A straight horizontal incision is created approximately 10 mm inferior to the anterior border of the clavicular fracture site (Figs. 38-3 and 38-4). This is done to reduce the likelihood of wound complications arising from an incision directly over the anterosuperior clavicular plate.
- Alternatively, a superior incision can be created directly on top of the clavicle. This incision can either be straight or slightly S-shaped, following the contour of the clavicle.

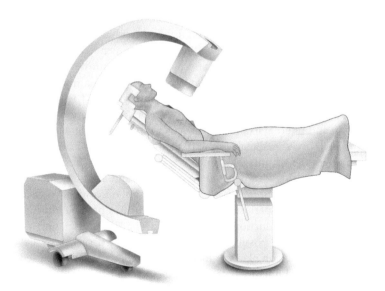

Figure 38-1 C-arm positioning for a midshaft clavicle fracture.

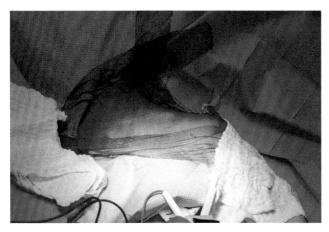

Figure 38-2 The clavicle is prepped and draped in a sterile fashion. It is important to drape widely so that both the proximal and distal clavicular ends are accessible.

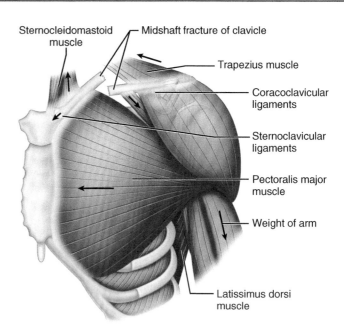

Figure 38-3 Anatomy of a midshaft clavicle fracture with displacing forces. The medial segment is displaced superiorly by the sternocleido-mastoid and superiorly/posteriorly by the trapezius, and the lateral segment is displaced anteriorly and rotated inferiorly by the weight of the arm and is displaced medially by the pectoralis major and latissimus dorsi muscles (acting through the humerus).

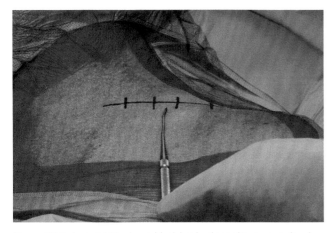

Figure 38-4 A straight horizontal incision is planned to expose the clavicle. The incision can either be made inferior to the anterior border of the clavicle or directly superficial to the clavicle.

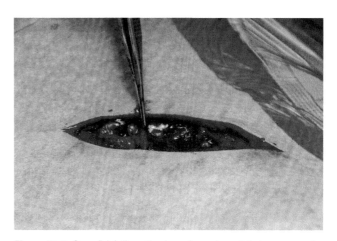

Figure 38-5 Superficial dissection is performed carefully to preserve the supraclavicular nerves (pointed to with pickups), which typically run superoinferiorly along the transverse incision.

Exposure of Clavicle and Fracture Site

- After the skin is incised, subcutaneous dissection should be bluntly performed to identify the supraclavicular nerves, which typically run superoinferiorly along the transverse incision (Fig. 38-5).
- Supraclavicular nerves should be protected when possible to prevent numbness over the anterior chest wall or painful dysthesias from developing.
- The platysma layer is encountered next and should be sharply incised along the anterior border to facilitate preservation of this layer for closure at the conclusion of the case.
- The fracture can be further exposed with a #15 blade scalpel, small curettes, and periosteal elevators (Fig. 38-6).

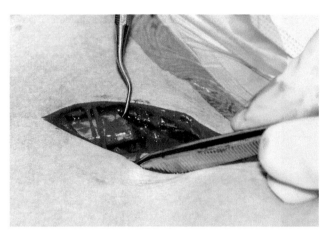

Figure 38-6 The clavicle fracture is exposed.

- Evaluation for concomittant muscle damage and perforation of the trapezial fascia is important.

Fracture Reduction

- Most midshaft clavicle fractures involve a spiral oblique pattern with a butterfly fragment.
- Length can be achieved on the fracture by gently extending the shoulder and arm.
- Pointed tenaculum clamps should be used for fracture reduction.
- K-wires are helpful to gain reduction.
- Reduction then can be maintained with a racking half-hitch cerclage suture because this obviates provisional fixation devices that block or restrict placement of the definitive plate fixation (see Millett PJ. *Plate fixation of midshaft clavicle fractures.* VuMedi-video, www.vumedi.com/video/plate-fixation-of-midshaft-clavicle -fractures-2/).
- In cases in which a large butterfly fragment is present, it can be joined with either the proximal or distal end with a mini-frag screw and plate construct, although the authors prefer to simply cerclage this with #2 Vicryl (Ethicon, Cincinnati, OH) sutures.
- If the fracture has a long oblique pattern, one to two lag screws (2.7-mm or 3.5-mm) may be placed perpendicular to the fracture site.
- Preliminary reduction can be held in place by lag screws, strategically placed pointed tenaculum clamps, racking half-hitch nonabsorbable suture, or a K-wire.
- In cases of severe comminution, bridge plating should be used.

Plate Fixation

- A 3.5-mm dynamic compression plate is generally preferred in most individuals, although a 2.7-mm dynamic compression plate may be used in younger patients.
- Locking plates are preferred in situations in which fixed angle construct stability is desired, such as excessive comminution or poor quality bone.
- A general rule of thumb is to place at least six cortices of purchase on either side of the fracture. More cortical sites of fixation may be desired in osteoporotic bone or when excessive comminution exists. In such cases, it is preferable to have eight cortices.
- The most biomechanically sound position for plate placement is on the anterosuperior or tension side of the clavicle fracture (Fig. 38-7), although superior placement is preferred with precontoured plates because they fit better in this location.
- Manual contouring of the clavicle plate may be necessary even if it has already been precontoured. Provisionally fixing the plate medially and laterally with K-wires or plate holding clamps ensures that the plate aligns properly.

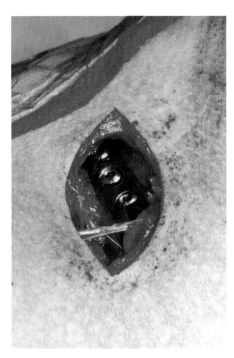

Figure 38-7 The plate should be placed on the anterosuperior side, or tension side, of the clavicle fracture because this is the most biomechanically sound position. If the supraclavicular nerve is in the way, the plate should be slid underneath it.

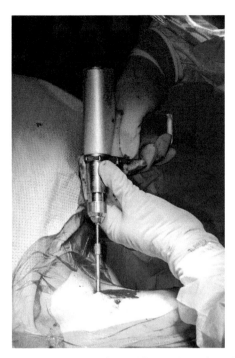

Figure 38-8 When drilling into the clavicle, avoid plunging inferiorly to prevent vascular damage. Use both hands to optimize control and to prevent overshooting of the drill bit.

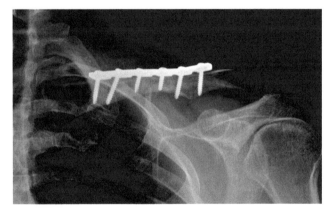

Figure 38-9 Postoperative x-ray of a midshaft clavicle fracture after open reduction and internal fixation.

- When drilling into the clavicle, avoid plunging inferior to the clavicle to prevent vascular injury (Fig. 38-8). This is most important in the medial third of the clavicle.
- Confirm appropriate screw length with depth gauge and fluoroscopy.
- Figure 38-9 shows postoperative x-ray of a midshaft clavicle fracture after open reduction and internal fixation.

Wound Closure

- The platysma layer should be carefully closed over all areas of the plate with a 0 Vicryl suture (Fig. 38-10). This is followed by a 2-0 Vicryl for the subcutaneous layer placed in an inverted, interrupted fashion. The epidermis is reapproximated with a running, subcuticular monofilament suture such as an absorbable 4-0 Monocryl (Ethicon, Cincinnati, OH).

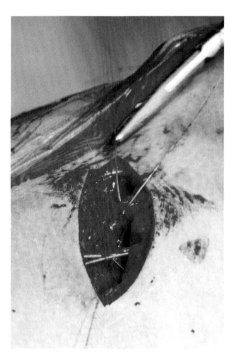

Figure 38-10 The platysma layer is carefully closed with an interrupted figure-of-8 stitch.

BRIEF SUMMARY OF SURGICAL STEPS

- Skin incision
- Exposure of clavicle
- Exposure of fracture site and removal of callus or hematoma
- Fracture reduction with or without lag screws or cerclage sutures to reconstitute the "tube"
- Placement of plate over fracture site with at least six cortices of fixation on either side of fracture
- Wound closure

REQUIRED EQUIPMENT

Appropriately sized anterosuperior 3.5-mm or 2.7-mm precontoured clavicular plate
2.7-mm lag screws
Fluoroscopy
Pointed tenaculum bone clamps
K-wires

TECHNICAL PEARLS

- Make an incision 1 cm distal to the anterior border of the clavicle to avoid placing the wound directly over the clavicular plate
- Look out for the supraclavicular nerve in the subcutaneous layer
- Incise the platysma sharply to allow for a clean layer for closure
- Use a pointed reduction clamp
- Use a 2.7-mm or 3.5-mm lag screw if the fracture pattern has a long oblique component to it
- If a large butterfly fragment exists, a mini-frag screw set may be helpful for reduction or cerclage sutures
- Do not plunge when drilling to avoid neurovascular injury

COMMON PITFALLS

(When to call for the attending physician)

- Inadvertently cutting of the supraclavicular nerve when it is avoidable
- Excessive soft tissue and periosteal stripping, which unnecessarily compromises healing
- Failure to achieve reduction
- Not centering the plate directly over the clavicle on both sides of the fracture
- Poor soft tissue coverage of the plate during wound closure

POSTOPERATIVE PROTOCOL

A sling is applied immediately after the surgery in an effort to reduce tension on the fracture site. Pendulums can be performed, but more aggressive range of motion is not necessary initially. The patient should be seen 1 week after surgery for clinical and radiographic follow-up. Full passive and active-assisted range of motion can be initiated at this point and should continue until 6 weeks after surgery. The patient then should begin more aggressive active range of motion and light lifting. Twelve weeks after surgery is typically when all restrictions are lifted, assuming radiographs show good healing of the fracture site.

POSTOPERATIVE CLINIC VISIT PROTOCOL

Patients are scheduled to return to the clinic for follow-up visits at 1 to 2 weeks, 6 to 8 weeks, and 12 weeks.

SUGGESTED READINGS

1. Celestre P, Roberston C, Mahar A, Oka R, Meunier M, Schwartz A. Biomechanical evaluation of clavicle fracture plating techniques: does a locking plate provide improved stability? *J Orthop Trauma*. 2008; 22(4):241-247.
2. Gardner MJ, Silva MJ, Krieg JC. Biomechanical testing of fracture fixation constructs: variability, validity, and clinical applicability. *J Am Acad Orthop Surg*. 2012;20(2):86-93.
3. Heuer HJ, Boykin RE, Petit CJ, Hardt J, Millett PJ. Decision-making in the treatment of diaphyseal clavicle fractures: is there agreement among surgeons? Results of a survey on surgeons' treatment preferences. *J Shoulder Elbow Surg*. 2014;23(2):e23-e33.
4. Jeray KJ. Acute midshaft clavicular fracture. *J Am Acad Orthop Surg*. 2007;15(4):239-248.
5. Leroux T, Wasserstein D, Henry P, et al. Rate of and risk factors for reoperations after open reduction and internal fixation of midshaft clavicle fractures: a population-based study in Ontario, Canada. *J Bone Joint Surg Am*. 2014;96(13):1119-1125.
6. Millett PJ, Hurst JM, Horan MP, Hawkins RJ. Complications of clavicle fractures treated with intramedullary fixation. *J Shoulder Elbow Surg*. 2011;20(1):86-91.
7. Postacchini F, Gumina S, De Santis P, Albo F. Epidemiology of clavicle fractures. *J Shoulder Elbow Surg*. 2002;11(5):452-456.
8. Rickert JB, Hosalkar H, Pandya N. Displaced clavicle fractures in adolescents: facts, controversies, and current trends. *J Am Acad Orthop Surg*. 2013;21(1):1.
9. Schulz J, Moor M, Roocroft J, Bastrom TP, Pennock AT. Functional and radiographic outcomes of nonoperative treatment of displaced adolescent clavicle fractures. *J Bone Joint Surg Am*. 2013;95(13): 1159-1165.
10. Smith SD, Wijdicks CA, Jansson KS, et al. Stability of mid-shaft clavicle fractures after plate fixation versus intramedullary repair and after hardware removal. *Knee Surg Sports Traumatol Arthrosc*. 2014; 22(2):448-455.
11. Millett PJ. *Plate fixation of midshaft clavicle fractures*. VuMedi-video <www.vumedi.com/video/plate-fixation-of-midshaft-clavicle-fractures-2/>. Accessed 04.12.15.

CHAPTER 39

ACROMIOCLAVICULAR JOINT RECONSTRUCTION

Joshua A. Greenspoon | Maximilian Petri | Peter J. Millett

Acromioclavicular (AC) joint injuries account for 9% to 12% of all shoulder injuries and are grouped according to the Rockwood classification system. Grades I and II injuries represent strain and partial tearing of supporting ligaments and are treated conservatively with excellent results. Surgical management is typically indicated for patients with grades IV to VI AC joint injuries. For patients with grade III injuries, controversy still exists regarding the optimal treatment strategy. In addition to patients with failed conservative treatment, some surgeons advocate early operative management for high-level athletes and manual laborers. However, complication rates of AC joint reconstruction have been reported to be as high as 80%, including hardware failure, graft ruptures, coracoid and clavicle fractures, adhesive capsulitis, and damage to the brachial plexus and axillary nerve.

A large variety of stabilization methods have been introduced for the AC joint, with 162 techniques described in 120 studies, including K-wire transfixation, hook plates, arthroscopic TightRope (Arthrex, Naples, FL), and suture anchors. No gold standard procedure has been established. The authors' preference is an arthroscopically assisted anatomic coracoclavicular ligament allograft reconstruction.

SURGICAL TECHNIQUE (Video 39-1)

Room Set-Up

- The operating room (OR) table is likely rotated from the initial position to allow ease in accessing the shoulder.
- Fluoroscopy should be positioned over the top and from the cephalad portion of the OR bed. Be sure to confirm that an anteroposterior view and axillary view are possible before draping.

Patient Positioning

- The patient is placed in the modified beach chair position (Fig. 39-1).
- The ipsilateral arm can be positioned in a specialized arm holder.

Prepping and Draping

- The index shoulder is prepped and draped in a sterile fashion.
- Wide draping is used so the distal clavicle and the AC joint area are free and accessible.

Diagnostic Arthroscopy

- The distal clavicle, AC joint, and acromion are palpated. Osseous margins are marked with a sterile pen (Fig. 39-2).

CASE MINIMUM REQUIREMENTS

- There are no ACGME case minimum requirements for acromioclavicular joint reconstruction.

COMMONLY USED CPT CODES

- CPT Code: 23550—Open treatment of acromioclavicular dislocation, acute or chronic.
- CPT Code: 23552—Open treatment of acromioclavicular dislocation, acute or chronic; with fascial graft (includes obtaining graft)

COMMONLY USED ICD9 CODES

- 840.0—Acromioclavicular joint sprain

COMMONLY USED ICD10 CODES

- S43.101 (A,D,S)—Unspecified dislocation of right acromioclavicular joint, initial encounter
- S43.102 (A,D,S)—Unspecified dislocation of left acromioclavicular joint
- S43.109 (A,D,S)—Unspecified dislocation of unspecified acromioclavicular joint
- S43.111 (A,D,S)—Subluxation of right acromioclavicular joint
- S43.112 (A,D,S)—Subluxation of left acromioclavicular joint, initial encounter
- S43.119 (A,D,S)—Subluxation of unspecified acromioclavicular joint
- S43.121 (A,D,S)—Dislocation of right acromioclavicular joint, 100%-200% displacement
- S43.122 (A,D,S)—Dislocation of left acromioclavicular joint, 100%-200% displacement

Continued

- S43.129 (A,D,S)—Dislocation of unspecified acromioclavicular joint, 100%-200% displacement
- S43.131 (A,D,S)—Dislocation of right acromioclavicular joint, greater than 200% displacement
- S43.132 (A,D,S)—Dislocation of left acromioclavicular joint, greater than 200% displacement
- S43.139 (A,D,S)—Dislocation of unspecified acromioclavicular joint, greater than 200% displacement
- S43.141 (A,D,S)—Inferior dislocation of right acromioclavicular joint
- S43.142 (A,D,S)—Inferior dislocation of left acromioclavicular joint
- S43.149 (A,D,S)—Inferior dislocation of unspecified acromioclavicular joint
- S43.151 (A,D,S)—Posterior dislocation of right acromioclavicular joint
- S43.152 (A,D,S)—Posterior dislocation of left acromioclavicular joint
- S43.159 (A,D,S)—Posterior dislocation of unspecified acromioclavicular joint

- Markings are made at planned portal positions (anterosuperior, anteroinferolateral, and posterior).
- Standard diagnostic arthroscopy is performed to identify and manage concomitant intraarticular injuries. The diagnostic arthroscopy should be performed even if an open reconstruction is planned because up to 30% of patients with AC dislocations have concomitant injuries.

Exposure of Coracoid and Distal Clavicle

- The rotator interval is opened, with care taken to preserve the superior and middle glenohumeral ligaments.
- The coracoid is identified, and its undersurface is débrided to a smooth surface with a radiofrequency ablator.
- An accessory inferolateral portal is established with an 8.25-mm cannula that allows access to the subcoracoid space.
- The distal clavicle is then exposed superiorly. A 2.5-cm inscision is made along Langer's lines and centered over the AC joint (Fig. 39-3).

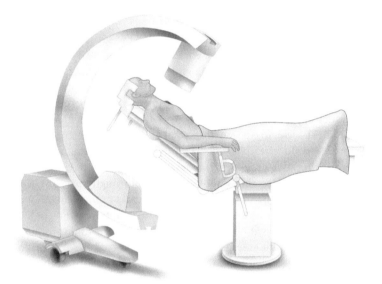

Figure 39-1 C-arm position for acromioclavicular joint reconstruction surgery.

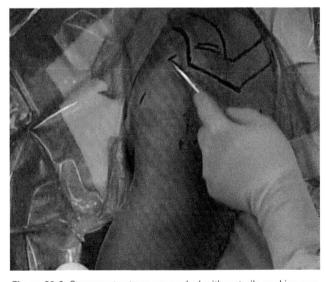

Figure 39-2 Osseous structures are marked with a sterile marking pen.

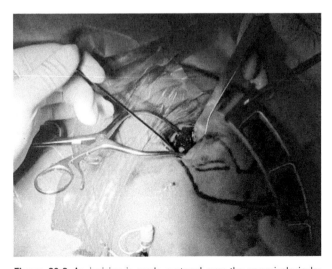

Figure 39-3 An incision is made centered over the acromioclavicular joint.

■ Superficial dissection is performed, incising the deltotrapezial fascia in line with its fibers while maintaining hemostasis.

■ Subperiosteal dissection is performed to faciliate adequate repair of the deltoid and imbrication of the superior AC joint capsule at the end of the procedures.

■ The distal clavicle should be preserved in most cases in light of evidence that suggests improved stability of the distal clavicle after AC reconstruction. However, if posttraumatic osteoarthritis is present, an 8-mm to 10-mm distal clavicle excision should be performed.

Coracoclavicular Ligament Reconstruction

■ A drill guide is used to place a 2.4-mm K-wire through the distal clavicle and through the central portion of the coracoid base.

■ Fluoroscopy should be used to confirm positioning (Fig. 39-4).

■ A cannulated 3.0-mm drill is used to overdrill the final bone tunnels.

■ The K-wire is removed, and a passing suture is placed through the cannulation of the drill. The drill then is removed, leaving the passing suture in place.

■ With the passing suture, four strands of suture tapes are shuttled through both the clavicle and coracoid bone tunnels from superior to inferior and pulled out the anteroinferolateral portal.

■ The first cortical fixation button is threaded onto the suture tapes and pulled into position at the inferior cortex of the coracoid base (Fig. 39-5).

■ A previously whipstitched 8-mm allograft is placed such that the medial limb reconstructs the conoid ligament and the lateral limb reconstructs the trapezoid ligament. To facilitate passage of the graft, soft tissue tunnels are created with a switching stick and a soft tissue dilator. The switching stick is guided from posterior to the distal clavicle to the inferomedial border of the coracoid with both arthroscopic and fluoroscopic visualization. An 8-mm cannula dilator is passed over the switching stick until it emerges medial to the coracoid base. The switching stick is removed, and a passing suture is advanced through the cannula dilator. The passing suture is retrieved through the anteroinferolateral portal. A similar procedure is performed to create a soft-tissue tunnel lateral to the coracoid.

■ The allograft then is passed posterior to the distal clavicle and through the medial soft-tissue tunnel until it emerges medial to the coracoid base. The allograft then is shuttled inferiorly and around the coracoid and superiorly through the lateral

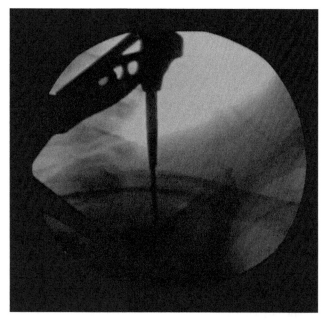

Figure 39-4 Fluoroscopy is used to confirm positioning during drilling.

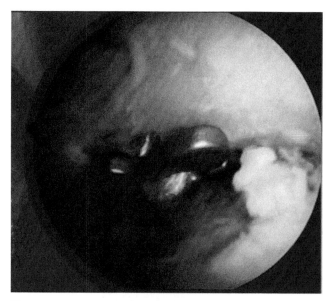

Figure 39-5 Arthroscopic view of the button placed on the inferior aspect of the coracoid.

soft-tissue tunnel with the passing suture that was previously placed through the lateral soft tissue tunnel.

Joint Reduction

- The joint then is reduced.
- The second cortical fixation button is threaded down the four stands of suture tapes that were previously placed until the button makes contact with the cortex of the distal clavicle (Fig. 39-6).
- While an assistant manually maintains AC joint reduction, the free ends of the suture tapes are knotted over the button and its remaining limbs are trimmed.
- The allograft then is cycled.
- The free ends of the allograft are looped together in an overhand configuration (Fig. 39-7).
- High-strength sutures are placed through the graft knot and tied for additional security (Fig. 39-8).
- Dynamic and fluoroscopic examination then is performed by observing the final construct while moving the arm through range of motion (Fig. 39-9).

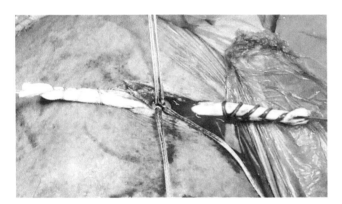

Figure 39-6 A second button is used to maintain reduction.

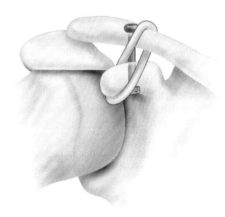

Figure 39-7 Acromioclavicular joint reconstruction with suture button fixation and allograft.

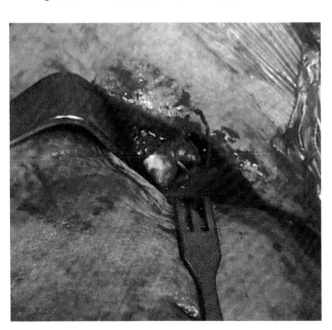

Figure 39-8 The two ends of the graft are tied together. High-strength sutures are used to reinforce the knot.

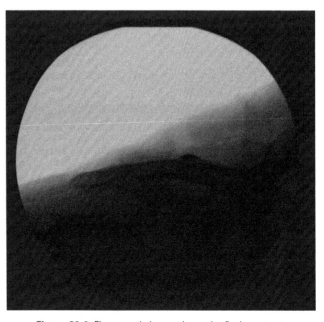

Figure 39-9 Fluoroscopic image shows the final construct.

BRIEF SUMMARY OF SURGICAL STEPS

- Diagnostic arthroscopy
- Débridement of the coracoid
- Exposure of the distal clavicle
- Bone tunnels drilled through the clavicle and the coracoid
- Cortical fixation button threaded onto suture tapes and pulled into position at the inferior cortex of the coracoid base
- 8-mm allograft used to reconstruct the conoid and trapezoid ligaments
- The allograft is passed posterior to the clavicle and then shuttled around the inferior coracoid base from medial to lateral
- Joint is reduced and second cortical fixation button threaded down the suture tapes
- Allograft tied in knot and high-strength sutures placed through the graft knot for additional security

TECHNICAL PEARLS

- Use a 70-degree arthroscopic camera to look medially from the posterior glenohumeral portal to see the undersurface of the coracoid
- Be sure to make the initial anterior glenohumeral portal slightly lower and more lateral to allow the instruments to more easily reach the undersurface of the coracoid
- Do not disturb the soft tissue distal to the tip of the coracoid; the musculocutaneous nerve pierces the coracobrachialis 3-cm to 8-cm distal to the tip of the coracoid in most people
- Drilling should be performed with arthroscopic and fluoroscopic guidance
- Reduction and initial fixation of the coracoclavicular ligaments should be performed with fluoroscopic guidance
- If the distal clavicle is arthritic or does not reduce properly, 8 to 10 mm of bone can be resected from the distal end
- Use a soft tissue dilator to create space for the allograft before passage around the clavicle
- In situations in which an allograft is not recommended because of lack of availability or patient preference, a hamstring autograft can be used instead

REQUIRED EQUIPMENT

| Arthroscopic equipment: 30-degree and 70-degree scope |
| 8-mm allograft (either anterior tibialis, posterior tibialis, or semitendinosus) |
| Two broad suture buttons for coracoclavicular fixation |
| Suture tape for coracoclavicular fixation |
| Fluoroscopy |
| Arthroscopic mechanical shaver |
| Arthroscopic mechanical burr |
| Arthroscopic radiofrequency wand |

COMMON PITFALLS

(When to call for the attending physician)

- Not using a 70-degree arthroscope to properly visualize coracoid
- Not making the anterior glenohumeral portal lateral enough to allow instruments to reach the undersurface of the coracoid
- Accidentally disturbing the musculocutaneous nerve 3 cm distal to coracoid tip
- Not properly exposing the undersurface of the coracoid
- Not appropriately reducing the acromioclavicular and coracoclavicular interfaces before fixation
- Failure to appropriately dilate the soft tissue before allograft passage
- Poor exposure of distal clavicle area

POSTOPERATIVE PROTOCOL

An abduction sling is applied immediately after surgery in an effort to reduce tension on the reconstruction. Passive range of motion is allowed at this time. Active and active-assisted range of motion is started at approximately 6 weeks after surgery. Shoulder strengthening exercises are begun at 8 weeks after surgery. Patients are usually cleared for full activities at 16 weeks; however, the rehabilitation period may be longer if concomitant intraarticular injuries were addressed during surgery.

POSTOPERATIVE CLINIC VISIT PROTOCOL

Patients are scheduled to return to the clinic for follow-up visits at 2 weeks, 6 to 8 weeks, and 12 weeks.

SUGGESTED READINGS

1. Beitzel K, Sablan N, Chowaneic DM, et al. Sequential resection of the distal clavicle and its effects on horizontal acromioclavicular joint translation. *Am J Sports Med*. 2012;40:681-685.
2. Beitzel K, Cote MP, Apostolakos J, et al. Current concepts in the treatment of acromioclavicular joint dislocations. *Arthroscopy*. 2013;29(2):387-397.
3. Ceccarelli E, Bondi R, Alviti F, Garofalo R, Miulli F, Padua R. Treatment of acute grade III acromioclavicular dislocation: a lack of evidence. *J Orthop Traumatol*. 2008;9(2):105-108.
4. Dias JJ, Steingold RF, Richardson RA, Tesfayohannes B, Gregg PJ. The conservative treatment of acromioclavicular dislocation. Review after five years. *J Bone Joint Surg Br*. 1987;69(5):719-722.
5. Martetschläger F, Horan MP, Warth RJ, Millett PJ. Complications after anatomic fixation and reconstruction of the coracoclavicular ligaments. *Am J Sports Med*. 2013;41(12):2896-2903.
6. Millett PJ, Braun S, Gobezie R, Pacheco IH. Acromioclavicular joint reconstruction with coracoacromial ligament transfer using the docking technique. *BMC Musculoskelet Disord*. 2009;10:6.
7. Nüchtern JV, Sellenschloh K, Bishop N, et al. Biomechanical evaluation of 3 stabilization methods on acromioclavicular joint dislocations. *Am J Sports Med*. 2013;41(6):1387-1394.
8. Rockwood CA. Injuries to the acromioclavicular joint. In: Rockwood CA, Green DP, eds. *Fractures in Adults*. Vol. 1. 2nd ed. Philadelphia: JB Lippincott Co; 1984.
9. Rolf O, Hann von Weyhern A, Ewers A, Boehm TD, Gohlke F. Acromioclavicular dislocation Rockwood III-V: results of early versus delayed surgical treatment. *Arch Orthop Trauma Surg*. 2008;128(10):1153-1157.
10. Tamaoki MJ, Belloti JC, Lenza M, et al. Surgical versus conservative interventions for treating acromioclavicular dislocation of the shoulder in adults. *Cochrane Database Syst Rev*. 2010;(8):CD007429.

CHAPTER 40

HIP HEMIARTHROPLASTY

Paul Hyunsoo Yi | Erik Nathan Hansen

emoral neck fractures are common injuries that most often result from low-energy falls in the elderly; however, they also can occur in young patients as a result of high-energy mechanisms, such as motor vehicle accidents. Although the commonly used Garden Classification is composed of four categories, femoral neck fractures can be thought of conceptually as either nondisplaced or displaced. Nondisplaced femoral neck fractures may present with benign clinical examination results, whereas displaced femoral neck fractures present with the affected leg shortened, held in external rotation and abduction. Radiographs are obtained initially, and magnetic resonance imaging and computed tomographic scan (fine-cut and three-dimensional) are obtained as necessary.

In terms of economic impact, hip fractures result in billions of healthcare dollars spent in the United States each year. This tremendous burden on the healthcare system and society is projected to increase significantly in the decades to come as the general population ages. In terms of morbidity and mortality, more than a third of patients with hip fractures die within 1 year of injury, and an even smaller proportion returns to their prior state of function. Although common, femoral neck fractures represent a potentially devastating injury that demands cost-effective and clinically effective treatment options.

Hip hemiarthroplasty has proven to be an effective treatment for displaced femoral neck fractures for more than 50 years, with low incidence rates of infection and dislocation. Typically indicated patients include the elderly with displaced femoral neck fractures without osteoarthritis and the medically infirm for whom the additional risks of a total hip replacement do not outweigh the functional benefits. Hip hemiarthroplasty is not without its disadvantages, perhaps most notably the risk of progressive acetabular erosion. Although its use has declined in recent years, with an increase in the utilization of total hip arthroplasty, hip hemiarthroplasty remains a staple in the general orthopaedic surgeon's arsenal in treatment of displaced femoral neck fractures and is one that every orthopaedic resident should know how to perform (Video 40-1).

SURGICAL TECHNIQUE

Room Set-Up

- A standard operating room table is placed in the center of the room with a pegboard or positioner to allow for lateral decubitus positioning (the authors' preferred approach is the anterolateral approach; Fig. 40-1).
- The appropriate radiographs are displayed in plain view of the surgical team. Templating of the planned femoral stem is completed if possible.

Patient Positioning

- Place the patient in the lateral decubitus position on either a pegboard or secured with hip grip positioners and ensure that all bony prominences are well-padded (Fig. 40-2).

CASE MINIMUM REQUIREMENTS

- 30 Hip fractures (minimum number required by Accreditation Council for Graduate Medical Education [total, not specifically hemiarthroplasty])

COMMONLY USED CPT CODES

- CPT Code: 27125—Hemiarthroplasty, hip, partial (e.g., femoral stem prosthesis, bipolar arthroplasty)

COMMONLY USED ICD9 CODES

- 820.00—Closed intracapsular femoral neck fracture
- 820.8—Closed femoral neck fracture (unspecified)

COMMONLY USED ICD10 CODES

- S72.00—Fracture of unspecified part of neck of femur
- S72.01—Unspecified intracapsular fracture of femur
- S72.02—Fracture of epiphysis (separation) (upper) of femur
- S72.03—Midcervical fracture of femur
- S72.04—Fracture of base of neck of femur
- S72.05—Unspecified fracture of head of femur
- S72.06—Articular fracture of head of femur
- S72.09—Other fracture of head and neck of femur

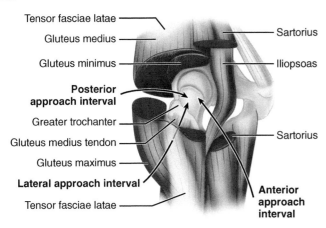

Figure 40-1 Surgical approaches for hip replacement.

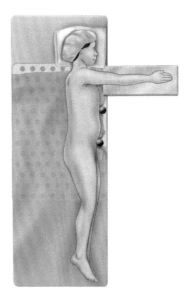

Figure 40-2 Patient positioning with a peg board.

- An axillary roll made of a 1-L bag of saline solution wrapped in cotton undercast padding is placed just inferior to the axilla.

Prepping and Draping

- Prep and drape the surgical leg in the usual sterile fashion.
- For the anterolateral approach, the hip drape should include an anterior leg bag because the leg needs to be lowered into the bag during hip dislocation.

Anterolateral Approach (Incision, Superficial, and Deep Dissections)

- Mark out the tip of the greater trochanter (GT) and the anterior and posterior borders of the femur with dots.
- Draw the incision centered over the GT and angled slightly posteriorly (Fig. 40-3).
- Make an incision sharply down to the fascia lata, followed by a fascial incision in line with the skin incision (Fig. 40-4). Identify the gluteus medius inserting into the GT and the vastus lateralis fibers originating from the vastus ridge.
- Next, make an incision through the anterior one third of the gluteus medius tendon (palpate the raphae at this junction); carry dissection distally through anterior fibers of vastus lateralis (Fig. 40-5).
- Continue to dissect anteriorly in a periosteal fashion, elevating the gluteus medius, minimus, and capsule in a single layer. It is often helpful to keep a proximal Hohmann retractor posterior to the femoral neck and a distal Hohmann retractor over the anterior femur to tension this musculocapsular flap (Fig. 40-6).
- As dissection proceeds further anteriorly, have the assistant on the opposite side of the table bring the leg into a figure-of-4 position to present more of the anterior femur into the wound (Fig. 40-7); this allows for adequate exposure of the femoral neck.
- Carefully place the retractors superior and inferior to the neck to protect the trochanter and abductors proximally and the lesser trochanter and vastus inferiorly (Fig. 40-8).

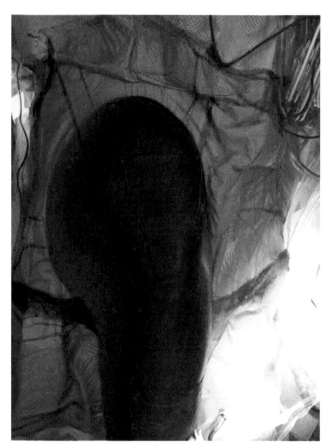

Figure 40-3 Incision for anterolateral approach.

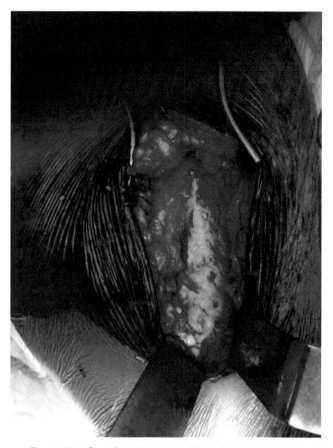

Figure 40-4 Superficial dissection with the fascia lata in view.

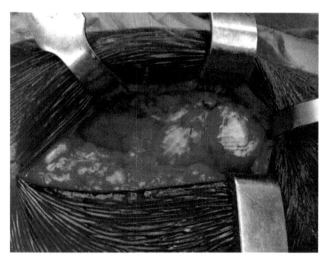

Figure 40-5 Incision through gluteus medius tendon and anterior fibers of vastus lateralis.

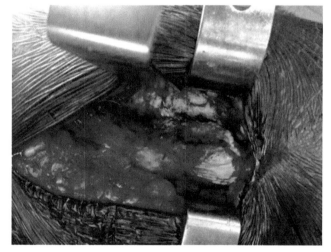

Figure 40-6 Hohmann retractor positioning (posterior to femoral neck and over anterior femur) to tension layer comprised of gluteus medius, gluteus minimus, and capsule.

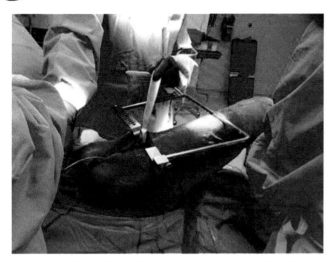

Figure 40-7 Figure-of-4 position to improves exposure of the femoral neck into the wound.

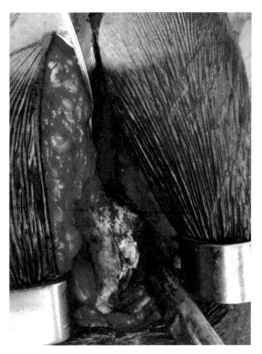

Figure 40-8 Retractor placement to protect greater and lesser trochanters, abductor muscles, and vastus lateralis during femoral neck osteotomy.

Neck Osteotomy and Femoral Head Sizing

- Plan the femoral neck osteotomy to start proximally from the saddle of the femoral neck (where the concavity of the lateral femoral neck meets the convexity of the greater trochanter) to a planned distance distally above the lesser trochanter (Fig. 40-9). This is often facilitated with preoperative templating. The napkin ring of bone can be removed with rongeur or towel clip.
- Next, use a corkscrew device to remove the femoral head from the acetabulum (Fig. 40-10). If necessary, transect the ligamentum teres with a Cobb elevator or other instrument to extract the femoral head.
- With the now osteotomized femoral head, size the hemiarthroplasty femoral head to be initially trialed (Fig. 40-11).
- To expose the acetabulum, extend the hip and externally rotate the leg at the knee. This helps translate the proximal femur posteroinferior to the acetabulum.
- Place retractors anteriorly and posteriorly at the capsulolabral junction. In contrast to a total hip replacement, the labrum is preserved in hemiarthroplasty cases to maintain suction seal of the hip joint (Fig. 40-12).
- With a trial femoral head on a "lollipop" handle, reduce the trial head into the acetabulum (Fig. 40-13).
- Take the trial head through a range of motion and then piston it. The appropriately sized femoral head trial should yield a suction seal sensation when attempting to "shuck" the femoral head.

Preparation of Femoral Canal, Trialing Components, and Implantation of Components

- To prepare the femur, place the leg into figure-of-4 position in the anterior leg bag.
- Place retractors along the medial calcar and lateral to the trochanter.
- Use a straight curette to determine the trajectory of the femur (Fig. 40-14).
- With a box cutter osteotome, remove any remaining lateral femoral neck to avoid varus malposition or undersizing of the stem (Fig. 40-15).

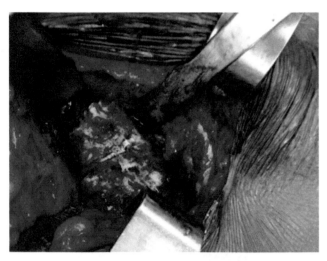

Figure 40-9 The femoral neck osteotomy site should start at the saddle proximally and end distally a planned distance above the lesser trochanter.

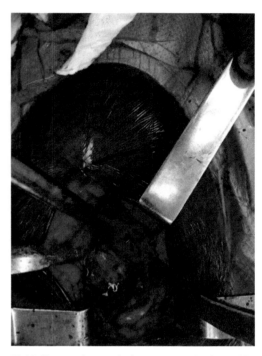

Figure 40-10 Use a corkscrew device to remove the femoral head from the acetabulum.

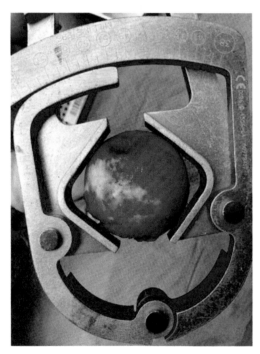

Figure 40-11 Use the femoral head to size the initial trial femoral head.

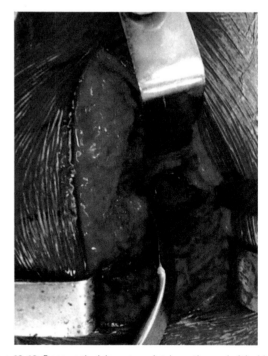

Figure 40-12 Preserve the labrum to maintain suction seal of the hip joint (in contrast to total hip arthroplasty).

- Sequentially broach the femur, attemping to fully lateralize the stem to avoid a varus malposition or undersized stem (Fig. 40-16).
- The appropriately sized stem is one that has both axial and rotational stability.
- Once the stem size has been determined, trial the femoral head that had been previously decided on. Reduction of the hip should be performed by the assistant on the opposite side of the table by placing the middle and index fingers around the trunnion and pulling longitudinally while the hip is extended and internally rotated.

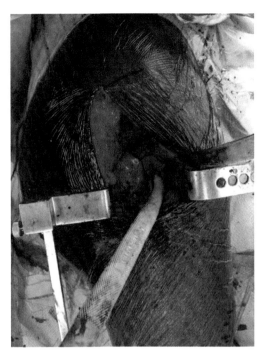

Figure 40-13 Use a lollipop handle to reduce the trial femoral head into the acetabulum.

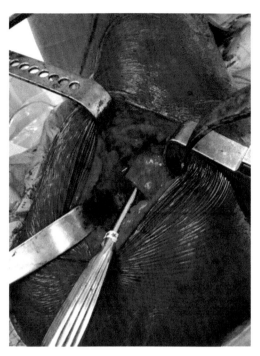

Figure 40-14 Use a straight curette to determine the trajectory of the femur.

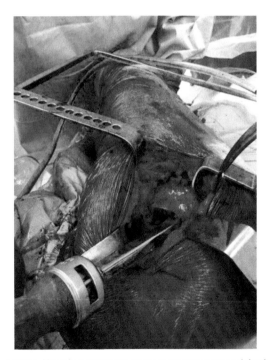

Figure 40-15 Use a box cutter osteotome to remove any remaining lateral femoral neck.

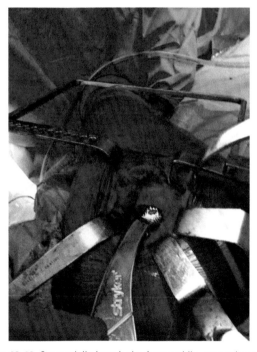

Figure 40-16 Sequentially broach the femur while attempting to fully lateralize the stem.

Often a femoral head pusher can be used by the surgeon to facilitate reduction by pushing the femoral head down into the acetabulum.

■ The hip then should be taken through a full arc of motion to test its stability. Specifically, posterior stability is assessed with flexion, adduction, and internal rotation of the hip until the femoral head begins to sublux out. Anterior stability is determined by hip extension, external rotation, and adduction. Longitudinal traction can be pulled through the hip to assess soft tissue tension or shuck.

- Instability can be addressed by increasing neck length or offset.
- Once you are content with the trial construct, the hip is atraumatically dislocated via traction, adduction, and external rotation. Sometimes a bone hook on the neck trunnion is necessary to generate sufficient traction to dislocate the hip. However, one should be careful not to torque the hip too much because this may cause a periprosthetic fracture.
- Next, choose a cement restrictor. Consider making radial cuts in the restrictor to allow for easier sitting. Plan to seat the restrictor approximately 2 cm distal to the tip of the stem.
- Use a pen to mark the cement restrictor inserter where the collar of the stem is expected to meet the proximal neck osteotomy and still allow for 2 cm of a distal cement mantle (Fig. 40-17).
- Irrigate the canal with a femoral canal brush with pulsative lavage, seat the restrictor in the femur at the planned depth, and then fill the canal with an epinephrine-soaked vaginal pack to minimize back bleeding (Fig. 40-18).
- Fill the canal with low viscosity cement in retrograde fashion with a cement gun. The cement should neither be too runny (which could result in blood laminations in cement and weakened mechanical strength) nor too doughy (preventing inter-digitation into cancellous bone).
- Insert the stem on its handle and hold in appropriate version while the cement hardens. The goal is to attempt to match the patient's native proximal femoral anteversion.

Closure

- Once the cement is hard, remove excess cement.
- Irrigate the wound.
- Close the abductor tendon and vastus lateralis fascia with one nonabsorbable, braided suture in figure-of-8 fashion. Some surgeons instead complete the abductor tendon repair with nonabsorbable, braided polyester suture/tape and bone tunnels in the trochanter (Fig. 40-19).
- The remainder of the wound is closed in routine multilayer fashion.

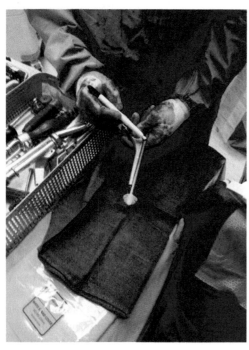

Figure 40-17 Use a pen to mark the cement restricter to allow for a 2-cm distal cement mantle.

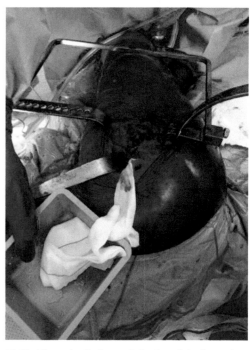

Figure 40-18 After pulsatile lavage irrigation of the femoral canal with a canal brush, fill the canal with an epinephrine-soaked vaginal pack to minimize back bleeding.

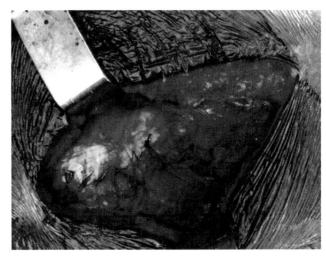

Figure 40-19 Close the abductor tendon and vastus lateralis fascia with one nonabsorbable, braided suture.

BRIEF SUMMARY OF SURGICAL STEPS

- Room set-up
- Position patient, prep, and drape
- Anterolateral approach
- Osteotomy of neck; size femoral head
- Broach femur
- Trial components
- Prepare the femoral canal
- Cement final implants
- Abductor repair and multilayer tissue closure

TECHNICAL PEARLS

- During fascial incision, abduct the leg to avoid injuring the underlying abductor and vastus lateralis
- Keep the deep dissection perpendicular to the abductor tendon rather than beveling (this allows for good tendon reapproximation at conclusion of case)
- During deep dissection of gluteus medius, minimus, and capsule, use a proximal Hohmann retractor posterior to the femoral neck and a distal Hohmann retractor over the anterior femur to tension the musculocapsular flap (see Fig. 40-4)
- As dissection proceeds further anteriorly, it is helpful to bring the leg into a figure-of-4 position to present more of the anterior femur into the wound (see Fig. 40-5)
- During the neck osteotomy, hold the leg in figure-of-4 position with the tibia straight up and down between the legs of the assistant on the opposite side of the table to allow for better exposure and determination of version
- During cementation, place a lap sponge in the acetabulum to prevent cement from inadvertently getting into the acetabulum

REQUIRED EQUIPMENT

Standard operating room table

Hip positioners (for anterolateral or posterior approach)

Hip hemiarthroplasty system

Low viscosity cement/cement gun/cement restrictor (if using cemented hemiarthroplasty system)

COMMON PITFALLS

(When to call for the attending physician)

- Calcar crack is noted during broaching the femur; requires removing broach, exposing distal extent of fracture, and passing cerclage cables
- Hip is a struggle to reduce; possibly too high a neck osteotomy requiring a recut or poor reduction technique
- Hip is a struggle to dislocate; possibly too tight a construct or poor dislocation techinque; may require use of bone hook
- Periprosthetic fracture is noted during difficult attempted reduction or dislocation; requires removing broach, exposing distal extent of fracture, and passing cerclage cables
- Cement hardens too quickly to fully seat the femoral stem; call for the cement removal devices
- Cement quantity insufficient to cement stem; quickly try to remove as much cement from canal by any means necessary; ask for an additional pack of cement and retry

POSTOPERATIVE PROTOCOL

After surgery, the patient is made weight-bearing as tolerated and is mobilized as soon as clinically possible (ideally beginning on postoperative day 0). There are typically no specific range of motion or weight-bearing precautions for an anterolateral approach and cemented hemiarthroplasty, which is why the authors prefer this mode of fixation and surgical approach. This cohort is typically frail and elderly, possibly with cognitive decline, which makes compliance with any type of restrictions difficult. Regardless of the patient's preinjury mobility, a walker is often needed in the early postoperative period for balance and gait training. Although the goal of physical therapy is to get the patient back to the preinjury level of ambulation and function, ample literature suggests that the functional level will decline to some degree.

Postoperative radiographs are often obtained in the recovery room, including a low anteroposterior pelvis and a frog leg lateral of the affected hip. These are scrutinized for restoration of anatomy (offset/leg length and stem position and cement mantle). The authors use the technique described by Barrack and colleagues to assess cement mantle. Reviewing these x-rays and the technical details of the case with the faculty member immediately after the surgery can be very educational and facilitates the learning curve for the trainee's subsequent case.

Perioperative antibiotics are continued for one postoperative dose to maintain Surgical Care Improvement Project (SCIP) compliance. The Foley catheter is discontinued on postoperative day 1 in the morning. Postoperative pain control is managed with a preference for oral medications and conservative use of narcotics given the propensity of this cohort for delirium and confusion and associated falls.

POSTOPERATIVE CLINIC VISIT PROTOCOL

Patients are scheduled to return to clinic for routine follow-up visits at 6 weeks, 12 weeks, 6 months, 1 year, and every year thereafter for repeat physical examination, and radiographs.

SUGGESTED READINGS

1. Barrack RL, Mulroy RD Jr, Harris WH. Improved cementing techniques and femoral component loosening in young patients with hip arthroplasty. A 12-year radiographic review. *J Bone Joint Surg Br.* 1992; 74(3):385-389. Available at: <http://www.ncbi.nlm.nih.gov/pubmed/1587883>.
2. Deangelis JP, Ademi A, Staff I, Lewis CG. Cemented versus uncemented hemiarthroplasty for displaced femoral neck fractures: a prospective randomized trial with early follow-up. *J Orthop Trauma.* 2012;26(3):135-140. Available at: <http://www.ncbi.nlm.nih.gov/pubmed/22198652>.
3. Keene GS, Parker MJ. Hemiarthroplasty of the hip: the anterior or posterior approach? A comparison of surgical approaches. *Injury.* 1993;24(9):611-613. Available at: <http://www.ncbi.nlm.nih.gov/pubmed/8288382>.
4. Langslet E, Frihagen F, Opland V, Madsen JE, Nordsletten L, Figved W. Cemented versus uncemented hemiarthroplasty for displaced femoral neck fractures: 5-year followup of a randomized trial. *Clin Orthop Relat Res.* 2014;472(4):1291-1299. Available at: <http://www.ncbi.nlm.nih.gov/pubmed/24081667>.
5. Macaulay W, Pagnotto MR, Iorio R, Mont MA, Saleh KJ. Displaced femoral neck fractures in the elderly: hemiarthroplasty versus total hip arthroplasty. *J Am Acad Orthop Surg.* 2006;14(5):287-293. Available at: <http://www.ncbi.nlm.nih.gov/pubmed/16675622>.
6. Taylor F, Wright M, Zhu M. Hemiarthroplasty of the hip with and without cement: a randomized clinical trial. *J Bone Joint Surg Am.* 2012;94(7):577-583. Available at: <http://jbjs.org/content/94/7/577.abstract>.

INDEX

Page numbers followed by "*f*" indicate figures, "*b*" indicate boxes, and "*t*" indicate tables.

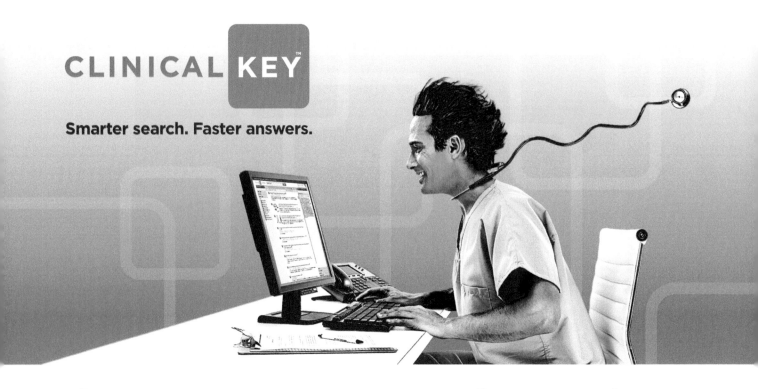

Printed and bound by CPI Group (UK) Ltd, Croydon, CR0 4YY

03/10/2024

01040305-0013